ATLAS OF ULTRASOUND MEASUREMENTS

Atlas of Ultrasound Measurements

X–RAY DEPT.
KINGS MILL
HOSPITAL

BARRY B. GOLDBERG, M.D.
Professor of Radiology
Director, Division of Diagnostic Ultrasound
Jefferson Medical College
Thomas Jefferson University
Philadelphia, Pennsylvania

ALFRED B. KURTZ, M.D.
Professor and Vice Chairman
Department of Radiology
Jefferson Medical College
Thomas Jefferson University
Philadelphia, Pennsylvania

YEAR BOOK MEDICAL PUBLISHERS, INC.
Chicago • London • Boca Raton • Littleton, Mass.

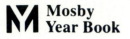

Mosby
Year Book

Dedicated to Publishing Excellence

95 96 97 98 99 / 9 8 7 6 5 4 3

Library of Congress Cataloging-in-Publication Data
Goldberg, Barry B., 1937-
     Atlas of ultrasound measurements / Barry B. Goldberg, Alfred B. Kurtz.
          p.   cm.
     Includes bibliographical references.
     ISBN 0-8151-3541-6
     1. Diagnosis, Ultrasonic—Atlases. 2. Ultrasonic imaging—
Atlases.   I. Kurtz, Alfred B.   II. Title.
     [DNLM: 1. Ultrasonic Diagnosis—atlases.   WB 17 G618a]
     RC78.7.U4G65   1990
     616.07′543—dc20   90-12159
     DNLM/DLC   CIP
     for Library of Congress

Sponsoring Editor: Bethany L. Caldwell/James D. Ryan
Associate Managing Editor, Manuscript Services: Deborah Thorp
Production Project Coordinator: Karen Halm
Proofroom Supervisor: Barbara M. Kelly

DEDICATION

To our families: their support is the foundation _____
upon which we create.

B.B.G. and A.B.K.

CONTRIBUTORS

ELIZABETH L. AFFEL, M.S.
Department of Visual Physiology
Wills Eye Hospital
Philadelphia, Pennsylvania

OKSANA H. BALTAROWICH, M.D.
Clinical Assistant Professor of Radiology
Jefferson Medical College
Thomas Jefferson University Hospital
Philadelphia, Pennsylvania

PETER N. BURNS, PH.D.
Associate Professor of Radiology
Director of Ultrasound Physics
Jefferson Medical College
Thomas Jefferson University
Philadelphia, Pennsylvania

WOLFGANG F. DÄHNERT, M.D.
Assistant Professor of Radiology
Jefferson Medical College
Thomas Jefferson University Hospital
Philadelphia, Pennsylvania

PAUL A. DUBBINS, M.D.
Consultant in Charge of Ultrasound
Plymouth General Hospital
Department of Diagnostic Ultrasound
Freedom Fields Hospital
Plymouth, England

STEVEN L. EDELL, D.O.
Chairman, Department of Radiology
Riverside Hospital
Wilmington, Delaware

BARRY B. GOLDBERG, M.D.
Professor of Radiology
Director, Division of Diagnostic
  Ultrasound
Jefferson Medical College
Thomas Jefferson University
Philadelphia, Pennsylvania

ALFRED B. KURTZ, M.D.
Professor and Vice-Chairman
Department of Radiology
Jefferson Medical College
Thomas Jefferson University
Philadelphia, Pennsylvania

LAURENCE NEEDLEMAN, M.D.
Assistant Professor of Radiology
Assistant Director
Division of Diagnostic Ultrasound
Jefferson Medical College
Thomas Jefferson University Hospital
Philadelphia, Pennsylvania

MATTHEW E. PASTO, M.D.
Clinical Associate Professor of Radiology
Department of Radiology
Jefferson Medical College
Thomas Jefferson University Hospital
Philadelphia, Pennsylvania

REBECCA G. PENNELL, M.D
Clinical Assistant Professor of Radiology
Division of Diagnostic Ultrasound
Jefferson Medical College
Thomas Jefferson University Hospital
Philadelphia, Pennsylvania

GORDON S. PERLMUTTER, M.D.
Director of Ultrasound
Department of Radiology
Reading Hospital and Medical Center
Reading, Pennsylvania

M. NATHAN PINKNEY, B.S.
President, Medical Imaging Consultant
Sonicor, Inc.
West Point, Pennsylvania

JOEL S. RAICHLEN, M.D.
*Assistant Professor of Medicine and
    Radiology*
Division of Diagnostic Ultrasound
Director, Noninvasive Cardiac Laboratory
Jefferson Medical College
Thomas Jefferson University Hospital
Philadelphia, Pennsylvania

MATTHEW D. RIFKIN, M.D.
Professor of Radiology and Urology
*Director, Division of Magnetic Resonance
    Imaging*
Jefferson Medical College
Thomas Jefferson University Hospital
Philadelphia, Pennsylvania

**LARRY D. WALDROUP, B.S.,
    R.D.M.S.**
Technical Manager
Division of Diagnostic Ultrasound
Jefferson Medical College
Thomas Jefferson University
Philadelphia, Pennsylvania

ALAN H. WOLSON, M.D.
Clinical Associate Professor of Radiology
Jefferson Medical College
Thomas Jefferson University Hospital
Philadelphia, Pennsylvania

PREFACE

The concept for this book occurred more than a decade ago. This was in response to the many questions from the sonographers and sonologists within the Division of Ultrasound at Jefferson Medical College, as well as from the numerous attendees at our ultrasound courses. In the 1960s, there were questions about the correct measurements of organs, fetal parts, etc., to which there would be the reply, "You have to develop your own table because there is nothing in the literature." Of course, in the ensuing years more data was collected and published regarding measurements in all areas of the body in which ultrasound could produce a satisfactory image.

The 1970s presented a new question: "Which table or graph should I use?" It was not surprising that as data was collected and published, discrepancies were found. This often meant that the examiner had to be lucky to select an appropriate chart or had to ask colleagues what they were using. Alternately, the examiner could conduct a scientific review of the literature, analyzing the data and choosing the most appropriate chart. However, this often required taking a new set of measurements to confirm what others had published. Certainly, large facilities had this ability, but with the dissemination of ultrasound, in both small and large hospitals as well as outpatient facilities and offices, this was not feasible. Also, it was not always possible to obtain a large number of patients, and it took considerable time and expertise to analyze the data.

During visits to other laboratories during the 1980s, we were astonished by the number of charts and tables that had been arbitrarily selected for use and how, in even some of the largest facilities, there was confusion relating to appropriate measurements. In addition, some of the seldom-used measurements were often difficult to find in the literature. Many seldom-used measurements appeared in journals that would not normally be read, as well as in foreign journals where translation would be a problem.

A thorough search of the world literature on articles relating to the measurement of structures within the body utilizing ultrasound, x-ray, CT, anatomy, and pathology was therefore conducted. This extensive research led to the accumulation of thousands of articles dating back to some of the original anatomical measurements from the 1800s and early 1900s. Using this data, categories were selected and assignments made to organize the information into a format that would be easy for readers to comprehend. In addition, the data was analyzed as to which tables or charts would be most appropriate to use. Although obstetrical measurements have been published in a separate book, this data has been included and updated, along with chapters covering all other areas of the body in which ultrasound measurements might be useful. It is obvious that not all possible tables and graphs could be included and that, even while this book was being written, new measurements were being published. However, we feel that the in-depth research, review, and analysis of available data on measurements is as complete as possible, taking into account the interval from writing to publication.

It is anticipated that this book should prove valuable to both sonologists and sonographers who now use ultrasound, as well as to those newly entering the field who wish to better understand ultrasound measurements. It is envisioned that this book will also be used as a reference manual, placed within reading areas for use whenever there is a question about what measurements should or could be used. This would prove particularly beneficial for those measurements that are not commonly used on a day-to-day basis. In addition, the measurements in this book could be helpful for those interested in establishing an ultrasound facility, to allow utilization of the most comprehensive measurements without referring to the extensive and often confusing and contradictory literature.

Barry B. Goldberg, M.D.
Alfred B. Kurtz, M.D.

ACKNOWLEDGMENT

Our special thanks to Phyllis R. Goldberg who performed the initial world literature search and organized it into specific sections, continuing the process on an ongoing basis. In addition, she edited the material contained in this book. Our thanks also to Liu Ji-bin, M.D., for his illustrative contributions and to Yu Ji-Wen for her assistance in organizing and duplicating the various materials. Also, we extend our thanks to Rosemarie Boccella, Dorothy Elitz, Joanne Gardner, and Emily Pompetti for their various contributions in the typing of the manuscripts. Finally, we wish to thank Fred Ross and Kenneth Goodman for their photographic assistance.

Barry B. Goldberg, M.D.
Alfred B. Kurtz, M.D.

CONTENTS

Chapter 1

Limitations of Ultrasound Imaging Measurements

Peter N. Burns, Ph.D.

Larry Waldroup, B.S., R.D.M.S.

M. Nathan Pinkney, B.S.

Good ultrasound measurements depend on an understanding both of the anatomy of the structures under study and of the nature of their depiction in the ultrasound image. The physical principles on which the ultrasound instrument relies also define the most important limitations of its precision. Although a detailed discussion of the physical basis of the ultrasound image is beyond the scope of the present chapter, we shall discuss certain factors which have the potential to influence the quality of measurements made from an ultrasound image.

FORMATION OF THE ULTRASOUND IMAGE

All ultrasound imaging instruments employ the pulse echo method. The image is composed of a multiplicity of lines, each of which depicts the stream of ultrasound echoes received after the emission of a single pulse. The location of dots along each line is determined by the time at which the echoes are received—and hence the depth at which the echo producing structures are situated. The intensity of each dot is governed by the strength of the corresponding ultrasound echo. It may be tempting to regard the image which is formed from the combination of these lines as a "picture" or "acoustic photograph" of the insonated tissues, and therefore the matter of measurement as a relatively straightforward one. The relationship, however, between the ultrasound echoes shown on the screen and the actual geometry of the structures under study is somewhat more complex. Measurements that are made without consideration to the principles which govern the generation and detection of echoes in the ultrasound image are prey to a variety of important sources of error.

Origin of Ultrasonic Echoes

Figure 1–1 shows that echoes tend to be produced at interfaces between soft tissue structures. In fact, any discontinuity in *acoustic impedance* of the tissue lying

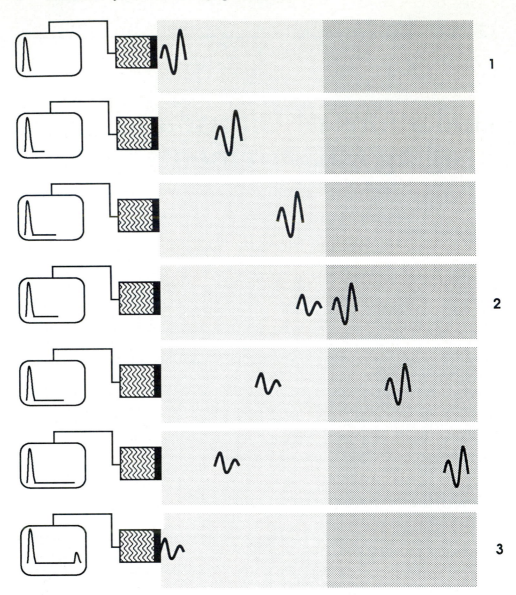

FIG 1–1.
The principle of a pulse echo imaging system. *1,* the pulse is emitted from the transducer. At the same time, the A-scan line (*left*) begins to move at a constant speed across the display screen. *2,* an echo is formed at a interface with a change in acoustic impedance. *3,* the echo reaches the transducer. A deflection on the A-line occurs at a point corresponding to the depth of the interface.

within the path of the ultrasound pulse will give rise to an echo. Acoustic impedance is defined as the product of the density and speed of sound in tissue. Factors which influence the acoustic impedance include tissue density, compressibility and temperature. For most interfaces between soft tissues, the majority of the energy contained in the ultrasound pulse is transmitted through the interface and only a small portion reflected as an echo. The size of this echo is dependent only on the difference in acoustic impedance, not on the tissue type. For this reason, different structures may be similar or identical in appearance on the ultrasound image, even though they are composed of different tissues.

Echoes from the parenchyma of soft tissue organs and fluids such as blood, on the other hand, arise by the process known as *Rayleigh scattering*. Variations in acoustic impedance occurring over a distance which is much smaller than the wavelength of the ultrasound (which lies between about 0.1 mm and 1.0 mm) act as point sources of weak echoes, which radiate in all directions. Some of these weaker echoes find their way back to the transducer. Radiating echoes from a multiplicity of such small scatterers interact with one another by a process known as *coherent interference*. One consequence of this interference is the distribution of local maxima and minima in the pattern of ultrasound echoes which return to the transducer, so resulting in the texture or *speckle pattern* which characterizes the appearance of solid soft tissues on an ultrasound image. Because the concentration and average distance between scattering centers is likely to be different for different organ structures, different kinds of tissue tend to have different characteristic speckle patterns. If speckle patterns are the sole basis for the identification of structures which are to be measured (e.g., in metastatic lesions of the liver), it should be borne in mind that speckle patterns are themselves dependent on acoustic factors such as the size and frequency of the transducer beam, and the focusing characteristics of the system in use. The speckle is a consequence of, not an image of, the acoustic structure of the organ. Thus measurements of structures which are defined only by changes in texture only (such as a liver metastasis) are limited in precision by speckle.

Image Geometry

Certain assumptions are implicit in the process which results in the ultrasound echo being written as a spot at a certain location on the screen. The first is that the velocity of sound in the tissues through which the pulses travel is constant. This velocity forms the basis of the calculation made by the instrument which relates the time of arrival of a specific echo to the distance between the transducer and the echo-producing structure (see Fig 1–1). Although it is known that the speed of sound in fact varies in different types of soft tissue, most instruments assume a constant velocity of 1,540 m/sec.

The second assumption is that all echoes received by the transducer arise from structures which lie in a straight line from the transducer pointing in the direction of its orientation. Thus, a structure which causes a deviation in the direction of the ultrasound beam will also result in incorrect registration of echoes on the image. Furthermore, as ultrasound beams extend beyond their central axis, both in the plane of the image and in the scan thickness plane, echoes which arise from structures that lie within the ultrasound beam, but not along its central axis, will be misregistered by the instrument to appear along the central axis.

Although an ultrasound image is a cross-sectional or tomographic image, it, like other tomograms, relies on information which is derived from a three-dimensional volume of tissue. The images shown are therefore projections of a series of cross sections that constitute a slice of finite thickness. This thickness will usually not be uniform for the depth of the image. As we shall see, this is one of several factors which together determine a fundamental limit of precision of a measurement made from an ultrasound image.

POTENTIAL SOURCES OF ERROR IN MEASUREMENT

1. Physical Limitations of the Image: Resolution and Contrast

Certain limitations to measurements are a fundamental consequence of the physics of the image itself: no amount of care on the part of the operator will alleviate these constraints. In particular, the resolution of the image determines the best precision of any measurement made from it. In ultrasound images, the resolution varies within each image, and between the three directions defined by the scan plane.

Axial Resolution.—Axial resolution is defined as the minimum separation of two targets in tissue in a direction parallel to the beam which results in their being imaged as two distinct structures. Figure 1–2 shows that the main factor which determines axial resolution is the length of the ultrasound pulse. Transducers have a tendency to "ring" after being excited by an electrical impulse, creating an acoustic pulse which has an extended length in space. The result is that even a point target produces an echo which is sustained in time. This is interpreted by the ultrasound scanner as a structure which is extended in axial length, and the result is an image which is smeared in the direction of the ultrasound beam. Highly dampened transducers are capable of producing pulses with a shorter spatial length, but require a more powerful impulse to achieve the same level of average acoustic energy in tissue. Moreover, shortening the length of an ultrasound pulse while keeping the total energy of the pulse constant results in a higher peak acoustic intensity. Thus a compromise is reached between the peak pressure to which tissue is exposed and the effective axial resolution of the ultrasound image.

Looking at Figure 1–2, it is clear that if the shortest pulse achievable was one solitary cycle, the length of this pulse, and hence twice the axial resolution, would be equal to the wavelength. In fact, the wavelength specifies the *best* resolution with which a pulse echo system is capable of defining an echo-producing structure, in axial, lateral, and slice thickness directions. The wavelength of ultrasound at 3 MHz (typical of that used in abdominal imaging) is about 0.5 mm; at 10 MHz it is 0.15 mm.

Lateral Resolution.—Lateral resolution is defined as the minimum separation of two targets in tissue aligned along a direction perpendicular to the ultrasound beam, which results in their being imaged as two distinct structures. Figure 1–3 shows that the principal determinant of lateral resolution is the width of the ultrasound beam. In general, the lateral resolution is inferior to, or at best comparable to, the axial resolution. Highly focused beams, such as the one shown in Figure 1–3 achieve good lateral resolution in the focal zone but poor lateral resolution in the near- and far-field regions. Thus the precision of a distance measurement made in the lateral direction varies according to depth, the size of the transducer, and the degree of focusing achieved. With array transducer systems, neither the focus nor the effective size of the transducer remains fixed. As echoes from different depths are received at different times, the focus of the beam created by the transducer array can be arranged to coincide with the precise depth from which the echoes at that particular time are originating. This is known as *swept focusing*. Thus, an image is created at which the echoes from every depth are detected with an optimally focused beam. The result is an image with more uniform lateral resolution than that illustrated in Figure 1–3. In general, narrower beams are obtained from using higher-frequency transducers, so that lateral resolution improves with increasing transducer frequency.

1. Short Pulse

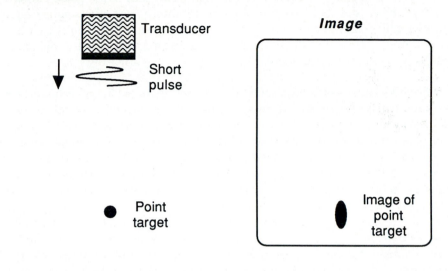

2. Long Pulse

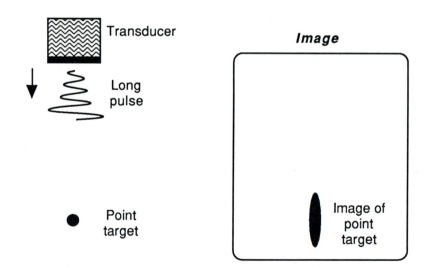

FIG 1–2.
Axial resolution of the ultrasound image is dependent on the length of the pulse emitted by the transducer.

Even if swept focusing is employed, the high bandwidth of the pulse emitted from the transducer and the tendency of tissue to absorb high ultrasound frequencies more rapidly results in a lowering of the center frequency of the pulse as it traverses tissue. The result is that there is always some degradation of both axial and lateral resolution with increasing depth.

   Slice Thickness.—The ultrasound instrument assumes that all echoes arise from the central axis of the beam. In reality echoes are produced by the full cross section of the beam. This leads to an inevitable uncertainty over the actual location from which an echo arises, causing what may be described as a "superimposition" effect. Echoes arising from tissues located near the edge of the beam are presented in the image as if they are located on the central axis of the beam. Therefore, any given point in the ultrasound image represents a summation of changes in tissue construction *across* a slice of tissue. When viewing the image, the observer is "looking through" a slice whose thickness is equivalent to the width of the beam which produced the image (Fig 1–4). This "slice thickness" is one source of the characteristic "fuzzy" edges of imaged spherical structures. Since most of the surfaces in the body are curved, the ultrasound image superimposes echoes from these curving surfaces, producing less well defined margins to structures.

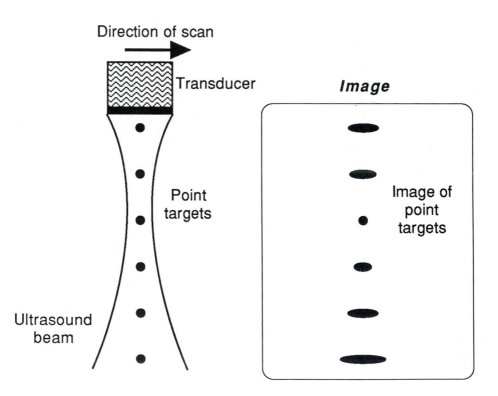

FIG 1–3.
Lateral resolution of the ultrasound image is dependent on the width of the ultrasound beam. This is rarely uniform over the depth of the image.

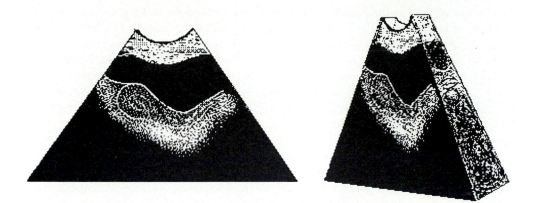

FIG 1–4.
The "thickness" of the ultrasound image is governed by the width of the acoustic beam which produced the image. This thick image is the reason edges of structures are rarely sharply defined in ultrasound images.

Contrast.—The effective resolution with which a structure can be delineated, and thus measured, from an ultrasound image is also affected by the strength of the echo itself. Several factors are involved. First, even a strong echo may arise from tissue sufficiently deep for attenuation to render it weak by the time it returns to the transducer: it only takes about 4 mm of muscle, for example, to reduce a 2.5-MHz echo to one-half of its amplitude. A weak echo requires more amplification from the receiver, but increasing the receiver gain also increases noise. If the echo is comparable in amplitude to the noise, it will be difficult or impossible to detect it on the image, and edges will be corrupted by randomly distributed signals that have the appearance of "snow" but are in fact artifactual consequences of a low signal-to-noise ratio. Second, the ultrasound beam does not have a uniform sensitivity pattern: at greater sensitivities, the beam is effectively wider. If the gain is increased enough to detect a weak echo, stronger echoes from the same depth will be "smeared" so as to reduce lateral resolution. Thus the *contrast resolution* is affected by echo amplitude and tissue attenuation. This provokes an inevitable conflict between raising the ultrasound frequency, which results in higher spatial resolution, and lowering it, which improves signal amplitude and hence often contrast resolution. The optimum frequency with which to carry out a specific measurement is thus always a compromise.

2. Technical Limitations: Engineering Precision of the Imaging System

A number of technical factors influence the technique and precision of ultrasound image measurements.

Detection of Edges.—As discussed above, the relative amplitude of an individual echo can influence its apparent size on the ultrasound image. However, if the beginning of the ultrasound pulse is sufficiently sharp (Fig 1–5), the axial location of the leading edge of the ultrasound echo will not be influenced by its amplitude. Thus, a basic technique of ultrasound measurement is to use the "leading edge" of the echo when making a measurement.

The use of the "leading edge to leading edge" method for making measurements implies, of course, that the leading edge is situated at the margin of the structure to be measured. It should be borne in mind, however, that it is a change in acoustic impedance which causes an echo, and there may be several of these in the immediate vicinity of an organ boundary. In addition, the image processing schemes used in many instruments frequently contain a degree of *differentiation*, a process which has the effect of artificially enhancing the leading edge of an echo, and decreasing its dependence on echo amplitude. Although this may help in the definition of a echo, it can potentially be misleading in the identification of the structure giving rise to the echo and confusion over what is actually being measured.

One example in which the strongest, and therefore the dominant, echoes on an image (which arise from the interface with the largest change in acoustic impedance) may not be the interface of interest for measurement is in the estimation of the lumen diameter of a blood vessel. Here, multiple echoes might occur at the wall of a blood vessel which include echoes between the blood and the intimal layer of the vessel wall, the intimal layer and contiguous parts of the vessel wall, and the vessel wall and its associated connective or fatty tissues. These echoes combine to create a single echo with a single leading edge: simply measuring between the two points at which the brightest echoes are observed will only provide an estimate of the lumen diameter if the largest change in acoustic impedance happens to be between the blood and the innermost layer of the vessel wall. This, then, is one example in which the leading edge approach to axial measurement is probably not the most accurate.

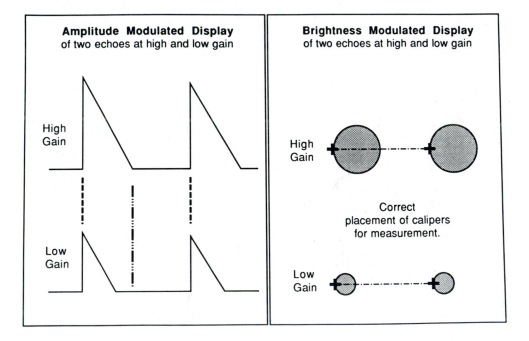

FIG 1–5.
The leading edge of echoes is affected by the location of the structure, but the trailing edge varies with amplitude.

a)

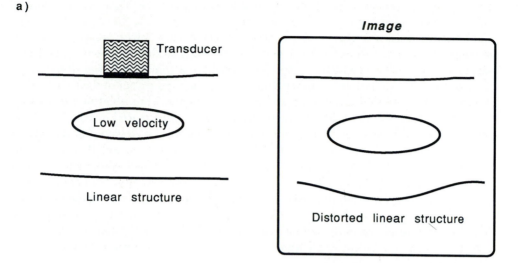

b)

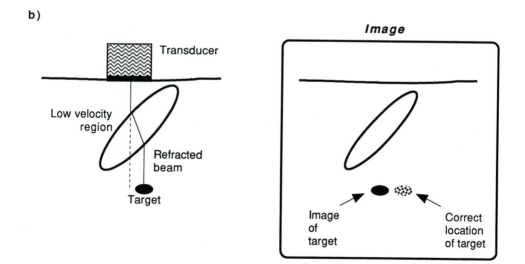

FIG 1–6.
a, a region of low velocity causes misregistration of distal structures and the potential for measurement error. *b,* nonperpendicular incidence on an interface between two regions of differing sound velocity gives rise to refraction and misregistration of echoes.

Velocity Calibration.—Virtually all ultrasound instruments are calibrated to an average speed of ultrasound in human soft tissue (1,540 m/sec). In most instruments, the velocity calibration is not open to adjustment by the user. There is, however, a significant variation between velocities in different soft tissues. The more dense and rigid tissues have a higher velocity, while fluids have a lower velocity than the average. The largest difference encountered clinically is that between fat and collagen, which can be as much as 12%. The effects of a region of tissue which has a different velocity all influence measurement: first, the axial extent of the region itself will be misrepresented because of the incorrect velocity. Thus a fatty tumor with a velocity of 5% below the calibration velocity will be overestimated in axial length by 5%. Second, any tissue interfaces distal to the tumor will be depicted in the wrong location, because of the transit time of the pulse having been lengthened by the region (Fig 1–6,*a*). Third, *refraction* will occur when the beam enters and leaves a low- or high-velocity region. This usually results in a deflection of the beam. As the scanner assumes ultrasound to travel in a straight line, and as the echoes return along the same path as the transmitted pulse, all structures distal to the refracting interface will be shown in the wrong location, and their spatial relationship to nearby structures which were imaged without refraction will be distorted (Fig 1–6,*b*).

Caliper Calibration.—In the days when most ultrasound systems were entirely analog, the measurement calipers usually comprised some sort of "overlay" on the image screen, which required regular testing and realignment. Today, most instruments are digital, and their calipers simply count pixels which have been set to represent fixed spatial locations. Caliper "drift" is no longer a matter for concern in these instruments.

Geometric Distortion.—While the calipers themselves may be accurate, the geometry of the measurement performed and the type of transducer used may introduce geometric errors. There are four basic scanning patterns used to generate a diagnostic ultrasound image: the rectangular, truncated wedge, sector, and curvilinear. With any of these approaches, measurements that are made along the axis of the sound beam are generally the most accurate. This is because axial measurements are based solely on the velocity calibration of the ultrasound system and the axial resolution of the system, which is usually superior to the lateral resolution. With proper scanning technique and equipment operation, axial measurements are preferred. If the angle used for measurements is not parallel to the axis of the sound beam, errors are more likely, and measurements that are made in a direction that is perpendicular or lateral to the ultrasound beam tend to have the greatest measurement error (Fig 1–7).

Some additional error can accrue from lack of precision of alignment of elements in a mechanically steered sector scanner. The electronic phased array transducer and the convex array (curvilinear) transducer use nonmechanical methods for beam steering and, when properly calibrated, will provide satisfactory measurements. Transducers that use internal mechanical components to steer the sound beam tend to become less accurate as they age, and have a tendency to introduce some degree of geometric distortion (and resultant measurement inaccuracy) near the edges of the sector display (Fig 1–8). This problem is easily corrected through recalibration by service personnel, so that the mechanical sector transducer should be checked more frequently for this problem.

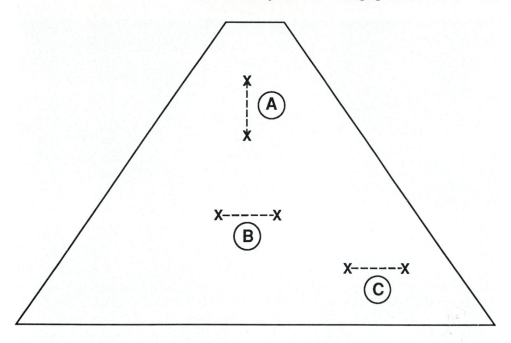

FIG 1–7.
In a sector scan, measurement *A,* parallel with the axis of the ultrasound beam, has the least measurement error. Measurement *B* is in the lateral direction and is likely to have a greater error. Measurement *C* is both deeper than *B* and toward the edge of the sector, both of which factors are likely to increase error further.

Display Monitor.—In spite of advances in practically all areas of ultrasound technology, the problems created by display monitors remain unchanged. The monitor is an analog, tube-type device, and is subject to user adjustments of its brightness and contrast levels as well as drift with age of its operating characteristics. The most significant problem introduced by display monitors has to do with their role in establishing gain levels used during the scan. Since the operator sets the instrument gain levels on the basis of an initial trial scan, if the monitor is misadjusted for brightness or contrast (due perhaps to an inappropriate ambient lighting level) the operator will tend to compensate by setting excessively high or low gain levels. Gain levels applied to the returning echoes will influence the accuracy of measurements in the ways already described. High gain levels cause interfaces to appear thicker than they actually are, and may obscure many of the lower-amplitude interfaces with overwritten acoustic noise. In addition, higher gain levels will often compress the range of the gray scale of the displayed echoes, because the strongest echoes are grouped into the highest gray level. Together, these two effects make it more difficult for the instrument operator to judge accurately the position of a specific anatomic interface, leading to possible measurement error. Excessively low gain levels create a different set of problems. If the power output/gain is set too low, some low-amplitude scattered echoes may not appear at all, leading to both measurement errors and mistaken conclusions about masses or fluid collections (e.g., lymphomatous masses misidentified as cysts).

Most ultrasound instruments provide some form of electronically generated on-screen display of the maximum range of gray shades which the instrument can display.

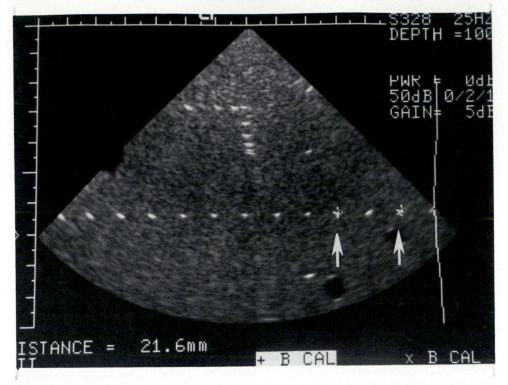

FIG 1–8.
Measurement of the distance between the two reflectors (*arrows*) in a test object filled with tissue-mimicking material. The actual distance is 20 mm. The measured distance of 21.6 mm shows the magnitude of potential error in lateral measurements.

With this gray-scale test pattern displayed, the user should adjust the display monitor brightness and contrast so as to provide an optimized display of the test pattern from full black to full white. Once set, these controls should only be adjusted to compensate for aging of the monitor. If the controls are readily accessible to the user, and especially if they might accidentally be moved, they should be clearly marked for the correct settings or taped in position to prevent inadvertent changes.

Hard-Copy Device.—The most commonly used hard-copy device for ultrasound imaging is the 8 × 10 cut-film camera (often referred to as a "format" or "multiformat" camera). This device contains an analog display monitor which is photographed to produce up to six small images on a single 8 × 10 sheet of radiographic film. If there is a discrepancy between the settings (brightness and contrast) of the hard-copy monitor and the instrument display monitor, the hard-copy image will not appear the same as the image which the instrument operator observed on the display monitor screen. Because of the potential measurement errors related to image quality, it is recommended that all measurements be made with on-screen calipers rather than after the fact from the hard-copy images. There are several reasons to do this:

1. The display monitor screen is usually larger than the hard-copy image; thus on-screen measurements are made from a larger image, using a calibrated electronic technique, with resultant improved accuracy.

2. Misadjustment of the hard-copy monitor will have no effect on the measurements.
3. Measurements are permanently recorded on the image for future reference.
4. The exact site where the measurement was taken will be apparent for future reference if follow-up is required.

3. Errors in Scanning Technique

Technique errors are directly attributable to the choices which the instrument operator must make when measurements are actually carried out. There are a host of possible errors related to technique, and proper training of personnel is therefore essential.

Failure to Select Correct Scan Plane.—Perhaps the most common error in technique is failure to select the correct anatomic plane for measurement. If only a single image is provided in the hard copy, the reading physician will have no way of knowing that the plane selected for measurement was not optimal. Training to use the appropriate anatomic landmarks and a clear and precise protocol for the measurement to be acquired will help eliminate this source of error.

Failure to Correctly Align Scan Plane.—A more subtle error of technique is the failure to correctly align the scan plane in relationship to the organ to be measured. The kidney, the fetal head, and the fetal abdomen are frequent sources of this type of error (Fig 1–9).

Error in Caliper Placement.—Once the scan plane has been optimized, the sonographer must then correctly position the calipers to obtain the desired dimension. Although this would seem to be a simple task, the nature of the ultrasound image is such that borders of organs are not always distinct. Accurate placement of the calipers requires a substantial level of judgment based on experience and a thorough understanding of the physical principles which underlie generation of the ultrasound image.

Failure to Confirm Initial Measurements.—For the reasons cited above, it is quite possible to obtain accurate measurements of an incorrect section of an organ or structure. After the initial measurement is obtained, the individual performing the scan should rescan and repeat the measurement. If the two measurements are not in agreement, the process should be repeated until the reason for the discrepancy is identified and successive measurements fall within an acceptable range of variation.

4. Errors in Interpretation

Anatomic Error.—It is sometimes difficult for an individual who is not involved in ultrasound to understand how an ultrasound image can provide detailed measurements for an organ which is not there! Those who practice ultrasound imaging know that such errors do indeed occur. Thus one might try to identify a missing ovary and inadvertently measure a piece of bowel which mimics the ovary. A less dramatic version of this error occurs when the contours of an organ must be extrapolated (Fig 1–10). A considerable degree of cognitive skill, as well as prior knowledge

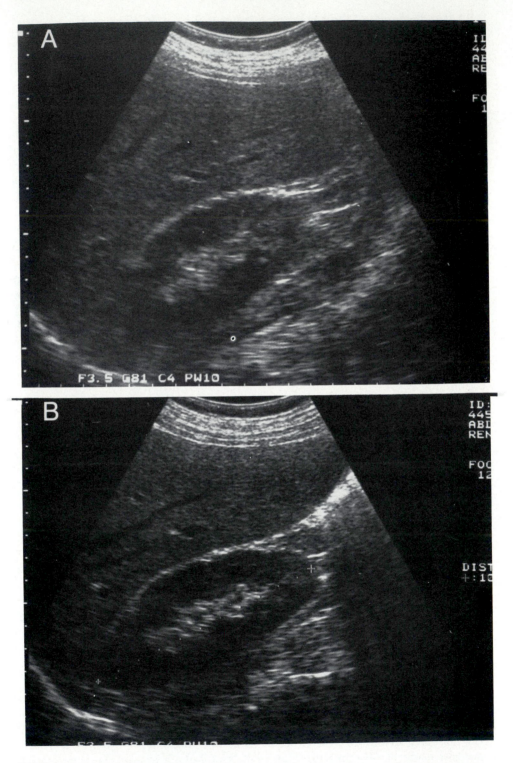

FIG 1–9.
In this sagittal image of the right kidney (**A**) the scan plane is not correctly aligned to the long axis of the organ. The ill-defined borders of the kidney suggest the presence of this error. Compare with the correct scan plane of the same kindey shown in **B**.

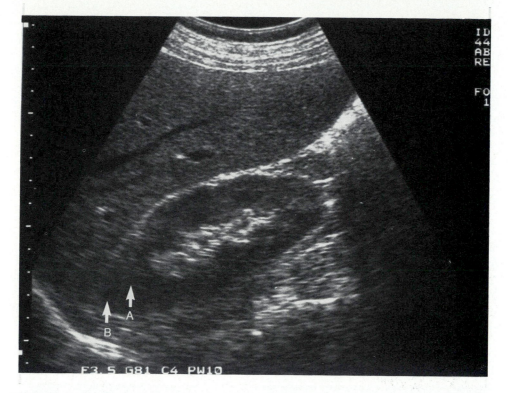

FIG 1–10.
A slightly different scan plane of the same kidney shown in Figure 1–9 illustrates the difficulty in selecting end points for measurement. Does point *A* or point *B* mark the upper margin of the kidney? This problem can only be solved during the real-time scan by sweeping the beam over the area in question until the instrument operator reaches a high level of confidence that the actual cephalad border of the kidney has been identified correctly.

of anatomy and pathology, is required to make sense of an ultrasound image. While this challenge is one of the exciting and rewarding aspects of diagnostic ultrasound, it must not be allowed to permit creation of a structure which is not really there. Careful technique and attention to anatomic relationships will help to avoid this particularly embarrassing error.

Edge Detection Error.—Another error is the tendency to "assign" borders in high-noise or low-resolution images or in images whose organ contours are obscured by (perhaps) overlying bone or gas (Fig 1–11). Figure 1–11 is an image which would *not* be acceptable for measurement of the sagittal axis of the kidney since neither the upper nor lower pole of the kidney is adequately demonstrated.

Reference Data Errors.—Once a measurement has been obtained, some assessment of the significance of that measurement must then be made. Most often, a table or graph is used to compare the obtained measurement with previously established normal values. Before using any particular set of normal values, the user should be aware of the types of errors which can be induced by the reference data themselves. These include the following:

1. Failure to use the same technique as was used to create the reference chart or table.
2. Failure of those who originated the data to specify technique and other parameters.
3. Different demographic characteristics of the reference data population to that under study.
4. Outdated data due to technology advance (e.g., improving resolution of ultrasound scanners has permitted development of more accurate reference data).

REPORTING MEASUREMENTS

No measurement can be perfectly precise. As we have seen, ultrasound measurements are prey to a number of errors, some of which depend on the operator, some on the machine, and some are an inescapable consequence of the physical behavior of sound in tissue. The best a sonographer can do is to report a measurement along with some indication of its accuracy. This is a prerequisite for, for example, the reproduction of the measurement by others. In doing so, one should be aware that different classes of error will affect their measurement differently.

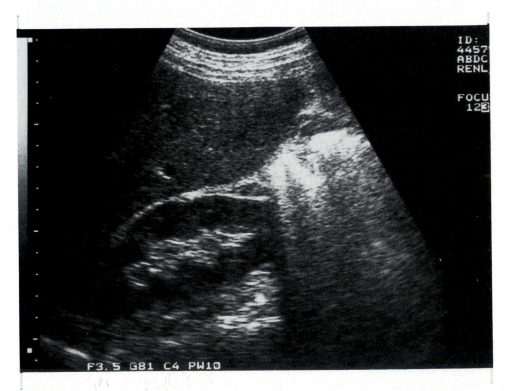

FIG 1–11.
Another sagittal scan of the same kidney shown in Figures 1–9 and 1–10. In this image the lower pole of the kidney is obscured by gas shadows, and the upper pole is inadequately delineated for caliper placement.

Two main types of error can influence accuracy. *Systematic error* (sometimes known as *bias*) will cause repeated measurements to be too high or low. There will be a physical explanation for this, of which the user may or may not be aware. Apart from careful physical analysis, the only way to detect systematic error is by calibration using some sort of standard. Thus a set of weighing scales might be compared to a laboratory standard in order to determine bias in its measurement of weight, and an ultrasound machine might be tested against a tissue equivalent measurement phantom in order to determine bias in its measurement of distance. However, there might still be systematic errors which result from the physics of the imaging itself, rather than the machine. Thus, for example, an area of reduced acoustic velocity lying in the region to be measured might be causing a systematic overestimation of axial length. Here only the velocity artifact which is present in the image will alert the sonographer that this measurement is unreliable.

Random error, on the other hand, is the result of the myriad of equipment, operator, observer, and patient variables which cause no two measurements to be alike. Random error can be estimated statistically. Many identical measurements are made, and it is inferred that the mean of the measurements is equal to the actual dimension under study. This is, of course, only an estimate, and the confidence with which such an estimate is made depends on the spread of values for the measurement. This spread decreases with an increase in the number of measurements, and is known as the *standard error of the mean*. It conveys to the reader how repeatable a measurement is.

It is not uncommon to use a further statistical method in ultrasound measurement. One measurement, for example, the biparietal diameter (BPD) of fetuses of 33 weeks gestation, is repeated for a number of *different* patients. These patients might be drawn at random from a larger *population*, which consists of *all* fetuses of 33 weeks gestation. The mean of these *sample* measurements is then taken as an estimate of the dimension in the population as a whole. Assuming no systematic bias in either the measurement technique or the selection of the sample exists, the confidence with which this inference can be made depends on variation within the sample and is expressed by a measure of variation such as the *standard deviation*. If the measurement varies in the population according to a *normal* (that is, bell-shaped) distribution, about 95% of the population will fall within 2 standard deviations above and below the mean value. This reasoning forms the basis of many of the anatomic charts against which the size of an anatomic structure is judged.

By estimating systematic error, by quoting the standard error of a measurement, and by giving the standard deviation of a sample taken from a population of subjects, ultrasonographers can ensure that their measurements are both interpreted correctly (not least by themselves) and capable of being reproduced independently.

SUMMARY

Unfortunately, it is impossible to respond to the question, How accurate are ultrasound measurements?, with a single answer. All ultrasound measurements are the result of a chain of processes, beginning with the interaction of an acoustic pulse with tissue and ending with a quantitative interpretation made by an observer. The precision of a given measurement is determined by each link in the chain, and in practice is likely to remain obscure to the person making the image. What one can do, however, is pay close attention to each link in the chain and thus ensure that the measurement made is the most accurate, and hence reproducible, that is possible. In summary:

1. No measurement can be more accurate than the axial or lateral resolution of the image at the point of measurement. In general, the axial is superior to the lateral resolution, so, if possible, linear measurements should be made in an axial direction.

2. Optimizing the resolution for a given scan is a matter of technique. Factors such as the choice of transducer configuration and frequency, image contrast, the scanning approach, and the machine power and gain settings will all influence the effective resolution. Resolution decreases with increasing depth in an ultrasound image; measurements are best as near to the focal zone of the transducer system as possible.

3. For measurement between two single similar echoes (such as a BPD measurement), the leading edge to leading edge approach is usually the most accurate, as it does not depend on system gain settings.

4. Variations in the speed of sound in an image (due to changes in intervening tissue type) will cause errors in registration and axial distance measurement. A scanning approach which avoids such regions is preferable.

5. It should be borne in mind when dealing with spherical structures such as cysts, that the slice thickness of an ultrasound beam is usually greater than the axial or lateral resolution.

6. Measurements should be made from the ultrasound imaging system's screen, rather than from hard copy.

7. The interpretation of a measurement is only as good as the reference data to which it is compared; it is worth taking the time to ensure that these are reliable and appropriate for the individual diagnosis and population under consideration.

8. Ultrasound measurements vary according to the machine and the operator, and between different scans by the same operator. Anatomic dimensions also vary among individuals in a population. For this reason it is essential to quote both the variation in an individual measurement and the variation within a population and to distinguish between the two when reporting a measurement. Only then will it be capable of reproduction or useful interpretation.

PART I

Head and Neck

Chapter 2

Ultrasound Measurements of the Central Nervous System

Matthew E. Pasto, M.D.

This chapter deals with measurements of the central nervous system. The chapter begins with a summary of the most useful measurements in the newborn, along with a discussion of obstructive versus atrophic hydrocephalus. For those seeking more comprehensive detail, the chapter continues with an overview of gross anatomy, the historical development of neurosonology, and further measurement techniques.

NEONATAL BRAIN

The most commonly used measurements are those of the frontal horn of the lateral ventricle and of the lateral ventricle itself, or its ratio to the intracranial hemidiameter. The frontal horn is best measured in a coronal view at the level of the foramen of Monro, the passageway between the third and lateral ventricles. The foramen is a fixed landmark that can be identified on follow-up scans to ensure accuracy and reproducibility. It is located at the level of the caudothalamic notch. The frontal horn is measured across its width, that is, the measurement is taken from the superior (superomedial) wall to the inferior wall at right angles to the longest dimension and at its midpoint—generally the widest point (Fig 2–1). In the newborn, up to 3 mm is normal.[1, 2] Generally, a measurement of 4 to 6 mm would constitute mild dilatation, 7 to 10 mm moderate dilatation, and greater than 10 mm marked dilatation.

The body of the lateral ventricle is measured in a transaxial view from its lateral edge to the midline, this being a "ventricular index," not truly the width of the lateral ventricle but rather the distance from the superolateral wall of the ventricle to the falx (Fig 2–2,A). This measurement should be less than 10 mm in the very premature infant, and 10 to 11 mm in the term infant[3] (up to 20 mm in the adult). The most common way of following ventricular size is using a ratio of ventricular size to cerebral diameter. The lateral ventricle (LV) and intracranial hemidiameter (ICHD) are measured in the transverse plane where the lateral walls of both ventricles are seen paralleling the midline echo (falx and interhemispheric fissure). The ICHD is measured perpendicular to the midline echo at its widest point. The ratio of the LV to the ICHD is 30% to 33% with dilatation absolutely documented at a ratio of 37% or above (Fig 2–2,B).[3, 4] The third ventricle in its transverse diameter should

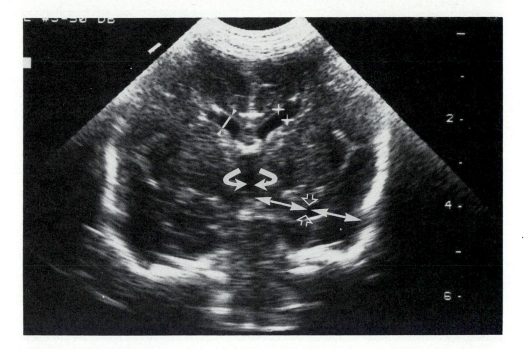

FIG 2–1.
Coronal view at the level of the foramina of monro. The frontal horns are measured perpendicular to their long axis and from bright wall to wall (distance between the crosses on viewer's right and the line shown on viewer's left). Note also the position of the medial wall of the temporal horn (denoted by *open arrows*), midway between the third ventricle (between *curved arrows*) and ipsilateral inner table.

be less than 4 mm in the newborn population, and up to 10 mm in the adult population[4, 5] (Fig 2–3).

Increased size of the lateral ventricles (ventriculomegaly) does not always constitute obstructive hydrocephalus. Configuration of the frontal horns and the third ventricle, in this author's opinion, will greatly assist in the diagnosis of obstructive versus atrophic dilatation when a borderline measurement is encountered. With obstructive dilatation, the walls are convex away from each other, whereas they remain mostly parallel with atrophic dilatation (Fig 2–4). This imparts a rectangular configuration to the frontal horns with atrophy as opposed to the ballooned or rounded configuration with obstructive hydrocephalus. A rounded dilatation of the temporal horns, as seen in the coronal view, also strongly favors obstruction, as this finding is very rarely found with atrophic dilatation. Clearly, follow-up measurements over time will further confirm or deny the presence of obstructive hydrocephalus. Indications for ventricular shunt placement may vary from institution to institution; therefore, these measurements need to be applied to each individual case. At the minimum, the obstructive posthemorrhagic dilatation must be documented to be increasing on three examinations over 7 to 10 days because (1) dilatation during resolution of hemorrhage is quite variable and rapidly changeable, and (2) a fairly persistent, moderate hydrocephalus may lessen or resolve months later.

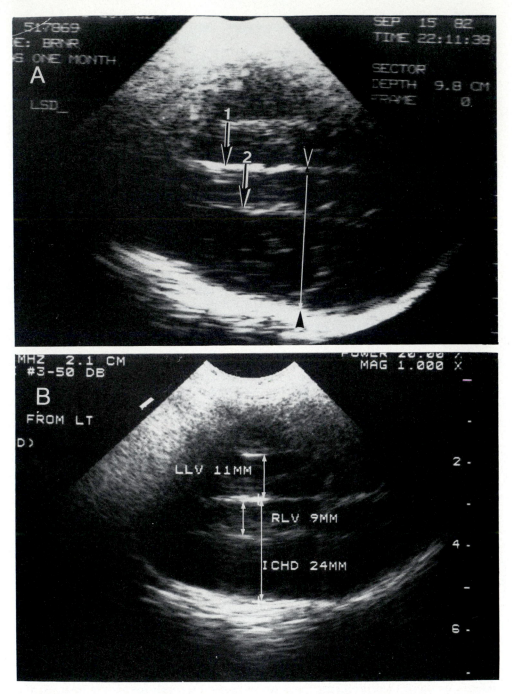

FIG 2–2.
Transaxial views of the lateral ventricles. **A,** the superolateral margins of the lateral ventricles are shown paralleling the midline. Measurements of both lateral ventricles can be made from the leading edge of the ventricle to the leading edge of the midline (*1*), thence to the leading edge of the far ventricle (*2*) (*arrows*). The ICHD is measured from the leading edge of the midline to the inner table at its widest point where the lateral ventricles are still visible on the scan plane (distance between *arrowheads*). **B,** dilatated lateral ventricles: near side 11/24 = 45.8%, far side 9/24 = 37.5% (assuming no midline shift, otherwise repeat the near side ICHD by scanning from the far side (i.e., reverse direction of sound travel to optimally visualize the ICHD as the near-side inner table is currently obscured by the near-field artifact).

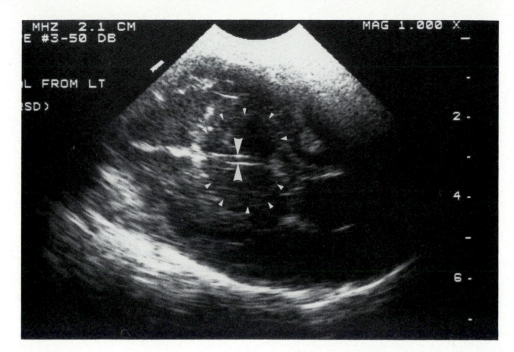

FIG 2–3.
Third ventricle and thalami, transaxial view. The most accurate way to measure the third ventricle is by scanning across its long axis, usually in the transverse plane as shown here, which would be the same approach used by A-mode. Measure the third ventricle across its widest axis (i.e, between the *arrowheads*) where it lies between the thalami (here outlined by *small arrowheads* as they would be traced for the thalamic area measurement).

GROSS ANATOMY

Anatomy[6] will be discussed from above downward, beginning with the intracranial contents. The largest components of the intracranial space are the cerebral hemispheres. These are paired structures with convex superior and lateral surfaces. The surfaces lie beneath bones that also correspond to segments of the hemispheres, which are: frontal lobe anteriorly, parietal lobes superiorly, occipital lobes posteriorly, and temporal lobes laterally. Medially within each hemisphere lies the lateral ventricle with segments correlating to the lobes in which they lie: frontal horn, occipital horn, and temporal horn. The midportion of the lateral ventricles is referred to as the body, and the trigone, or atria, is the portion where the temporal and occipital horns merge into the body. The sylvian fissure, or sulcus lateralis, is a well-marked groove on the lateral surface separating the frontal and parietal regions from the temporal region. The most medial extent of this fissure borders on the insula, a portion of the hemisphere lateral to the basal ganglia.

Under the occipital lobes lies the tentorium cerebelli, two fibrous bands which form the roof of the posterior fossa. Posterior to the brainstem, which will be described subsequently, lies the cerebellum. This is composed of a small median component, the vermis, and two lateral hemispheres. The fourth ventricle is a landmark separating the brainstem from the remaining posterior fossa contents.

The remaining structure within the cranium is the brainstem. This extends from just below the thalami down to the spinal cord. The thalami are the most central of the basal ganglia and lie immediately above the midbrain. The midbrain is a relatively short segment that is composed mainly of the cerebral peduncles, with a dorsal portion composed of the corpora quadrigemina (tectum of the midbrain). Embryologically, this is a separate portion of the brain from the remaining brainstem whose next portion inferiorly is the pons. The pons is recognized by a large ventral, rounded protuberance. Posteriorly, at this level, the cerebellar peduncles joint the brainstem. The lowest portion of the brainstem is referred to as the medulla oblongata. This contains the foramen of Magendie, the inferior (and medial) outlet of the fourth ventricle.

Extracranially, the central nervous system extends inferiorly (below the foramen magnum) as the spinal cord or medulla spinalis. In the adult it extends to the level of the first or second lumbar vertebral body. At this point it tapers, forming the conus medullaris. A delicate filament continues down from the apex of the conus to the first segment of the coccyx. This filum terminale is approximately 20 cm in length. The cord itself is slightly flattened dorsoventrally, and its surface is divided by a ventral median fissure and a dorsal median sulcus. A less apparent dorsolateral sulcus is present corresponding to the attachments of the dorsal roots. Thirty-one pairs of spinal nerves originate from the cord. The diameter of the cord is approximately 1 cm but there are fusiform enlargements in the cervical and lumbar regions compared with the remaining segments.

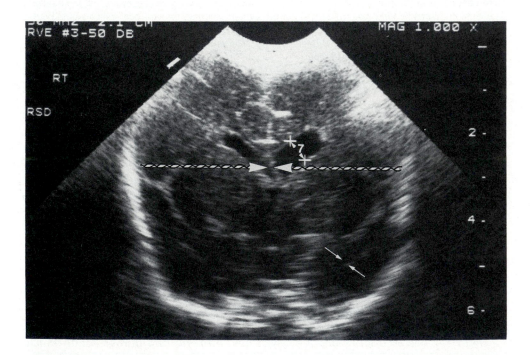

FIG 2–4.
Unilateral atrophic ventricular dilatation, coronal view. The frontal horn measures 7 mm, moderate dilatation, but its walls are parallel (giving it a roughly rectangular shape) and there is no temporal horn dilatation (*arrows* mark its position). The hemispheres are equal in width (*wavelike lines*) so there is no midline shift.

IMAGING TECHNIQUES AND BACKGROUND

Ultrasonic sounding (range or distance determination) was first used in navigation.[7] In the 1930s, industry began to use ultrasonic techniques to detect flaws in iron castings. As early as 1942, it was suggested that ultrasound might be used to locate lesions of the brain.[8] Early endeavors were directed at analyzing transmitted ultrasound. This, however, was of little use since the attenuation of sound passing through the skull was nearly 30 times greater than that passing through the brain; therefore, minimal variations in bone thickness would obscure slight differences in acoustic transmission of pathologic lesions. In 1951, reflections of intracranial structures were not recordable.[9] However, a suprasonic reflectoscope was invented using a pulsed echo technique.[10] A Japanese-language paper by Tanaka et al in 1952 was probably the first to document its use in the diagnosis of intracranial disease.[11] Their work did not receive much attention until later work was published in English. Other authors concurrently developed ultrasonic equipment to demonstrate the position of midline intracranial structures, and echoencephalography was born.[12]

Echoencephalography progressed rapidly throughout the 1960s; documentation of midline shifts, ventricular enlargement and displacement, and even mass detection became popular.[5, 13, 14]

Readers interested in more details regarding two-dimensional (B-scan) development in the late 1960s are referred to part IV of *Proceedings in Echo-Encephalography*.[14] Great progress had been made in waterpath scanning and contact B-scanning methods for mass detection and for ventricular landmarks and configuration. Before this time, x-rays had been used to obtain images of the calvarium. Bone or calcium was necessary to be measured radiographically; therefore, measurements were restricted to the cranial vault, sella turcica, pineal gland (when calcified), and rarely a calcified falx. With the birth of the specialty of neuroradiology, air (pneumoencephalography) and water-soluble contrast materials were instilled into the ventricular system, allowing better visualization on radiographs. Linear measurements and ratios, which suffer less from the magnification inherent in radiography, have been widely published. Cerebral angiography added little to the existing measurements, but new angiographic points were described, allowing improved localization of intracranial masses. These latter points are not generally identified by ultrasound, and will not be discussed in this chapter.

Since the 1970s, computed transaxial tomography (CT) has begun a new era in the imaging of the central nervous system. Images are routinely obtained in the transaxial view, angled 15 degrees to Reid's baseline, but coronal planes and reformated sagittal planes can also be obtained. Images are presented on a two-dimensional matrix. Sensitivity to differences in tissue radiographic density is nearly 100 times that of simple radiographs. This allows detailed differentiation of the surface and cisterns of the brain, as well as differentiation of solid areas whose radiographic attenuation differs by 10 to 15 Hounsfield units or more. Ventricles and most midline structures can be measured without added contrast. Currently, magnetic resonance imaging (MRI) of the brain is providing even more detail, and in planes limited only by the imagination. Even though the method of obtaining images is changing, it is not likely that the currently published measurements will be changed, as the computer reformating of the data in these modalities is free from magnification and parallax artifacts.

This is also true for ultrasound. As experience grew with A-mode ultrasound, the sylvian fissures, internal capsule, cavum septi pellucidi, and temporal horns were also identified in addition to the lateral ventricles and midline.[5] The majority of the work has been in the transaxial plane, although some sagittal visualization of the brainstem has been reported. Gray-scale imaging has added more substance to the images, but not a significant increase in measurement accuracy. What has increased greatly with real-time imaging is the speed and accuracy of localizing the proper image plane and identifying the anatomic structures to be measured. Gray-scale imaging of the adult brain reveals only the midline and lateral ventricles due to the great attenuation of the skull. Real-time imaging has been performed with the 1-MHz transducer. A-mode encephalographs employ 1- or 2-MHz transducers.

Sonography is the method of choice for imaging the neonatal brain. Five-megahertz and 7.5-MHz transducers can be used in the neonate through the open fontanels and cranial sutures. The ventricles are easily identified as are most anatomic structures. Reliable measurements can be made in multiple image planes to determine ventricular size, and to follow the course of ventricular dilatation, whether it be from obstruction or atrophy, and its response to shunt therapy.

In infants, the spinal cord can be visualized directly through the not yet totally ossified posterior neural arch. In adults, an anteroposterior (AP) measurement of the interosseous canal can be performed, but further evaluation of the cord can only be performed through laminectomy defects.

INTRACRANIAL DIAMETERS

Sounding of the skull size is done routinely in the fetus. This has been performed to a limited extent in adults with A-mode and in children with either A-mode or real-time imaging. Due to the less well developed ossification of the skull in the neonate, 5 MHz can adequately penetrate the bone to determine the distance to the falx, and its relationship to the diameter of the skull. Length can also be easily determined in the sagittal plane, that is, the fronto-occipital distance. In the very premature infant, 7.5 MHz is often adequate to penetrate the sutures.

MIDLINE

From above downward, the midline is marked by the falx cerebri, the septum pellucidum (or cavum septi pellucidi in neonates), the third ventricle, and the aqueduct and fourth ventricle. The brainstem itself is also a midline structure, and some attention has been paid to it with A-mode equipment. However, CT and MRI scanning have completely replaced ultrasound in visualizing the brainstem in adults. In children, however, brainstem and other central structures are easily visualized through the fontanel and, therefore, shifts in their position, enlargement, and other abnormalities can be visualized ultrasonically.

Midline echoencephalography was used primarily to determine a shift caused by a mass effect, either from a subdural hematoma or a unilateral mass. As the falx is fibrous, it is more rigid than the other structures and would shift less in pathologic conditions. Most soundings for mass effect were through the third ventricle and the septum pellucidum. An offset of the midline echo of more than 4 mm, that is, an absolute shift of 2 mm in either direction, was considered positive on A-mode scans.[5, 12, 13]

In the neonate, coronal scans through the anterior fontanel often demonstrate both temporal bones and, often, the lower parietal bones, so that the midline can be verified to be in its proper location by a transverse measurement (see Fig 2–4). Transaxial views can also be obtained throughout the period of infancy using 5-MHz or, on occasion, 3-MHz scans through the temporoparietal squamosa or through the coronal suture (see Fig 2–2).

The third ventricle can also undergo dilatation from obstruction or from atrophy. Its width can be measured reliably in the transaxial plane with either A-mode of gray-scale sonography (see Fig 2–3). The third ventricle should be normally 4 mm or less in transverse diameter in the pediatric population.[4] With atrophy, the walls of the third ventricle tend to remain parallel. However, with obstruction at the aqueduct or lower, the third ventricular walls are generally convex away from midline.

LATERAL VENTRICLES

Most of the mensuration of the lateral ventricles has focused on dilatation. These are indeed critical measurements in the follow-up of obstructive hydrocephalus as well as following ventricular response to shunt therapy. Atrophic dilatation, slower in its course, can also be documented. In adults, this is done with A-mode. However, real-time sector scanning is generally employed in children. The coronal views commonly used in children allow more measurements than the standard transaxial view of the lateral wall of the lateral ventricle.

Transverse views of the lateral ventricles reveal a top maximum diameter of 20 mm in the adult. This is a measurement from the lateral echo of the lateral ventricle to the midline. In infants this measurement is generally 10 to 11 mm, 8 to 10 mm in prematures, but the LV/ICHD ratio is more commonly used (see Fig 2–2). This ratio should be 30% to 33%,[3, 4] with dilatation diagnosed at 37% or greater. The same measurement can be obtained in the coronal projection by dividing the distance from the lateral wall of the lateral ventricle to the midline by the distance from midline to the inner table. This can be done for either side individually or as a combination of the biventricular distance divided by the widest intracranial diameter visualized in the coronal plane at the level of the superolateral margins of the lateral ventricles.

Additionally, in infants, the frontal horns can be measured across their diameter. Usually this is done at the level of the foramina of Monro. Normal measurements are up to and including 3 mm, with dilatation diagnosed at 4 mm or more across the frontal horns (see Fig 2–1).[1, 2] This measurement is apparently more sensitive to minor degrees of ventricular dilatation, as rounding of the ventricles is an early sign of obstruction. Significantly more dilatation is required to move the lateral margin of the lateral ventricle farther from midline, which would then make the LV/ICHD ratio abnormal.

Occasionally, the lateral ventricles of a newborn will appear empty of "slitlike," that is, there will be no fluid space within them and, therefore, an internal diameter cannot be measured. This configuration may be seen in up to 30% of normals but is seen in nearly all newborns who were passively addicted to narcotics in utero.[15] Slitlike ventricles may also be present with cerebral edema, but this diagnosis can usually be made by changes in white matter echogenicity.

A-mode studies in adults have also revealed the temporal horn position. The echo of the temporal horn normally lies midway between the third ventricle and inner table (see Fig 2–1).[5] A-mode sounding is done just above the petrous bone and behind the sella turcica.

THALAMUS

Transverse views of the thalami can be obtained through the temporal squamosa (see Fig 2–3). Pilot studies of control term infants have been performed to measure thalamic areas. This is done by tracing the thalamic margins with the map reader. In term infants, the average thalamic area is 241 mm² at birth, 333 mm² at 1 month, and 384 mm² at 6 months of life.[16]

INSULA AND INTERNAL CAPSULE, TRANSVERSE VIEW

The insula, also called the island of Reil, is cortical hemispheric tissue at the medial base of the sylvian fissure. On transaxial views, the insula-sylvian fissure complex generally is a fairly broad echo found 2 to 2.5 cm from the far inner table in the adult.[5] There is, generally, a pulsatile echo due to branches of the middle cerebral artery coursing through the sylvian fissure. With central masses and obstructive hydrocephalus, this insula is displaced laterally. With atrophic dilatation of the lateral ventricles, the insula is generally displaced medially.

The internal capsule is a band of white matter which lies immediately lateral to the basal ganglia. The basal ganglia, themselves, are very hypoechoic. However, the internal capsule serves as a margin. Echoes from the internal capsule are generally seen at the level of the third ventricle, and are 2 to 2.5 cm on either side of the midline.[5] Symmetry of these echoes is important for evaluation of central cerebral masses.

BRAINSTEM, SAGITTAL VIEW

From the posterior parietal region in the midline, a sagittal view can be obtained with A-mode coursing through the brainstem and fourth ventricle. The distance from the fourth ventricle to the clivus or dorsum sellae can then be obtained. The echo of the superior portion of the fourth ventricle or aqueduct should be within 2 mm of one-third the distance from the dorsum sellae to the posterior parietal bone. This measurement is of use when the brainstem is displaced by deep-seated intracranial masses. It may be possible to use this measurement in the pediatric population on the midline sagittal sonogram (Fig 2–5). In the newborn population, the fourth ventricle should be 2.9 mm deep when measured from the posterior fontanel approach, and 3.5 mm high in the coronal view.[4]

SPINAL CANAL

Measurements of the spinal canal have been obtained both in vivo and postmortem subjects by radiography. More recently, CT examination has also measured the spinal

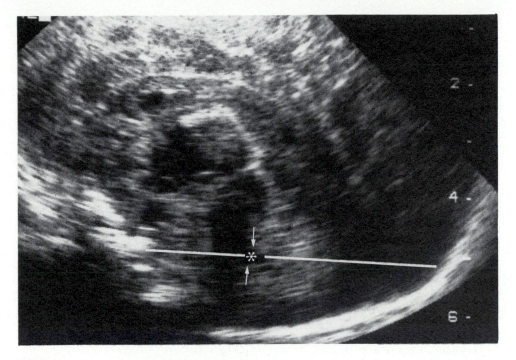

FIG 2–5.
Midline, sagittal view. The position of the fourth ventricle (*) is one-third the distance from the dorsum sellae to the posterior parietal bone (just above the posterior fontanel). The height of the fourth ventricle can be estimated on this view also (distance between *arrows*).

canal. Ultrasonically, a slightly oblique AP view angled 15 degrees from the true sagittal plane can be performed through the soft tissues of the back. Measurements of the canal in this fashion have been published and their relationship to the true AP dimension of a normally formed canal worked out.[17] In the operative suite, the diameter of the dural sac can be measured directly once the lamina have been removed. Transverse and sagittal planes are possible. Examining the intact adult spine is often limited by posterior spurring, narrow interlaminar distances, and ossification in the posterior soft tissues or ligamentum flavum. None of these problems are present in children, whose not-yet-completely ossified neural arch provides an ample window for visualizing the spinal canal.

The spinal cord itself has been measured by postmortem radiography, myelographic techniques (both post mortem and in vivo) and by CT scans, both with and without contrast material. Ultrasonic visualization of the cord itself is somewhat limited due to the surrounding bones and poor penetration of sound in the adult patient. The cord can be seen in newborns and in the postlaminectomy state. In these patients, measurements are of value in determining the normalcy of the spinal cord. Enlargements of the cord from swelling, masses, or cysts are easily differentiated from the small atrophic cords. Also, masses within cords whose overall dimension is normal may then imply atrophy with a superimposed space-occupying process.

Newborn spinal sonography can also verify the position of the conus, which should be no lower than the third lumbar vertebral body at birth and gradually reach its final level (at the first lumbar disk) by 10 months of age. An unusually low conus, or one which does not ascend during the first year of life, is diagnostic of the tethered cord syndrome.

REFERENCES

1. Fiske CE, Filly RA, Callen PQ: Sonographic measurement of lateral ventricular width in early ventricular dilatation. *J Clin Ultrasound* 1981; 9:303–307.
2. Perry RNW, Bowman ED, Roy RND, et al: Ventricular size in newborn infants. *J Ultrasound Med* 1985; 4:475–477.
3. Graziani LJ, Pasto ME, Stanley C, et al: Cranial ultrasound and clinical studies in preterm infants. *J Pediatr* 1985; 106:269–276.
4. Helmke K, Winkler P: Ultrasonic measurements of the normal intracerebral ventricular system in the first year of life. *Monatsschr Kinderheilkd* 1987; 135:148–152.
5. Tenner MS, Woodraska GM: *Diagnostic Ultrasound in Neurology*. New York, John Wiley & Sons, 1975.
6. Gross CM (ed): *Gray's Anatomy*, ed 28. Philadelphia, Lea & Febiger, 1966, pp 781–863.
7. Langevin MP: Les ondes ultrasonores. *Rev Gen Electr* 1928; 23:626–634.
8. Dussik KT: Ueber die Möglichkeit brochfrequente mechanische Schwingungen als diagnostisches Hilfsmittel zu verwerten. *Z Gesamte Neurol Psychiatr* 1942; 174:153–168.
9. Ballantine HT Jr, Bolt RH, Heuter TF, et al: On the detection of intracranial pathology by ultrasound. *Science* 1950; 112:525–528.
10. Firestone FA: The supersonic reflectoscope for interior inspection. *Metal Prog* 1945; 48:505.
11. Tanaka K, Kikuchi Y, Uchida R: Detection of intracranial anatomical abnormalities by ultrasound. *J Acoust Soc Jpn* 1952; 8:111–112.
12. Leksell L: Echoencephalography: 1. Detection of intracranial complications following head injury. *Acta Chir Scand* 1955; 110:301–315.
13. Uematsu S, Walker AE: *A Manual of Echoencephalography*. Baltimore, Williams & Wilkins Co., 1971.
14. Kazner E, Schiefer W, Zulch KJ (eds): *Proceedings in Echo-Encephalography*. New York, Springer-Verlag, 1968.
15. Pasto ME, Graziani LJ, Tunis SL, et al: Ventricular configuration and cerebral growth in infants born to drug-dependent mothers. *Pediatr Radiol* 1985; 15:77–81.
16. Pasto ME, Deiling JM, Graziani LJ, et al: Disparity in hemispheric and thalamic growth in infants undergoing abstinence, in NIDA *Research Monographic Series. Proceedings of the 47th Annual Scientific Meeting*, Vol 67. 1985, pp 342–348.
17. Kadziolka R, Asytely M, Hanai K, et al: Ultrasonic measurements of the lumbar spinal canal. *Bone Joint Surg* 1981; 63:504–507.

Chapter 3 _____

Ophthalmic Ultrasound: Axial Length Measurements

Elizabeth L. Affel, M.S.

The A-scan was first used in ophthalmology in the late 1950s.[1] It was used to determine axial length measurements as well as to aid in the diagnosis of ophthalmic pathologic conditions. In the United States, the ultrasound axial length was first used in 1974 to calculate intraocular lens powers. Since that time, these scans have become routine in the preoperative testing of a patient for cataract surgery.

The B-scan was introduced to ophthalmology not long after the A-scan. Early A- and B-scanning was performed with an immersion system. In the late 1970s a portable A- and B-scan unit was developed utilizing a contact B-scan. Ophthalmic B-scanning became more popular as a diagnosis tool due to the ease of its use.

The B-scan is ordered by the ophthalmologist when there is no view of the retina. Common causes for this are hemorrhage, mature cataract, corneal scarring, and trauma. The B-scan is used to rule out the presence of a retinal detachment, intraocular tumor, choroidal detachments, and other vitreoretinal conditions.

ANATOMY OF THE EYE IN RELATION TO THE A-SCAN

With the A-scan, the axis of the sound waves appears as a horizontal line on the oscilloscope. As the sound waves are emitted from the probe, and interface various acoustic structures, vertical deflections on the oscilloscope baseline appear. These are called echo spikes. The location, size, and number of spikes identify the acoustic structures involved[2] (Fig 3–1).

In the normal eye, the cornea, lens (anterior and posterior capsules), vitreoretinal interface, and orbital fat produce clear, identifiable echo spikes. The anterior chamber, the lens interior, and the vitreous cavity produce no echo return and, therefore, are seen as baseline.[1]

The axial length is determined as the distance from the corneal spike to the vitreoretinal interface. The probe must be aligned to assure axiality. This is accomplished by adjusting the probe until all spikes are at their maximum height. The retinal spike and corneal spike should be equal. The use of these criteria will greatly reduce errors in alignment.[3]

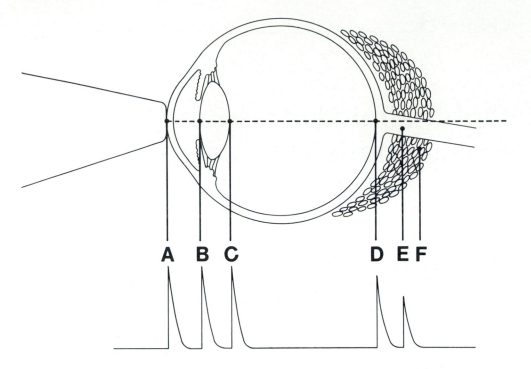

FIG 3–1.
Proper probe positioning and resultant echoes. *A* = corneal spike; *B* = anterior lens capsule; *C* = posterior lens capsule; *D* = retina; *E* = optic nerve; and *F* = orbital fat.

AXIAL LENGTH MEASUREMENTS

Numerous studies have been conducted to investigate the average anterior chamber depth and average axial length. As with many organs that change in size with development, there is no one standard of axial length and anterior chamber depth.

Normative pediatric data give axial length ranges of 17.0 to 20.1 mm at birth, 19.1 to 21.9 mm at 6 months, 19.8 to 22.4 mm at 1 year, and 20.5 to 23.1 mm at 2 years of age.[4] Blomdahl[4] found the average anterior chamber depth in newborn infants ranged from 2.4 to 2.9 mm with a mean axial length of 2.6 mm. He also measured the lens thickness in the infants. These measurements ranged from 3.4 to 3.9 mm with a mean of 3.6 mm.[4]

The lens thickness increases with aging. Weekers et al.[5] found a normal lens thickness of 3.91 ± 0.31 mm for 20- to 29-year-olds. This value increased to 4.33 ± 0.35 mm for the 40- to 49-year age group, and to 4.87 ± 0.66 mm for normal patients in their sixth decade.

The mean anterior chamber depth has been measured to be 2.91 ± 0.31 mm.[6]

Studies of ultrasonic axial length indicate a range from 23.37 (±0.75) to 23.65 (±1.35) mm in Western adult populations.[7, 8] Cross-culturally, the difference may be slight. Yu et al. studied 1,789 normal Chinese young adults and found a mean axial length of 23.74 (±1.24) mm.[9]

The axial length is usually constant in normal adult eyes. The anterior chamber depth has a positive correlation to the axial length.[7] Short, or hyperopic, eyes have shorter anterior segments and longer, or myopic, eyes have larger anterior chamber depth.

Francois and Goes found the thickness of the lens is independent of the axial length of the eye.[7] As the lens ages, the lens thickens and so correlates positively with age, rather than eye length.[5]

REFERENCES

1. Gitter K: Ophthalmic ultrasound: in *Proceedings of the Fourth International Congress of Ultrasonography in Ophthalmology.* St Louis, CV Mosby Co, 1969, pp 1—4, 158—164.
2. Ossinig K: Echography of the eye, orbit and periorbital Region, in Arger PH (ed): *Orbit Roentgenology* New York, John Wiley & Sons, Inc, 1977.
3. Hoffer KJ: Preoperative cataract evaluation: Intraocular lens power calculation. *Int Ophthalmol Clin* 1982; 22:37–75.
4. Blomdahl S: Ultrasonic measurements of the eye in the newborn infant. *Acta Ophthalmol* 1989; 57:1048–1056.
5. Weekers R, et al: Biometrics of the crystalline lens, in Bellows JG (ed): *Cataract and Abnormalities of the Lens* New York, Grune & Stratton, Inc, 1980.
6. Hoffer KJ: Accuracy of ultrasound intraocular lens calculation. *Arch Ophthalmol* 1981; 99.1819–1823.
7. Francois J, Goes F: Ultrasonographic study of 100 emmetrophic eyes. *Ophthalmologica* 1977; 175:321–327.
8. Hoffer KJ: Biometry of 7500 cataractous eyes. *Am J Ophthalmol* 1980; 90:360, 890.
9. Yu CS, Kao D, Chang CT: Measurement of the length of the visual axis by ultrasonography in 1,789 eyes. *Chung Hua Yen Ko Tsa Chih* 1979; 15:45.

Chapter 4

Ultrasound Measurements of the Thyroid

Laurence Needleman, M.D.

Two types of thyroid measurements are available: linear measurements of length and width, and volume measurements.

LINEAR MEASUREMENTS

A standard anatomic source quotes the average thyroid lobe size as 5 cm in length, 3 cm in width, and 2 cm in anteroposterior dimension.[1] There is no study of these dimensions in the normal population using ultrasonic measurements. Tong and Rubenfeld[2] did determine the linear measurements of the normal thyroid by nuclear medicine iodine 131 scans (Table 4–1).

VOLUME MEASUREMENTS

The volume of the thyroid is a useful clinical measure, particularly in determining the dosage of radioiodine therapy. Sonography has been used to determine thyroid volume in several studies.[3–6] In one, sonography was used in conjunction with nuclear medicine.[7] The methods all show good correlation between the calculated volume and either the measured volume[3, 5] or weight[4, 6, 7] of the gland. They indicate that there is a one-to-one relationship between thyroid volume in cubic centimeters and its weight in grams.

The calculation of thyroid volume generally requires a static scanner and either a planimeter or a scanner that permits on-line determination of area. A series of transverse scans are obtained at 0.1- to 0.5-cm intervals. The area of the thyroid at each level is determined (Fig 4–1). The volume of each level is determined by multiplying the traced area by the thickness. The entire volume is the sum of all of the slices.[6]

The volume of the gland can also be calculated by means of more complicated integration formulas as described by Rasmussen and Hjorth.[3] Using this method Hegedus et al.[5] determined the thyroid volume in normal subjects. Table 4–2 shows

TABLE 4–1.
Normal Thyroid Measurements by Iodine 131 Scans

Measurement	Size ± 2 SD (cm)
Right lobe, longitudinal length	4.8 ± 1.8
Left lobe, longitudinal length	4.7 ± 2.0
Whole thyroid, width	5.2 ± 1.4
Right lobe, width	2.3 ± 1.0
Left lobe, width	2.3 ± 1.2
Isthmus, height	1.7 ± 1.6

the normal volume of thyroid in milliliters per kilogram of weight (volume = weight ratio) for different age groups and sex.

Brown and Spencer[7] used a simple formula and a combination of the thyroid nuclear medicine scan and the sonogram to determine volume. The maximum size of the gland, on transverse images, was selected and the long axis determined. The longest length perpendicular to this was selected. These two diameters were measured. The length of the gland was obtained from the nuclear scan. Volume was calculated by the formula: Volume of an ovoid = $(\pi/6)$ length × width × height. This method had good correlation with surgical estimates of gland mass ($r = .92$). Although the length of the thyroid can be determined on sagittal sonograms there is no study which has investigated thyroid volume using sonographically derived length, width, and height.

TABLE 4–2.
Normal Thyroid Volume-Weight Ratio*

Sex	Age Range (yr)	Volume-Weight Ratio (Mean ± 2 SD) (mL/kg)
F	13–39	0.269 ± 0.122
M	14–29	0.249 ± 0.114
F	30–49	0.288 ± 0.120
M	30–49	0.275 ± 0.100
F	50–69	0.267 ± 0.086
M	50–69	0.279 ± 0.084
F	71–91	0.319 ± 0.136
M	72–91	0.293 ± 0.096

*From Hegedus L, Perrild H, Poulsen LR, et al: *J Clin Endocrinol Metab* 1983; 56:260–263. Used by permission.

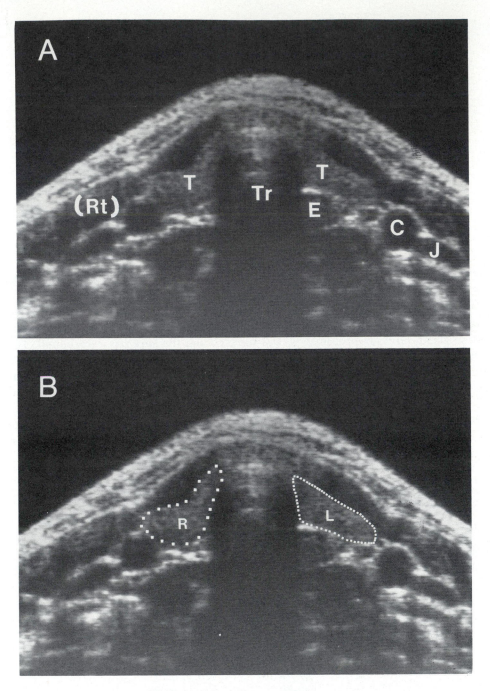

FIG 4–1.
Sonographic measurement of thyroid area. **A,** transverse sonogram of the neck. The right and left lobes of the thyroid (*T*) abut either side of the tracheal air column (*Tr*). The esophagus (*E*), carotid artery (*C*), and jugular vein (*J*) can also be identified. (*Rt*)-toward patient's right. **B,** the area of each lobe is determined and calculated by an off-line planimeter or on-line calculation of area. *L*-area of left thyroid lobe bounded by narrowly spaced dots; *R*-area of right thyroid lobe bounded by widely spaced dots.

REFERENCES

1. Williams PL, Warwich R: Endocrine glands, in *Gray's Anatomy,* ed. Philadelphia, WB Saunders Co, 1980, pp 1437–1464.
2. Tong ECK, Rubenfeld S: Scan measurements of normal and enlarged thyroid glands. *Am J Roentgenol* 1972; 115:706–708.
3. Rasmussen SN, Hjorth L: Determination of thyroid volume by ultrasonic scanning. *J Clin Ultrasound* 1974; 2:143–147.
4. Tannahill AJ, Hooper MN England M, et al: Measurement of thyroid size by ultrasound, palpation and scintiscan. *Clin Endocrinol* 1978; 8:483–486.
5. Hegedus L, Perrild H, Poulsen LR, et al: The determination of thyroid volume by ultrasound and its relationship to body weight, age, and sex in normal subjects. *J Clin Endocrinol Metab* 1983; 56:260–263.
6. Yokoyama N, Nagayama Y, Kakezono F, et al: Determination of the volume of the thyroid gland by a high resolutional ultrasonic scanner. *J Nucl Med* 1986; 27:1475–1479.
7. Brown MC, Spencer R: Thyroid gland volume estimated by use of ultrasound in addition to scintigraphy. *Acta Radiol (Oncol)* 1978; 17:37–41.

Ultrasound Measurements of the Parathyroid

Laurence Needleman, M.D.

There is no established sonographic size for the parathyroid gland. Sonographic visualization of normal glands is rare.[1] Most reports describe abnormally enlarged glands.[1-4] The major problem of parathyroid sonography is identifying the parathyroids rather than falsely calling normal glands enlarged. In practice, structures mistakenly called the parathyroid tend to be other structures, such as lymph nodes or the thyroid, rather than normal glands.

Wang described the average normal parathyroid gland to measure $5 \times 3 \times 1$ mm.[5] The largest normal gland in his group was $12 \times 2 \times 1$ mm and the smallest was $2 \times 2 \times 1$ mm. The vast majority of people (98%) have four glands.[5]

Simeone et al. have identified a normal 5- $\times$ 3- $\times$ 1-mm gland with ultrasound.[1]

In clinical hyperparathyroidism, the diagnosis of the enlarged gland is based on the identification of the gland rather than its size. The length and anteroposterior (AP) diameter are measured from sagittal scans (Fig 5–1), and the width, at right angles to the largest length on transverse section. Usually glands are not visualized unless they are 5 mm or more in size. Sonographically enlarged glands tend to be oval (see Fig 5–1).

REFERENCES

1. Simeone JF, Mueller PR, Ferrucci JT Jr, et al: High-resolution real-time sonography of the parathyroid. *Radiology* 1981; 141:745–751.
2. Crocker EF, Bautovich GJ, Jellins J: Gray-scale echographic visualization of a parathyroid adenoma. *Radiology* 1978; 126:233–234.
3. Reading CC, Charboneau JW, James EM, et al: High-resolution parathyroid sonography. *AJR* 1982; 139:539–546.
4. Stark DD, Gooding GAW, Moss AA, et al: Parathyroid imaging: comparison of high-resolution CT and high-resolution sonography. *AJR* 1983; 141:633–638.
5. Wang C-A: The anatomic basis of parathyroid surgery. *Ann Surg* 1976; 183:271–275.

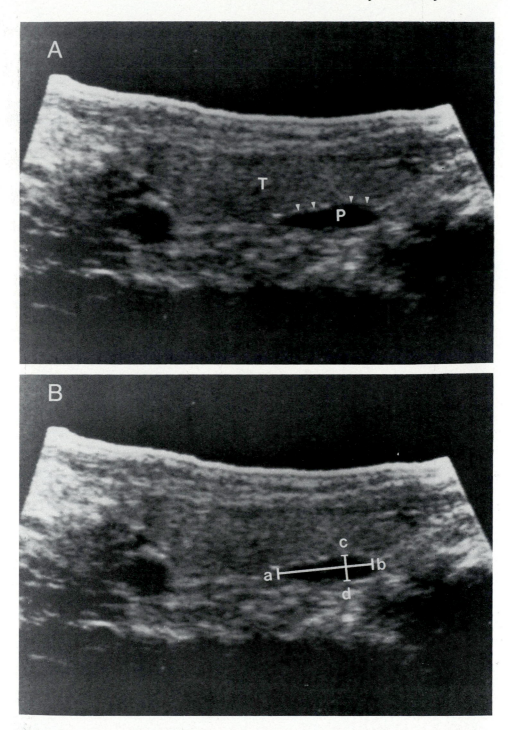

FIG 5–1.
Sonographic measurement of the parathyroid. **A,** longitudinal sonogram of the thyroid (*T*) shows the less echogenic parathyroid adenoma (*P*) posterior to the echogenic thyroid capsule (*arrowheads*). **B,** the length of the gland is measured parallel to the long axis (*line* from *a* to *b*) and at right angles to the long axis for the AP dimension (*line* from *c* to *d*).

PART II

Echocardiography

Chapter 6

Echocardiographic Measurements

Joel S. Raichlen, M.D.

Measurements of cardiac structures are made to aid in the diagnosis and monitoring of patients with heart disease. The first technique that enabled measurement of heart size was the chest x-ray.[1, 2] This inexpensive noninvasive technique has been most commonly applied to the measurement of the cardiothoracic ratio, the ratio of the maximum transverse diameter of the heart to the maximum transverse diameter of the thorax. Cardiac enlargement was diagnosed if heart size exceeded the normal range of 0.4 to 0.5. The posteroanterior and lateral views of the heart were used to generate estimates of cardiac volume from measurements of three orthogonal cardiac diameters, and estimates of specific chamber sizes could be made by combining these with oblique views. Although these measurements provided some previously unavailable estimates of heart size and volume, they were extremely limited due to poor resolution, the overlap of cardiac chambers, and size variations introduced by the specific timing of x-ray images within the cardiac and respiratory cycles. The use of x-rays was further limited by the inability to generate quantitative estimates of the size of specific cardiac chambers.

The development of cineangiography provided the first means of quantitatively assessing ventricular function and the consequences of valvular dysfunction. The injection of radiographic contrast material directly into the left ventricle enabled assessment of global and regional myocardial wall motion. By applying geometric assumptions about the shape of the left ventricle, Sandler and Dodge and co-workers developed a means of estimating left ventricular volume from single-plane or biplane cineangiograms.[3, 4] Measurement of the maximum and minimum myocardial volume enabled estimation of left ventricular end-diastolic volume, end-systolic volume, stroke volume, and ejection fraction. By examining ventricular volume as a function of time, one could obtain estimates of the rates of systolic ejection and diastolic filling. The major limitation of the technique was that it was invasive, required moderate x-ray exposure, and necessitated the use of radiographic contrast material. In addition, the images that were generated represented only a silhouette of the heart, requiring the application of geometric assumptions in order to make estimates of left ventricular volume.

Ventricular angiograms have also been obtained noninvasively using nuclear cardiology techniques. Radionuclide ventriculograms can be obtained from equilibrium gated blood pool studies of the heart. By viewing images acquired from different portions of the cardiac cycle in rapid succession, one can examine regional wall motion within the left and right ventricles. Inasmuch as the images are made from radioisotope-labeled red blood cells, the assessment of segmental left ventricular wall motion is limited due to the overlap of blood-containing structures such as the right ventricle, the atria, and the great vessels. An advantage provided by the use of labeled red blood cells is in the assessment of left ventricular volume and ejection fraction. Since the scintigraphic counts detected in the region of the left ventricle are generated from the presence of red blood cells, assessments of ventricular volume are based on the volume of red blood cells and require no geometric assumptions.[5-8] Using relative or absolute estimates of ventricular volume, one can obtain highly accurate estimates of left ventricular ejection fraction using this technique. One of the major limitations of equilibrium gated blood pool scans is the requirement of summing information from hundreds of cardiac cycles in order to create the images of the heart. As a consequence, this technique provides reliable information only when acquired during periods of regular cardiac rhythm and, under the best circumstances, results in estimates of left ventricular ejection fraction that are accurate to within 5%. Examining time activity changes within the left ventricle enables determination of rates of systolic ejection and diastolic filling of the left ventricle. Although offering the advantage over contrast ventriculography of being a noninvasive technique, gated blood pool scans do not avoid exposure to ionizing radiation.

Several newer noninvasive techniques are being applied to image the heart and quantify cardiac size and function. Digital subtraction radiographic techniques enable the generation of images of the left ventricular cavity after an intravenous (IV) injection of radiopaque contrast material.[9, 10] This technology eliminates the necessity of directly injecting contrast material into the left ventricular cavity, as is required in standard contrast ventriculography. When the two techniques are combined, digital subtraction angiography can produce high-quality images of the left ventricular cavity following intracavitary injection of relatively small quantities of contrast material.

X-ray computed tomography (CT) is now a standard imaging technique for obtaining tomographic views of stationary structures.[11, 12] Recently, rapid acquisition systems have been developed which can generate tomographic images in 50 ms. By gating to the electrocardiogram (ECG) and obtaining sequential images after injection of IV contrast material, a moving picture of the heart can be generated. From this, direct measurements of myocardial wall thickness and cavity dimension can be made.

The most recent imaging technique being applied to the heart is nuclear magnetic resonance imaging (MRI). Like CT, serial parallel images of the heart can be obtained in preselected orientations, gating to the ECG. In contrast, MRI images can be obtained without injecting radiographic contrast material. This technique has great promise for generating high-resolution noninvasive images that permit measurement of cardiac chamber size, wall thickness, and myocardial mass.[13-15]

The above techniques have the potential of providing estimates of cardiac size and function but all have major limitations in that they are invasive, require IV contrast media, do not provide beat-to-beat information about cardiac function, or require very expensive imaging equipment. Ultrasound offers an important imaging modality that is well suited for cardiac evaluation inasmuch as it is an inexpensive noninvasive technique that not only provides beat-to-beat information about cardiac

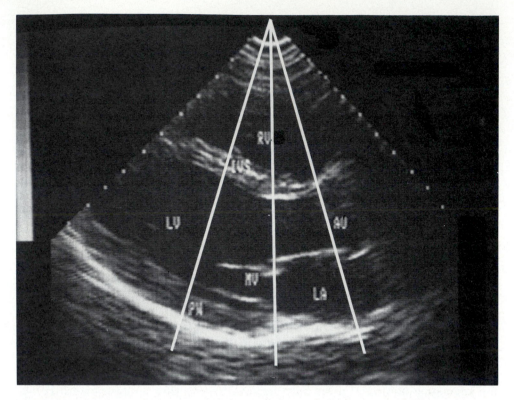

FIG 6–1.
Parasternal long-axis view of the heart showing the positions of the M-mode cursor used for generating M-mode echocardiograms. The left line traverses the right ventricle (*RV*), the interventricular septum (*IVS*), the cavity of the left ventricle (*LV*), and the posterior wall (*PW*). The middle line shows the position for imaging the motion of the mitral valve (*MV*). The right line shows the position of the M-mode beam as it traverses the outflow portion of the RV, the anterior wall of the aortic root, the aortic valve (*AV*), the posterior wall of the aortic root, and the cavity and posterior wall of the left atrium (*LA*).

size, function, and wall thickness, but also enables direct visualization of the cardiac valves which can be assessed qualitatively and quantitatively.

M-MODE ECHOCARDIOGRAPHY

M-mode echocardiography was the first noninvasive technique to enable real-time imaging of cardiac structures that enabled recording of the thickness and motion patterns of the walls and valves of the heart. The technique provided a means of obtaining quantitative measurements of the thickness and motion of the left ventricular septum and posterior wall, the size of the cardiac chambers and aorta, and the thickness and excursion of the cardiac valves. Before the advent of two-dimensional imaging, M-mode tracings were recorded using nonimaging transducers. Current recording technique utilizes two-dimensional images of the heart to direct the M-mode cursor into proper position (Fig 6–1). In 1978, the American Society of Echocardiography evaluated methods of generating M-mode echocardiographic measurements and made recommendations based on the techniques that yielded the most reproducible measurements of each parameter.[16] The following outline of M-mode echocardiographic measurements is based on those recommendations along with additions and alternatives derived from physiologic and practical considerations.

Measurements at the Base of the Heart

M-mode echocardiograms are recorded from the left parasternal acoustic window. Figure 6–2 shows a two-dimensional echocardiographic image of the long axis of the left ventricle obtained from this location. The dotted line through the base of the heart shows the position of the cursor that is used to generate the M-mode tracings. To the left of the two-dimensional image is the resulting M-mode echocardiogram. This tracing is used to measure the diameter of the proximal aortic root, the excursion of the aortic valve, and the size of the left atrium.

Aortic Root.—The aortic root is measured from the leading edge of the anterior wall of the aortic root to the leading edge of the posterior wall of the aortic root (Fig 6–3). Maximum reproducibility is obtained when measurements are made during the period of diastole rather than during systole. Therefore, measurements should be made either at the onset of the QRS complex of the ECG, or preceding that point, during the time that the anterior and posterior walls of the root appear horizontal. This measurement is made in the region of the tracing where the aortic cusps are visualized. If the cursor is positioned using the parasternal cross-sectional view at the level of the aortic valve, one can ensure that the M-mode beam traverses the center of the aortic root (Fig 6–4), thus making the measured diameter more accurate. The normal aortic root dimension ranges from 1.9 to 4.0 cm in adults (see Table 6–1). Increased aortic root dimensions are found in primary abnormalities of the aortic

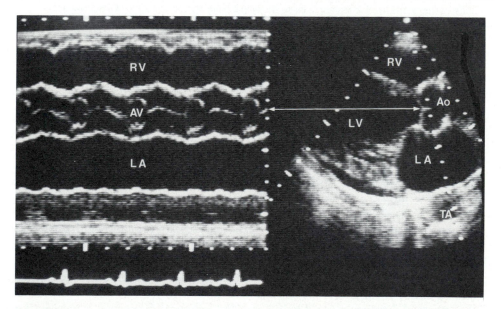

FIG 6–2.
An M-mode tracing at the level of the aortic valve (*AV*). The right image is a two-dimensional long-axis view of the heart showing the position of the M-mode cursor for obtaining the tracing (*dotted line*). The *horizontal line* shows the position of the AV on the M-mode and two-dimensional echocardiograms. *Ao* = proximal aortic root; *LA* = left atrium; *LV* = left ventricle; *RV* = right ventricle; *TA* = descending thoracic aorta.

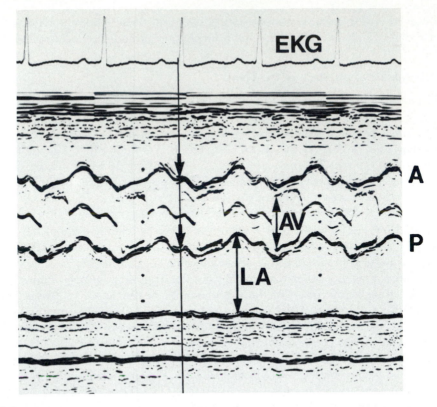

FIG 6–3.
M-mode tracing at the level of the aortic valve showing the timing and positions at which measurements are made. The *vertical line* is drawn at the beginning of the QRS of the electrocardiogram (*EKG*) which is taken as end-diastole. The aortic root may be measured at this time (*downward arrows*) from the leading edge of the anterior wall of the aortic root (*A*) to the leading edge of the posterior wall of the aortic root (*P*). The aortic valve (*AV*) is measured at the point of maximal excursion (*short bidirectional arrow*). The left atrium (*LA*) is measured from the leading edge of the posterior wall of the aortic root to the leading edge of the posterior wall of the left atrium (*long bidirectional arrow*).

root such as Marfan's syndrome, or in secondary abnormalities such as poststenotic dilatation associated with aortic stenosis.

Left Atrium.—The left atrium lies immediately posterior to the proximal aortic root. Its dimension should be measured in the same region of the M-mode tracing that is used to measure the aortic root. The left atrium is measured from the leading edge of the posterior wall of the aortic root to the leading edge of the posterior wall of the atrium. If a two-dimensional image is not available for orientation, the posterior wall of the left atrium may be identified using an M-mode sweep from the region of the left ventricle since the posterior walls of the atrium and ventricle are in continuity (see Fig 6–1). The left atrial dimension is measured at its maximum which occurs at end-systole when the atria reach maximum volume (Fig 6–3). The normal range of the left atrial dimension is 1.9 to 4.0 cm. The left atrial dimension is increased in diseases of the mitral valve and in disease states associated with decreased left ventricular compliance.

Aortic Valve.—At any given time, the M-mode beam traverses only two of the

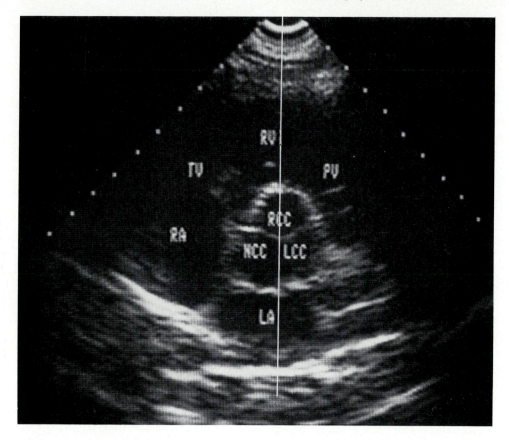

FIG 6–4.
Parasternal cross-sectional view of the heart at the level of the aortic valve showing the position of the M-mode cursor through the middle of the aortic root and valve (*solid line*). LA = left atrium; *LCC* = left coronary cusp; *NCC* = noncoronary cusp; *PV* = pulmonic valve; *RA* = right atrium; *RCC* = right coronary cusp; *RV* = right ventricle; *TV* = tricuspid valve.

TABLE 6–1.
Adult M-Mode Measurements

Parameters	Normal Ranges
Aortic root dimension	1.9–4.0 cm
Left atrial dimension	1.9–4.0 cm
Aortic cusp separation	1.5–2.6 cm
Mitral valve excursion	1.6–3.0 cm
Mitral valve EF slope	70–150 mm/sec
E-point septal separation	<1 cm
Right ventricular end-diastolic dimension	0.7–2.7 cm
Interventricular septal thickness	0.6–1.2 cm
Left ventricular posterior wall thickness	0.6–1.2 cm
Left ventricular end diastolic dimension	3.5–5.7 cm
Left ventricular ejection fraction	>55%
Left ventricular fractional shortening	>25%
Velocity of circumferential fiber shortening	>8.85 circumference/sec

three leaflets of the aortic valve. From the parasternal acoustic window, the more anterior right coronary cusp and the more posterior left or noncoronary cusp are imaged. These leaflets normally appear as thin linear echodensities that separate in a boxcar configuration in systole (see Figs 6–2 and 6–3). They open following the QRS complex of the ECG and close at end-systole, which occurs during the T wave portion of the ECG. Aortic cusp separation is measured in early systole when the leaflet separation is greatest. Measurements are made from the leading edge of the anterior right coronary cusp to the leading edge of the more posterior cusp. Normal aortic cusp separation ranges from 1.5 to 2.6 cm. In the normal valve, optimal positioning of the M-mode cursor may be made by directing the beam using the two-dimensional parasternal cross-sectional view (see Fig 6–4). This enables recording of the maximum separation of the valve leaflets. In the presence of a low cardiac output or significant mitral regurgitation, the leaflet opening may be normal initially, with gradual narrowing through systole. In aortic stenosis the leaflets appear thickened and/or calcified and have reduced cusp separation throughout systole. In aortic stenosis, systolic doming of the valve may be observed. When this occurs, sampling errors may suggest that cusp separation is relatively wide because the M-mode cursor is not directed through the leaflets at the orifice of the valve. Correct sampling can be assured by utilizing the parasternal long-axis image to ensure that the M-mode cursor is directed through the narrow orifice of doming aortic valve leaflets.

Although not a part of the routine clinical echocardiographic examination, left ventricular systolic time intervals may be measured from M-mode tracings of the aortic valve. The most useful of these is the left ventricular ejection time (LVET). This can be determined directly by measuring the time (in milliseconds) between aortic valve opening and aortic valve closure. The preejection period (PEP) can also be measured from this tracing. This parameter represents the time duration from the onset of the QRS until the time of aortic valve opening. It is the sum of the duration of the electromechanical delay and the isovolumic contraction period of the left ventricle. These systolic time intervals can be compared to normal values by correcting for sex and heart rate using standard regression equations.[17] The PEP/LVET ratio has proved to be a useful parameter reflecting left ventricular dysfunction.

Another measurement that may be made is the eccentricity index, which reflects the relative position of the aortic valve leaflets within the aortic root during diastole. The normal position of the closed aortic valve is in the central portion of the aortic root. In the case of a bicuspid aortic valve, the closure line may be eccentric, lying closer to one wall of the aortic root than the other. The eccentricity index is the ratio of the distance between the anterior wall of the aortic root and the closure line of the aortic valve, to the distance from the closure line to the posterior wall of the aortic root. Variation in beam orientation can artificially cause the appearance of an eccentric closure line in a normal tricuspid aortic valve, and similarly, a bicuspid aortic valve may appear to have a midposition closure line. Due to these limitations, this parameter is not routinely measured in clinical laboratories.

Measurements at the Level of the Mitral Valve

The M-mode image of the mitral valve is obtained by sweeping the M-mode beam inferiorly from the level of the aortic root, or superiorly from the level of the left ventricle. In continuous tracings, the anterior leaflet of the mitral valve appears contiguous with the posterior wall of the aortic root, and the posterior leaflet of the

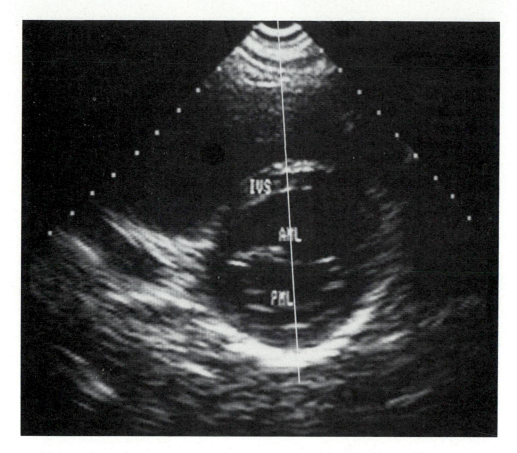

FIG 6–5.
Parasternal cross-sectional view at the level of the mitral valve showing the position of the M-mode cursor (*solid line*) through the interventricular septum (*IVS*), the anterior leaflet of the mitral valve (*AML*), and the posterior leaflet of the mitral valve (*PML*).

mitral valve appears contiguous with the posterior wall of the left atrium. Optimal positioning of the M-mode cursor through the midportion of the mitral valve leaflets can be made using a cross-sectional image of the valve (Fig 6–5).

Each inflection along the tracing of the mitral valve echocardiogram is labeled alphabetically beginning with the a wave (Fig 6–6). The a wave occurs in late diastole following electrical excitation of the atrium (P wave) and is labeled *A*. The point of closure at which the anterior and posterior mitral leaflets coapt is labeled *C*. If there is an interruption in the closure line between points A and C, it is labeled *B* and referred to as a B notch or B bump. This finding has been associated with an increase in left ventricular end-diastolic pressure. The point in diastole at which the anterior and posterior leaflets separate is labeled *D* and the maximum anterior excursion of the anterior leaflet is labeled *E*. The excursion of the mitral valve is measured as the vertical distance in centimeters from the D point to the E point (Figs 6–6 and 6–7). Normal values range from 1.6 to 3.0 cm. Following the E point, the anterior and posterior leaflets move toward one another. The point at which the anterior leaflet stops moving rapidly in a posterior direction is labeled *F*. The slope of the line made by the anterior leaflet as it moves from the E point to the F point is the

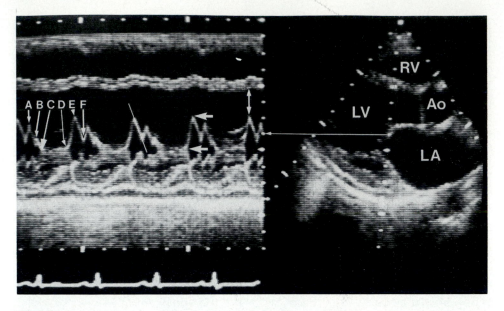

FIG 6–6.
Parasternal long-axis view of the heart showing the position of the M-mode cursor through the mitral valve (*dotted line*) and its associated M-mode tracing. The *horizontal line* shows the position of the mitral valve on the M-mode and two-dimensional echocardiograms. Each inflection of the anterior leaflet of the mitral valve is labeled in alphabetical order (*A–F*) beginning with the atrial "kick." The positions for measuring the EF slope, the mitral excursion, and the E point-septal separation are indicated in sequential diastoles (see text). *Ao* = proximal aorta; *LA* = left atrium; *LV* = left ventricle; *RV* = right ventricle.

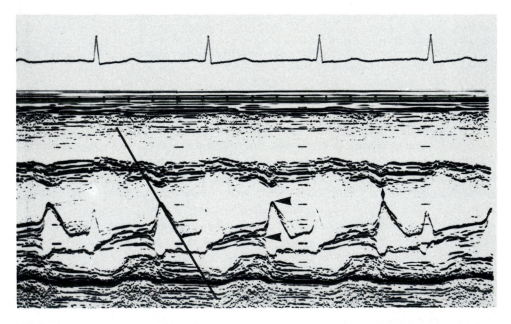

FIG 6–7.
M-mode tracing showing the positions for making measurements of the anterior leaflet of the mitral valve. The *straight line* indicates the position for measuring the EF slope. The *arrowheads* indicate the positions for measuring the excursion of the anterior leaflet. The vertical points indicate the position for measuring the E point-septal separation.

EF slope. It may be taken as the maximum slope, or as the slope of the line connecting the E point to the F point. The normal value of the EF slope is 70 to 150 mm/sec. In low-output states, the excursion of the mitral valve may be depressed due to the diminished stroke volume, but the EF slope remains within normal limits. This contrasts with the findings of mitral stenosis in which both the excursion of the thickened anterior leaflet and its EF slope are diminished. These measurements may also be reduced if the anterior leaflet motion is impeded by striking the interventricular septum or by being displaced posteriorly by a large regurgitant jet stream from an incompetent aortic valve.

The distance from the E point of the anterior mitral leaflet to the left side of the interventricular septum has been reported to have a normal value of 0.5 cm or less.[18] In our laboratory, the E point septal separation is measured at the time of the E point, and considered abnormal only if its exceeds 1 cm in the absence of left ventricular dilatation, mitral stenosis, or aortic insufficiency. The significance of this finding is similar to that of a low-profile mitral valve, both indicating the presence of left ventricular dysfunction.

Measurements at the Chordal Level of the Left Ventricle

M-mode echocardiographic measurements of the ventricles are made at the level of the chordae tendineae (Fig 6–8). Care must be taken to assure that the M-mode cursor is below the level of the mitral valve and above the level of the papillary muscles (Fig 6–9: two-dimensional image.) The majority of measurements are made at end-diastole, which is taken at the onset of the QRS of the ECG (Fig 6–9: M-mode tracing), or at the time that the left ventricle reaches its maximum diameter (Fig 6–10).

Right Ventricle.—When the epicardial and endocardial surfaces of the right ventricular free wall are clearly demonstrated, a measurement can be made of right ventricular wall thickness. In this circumstance, the right ventricular end-diastolic dimension is measured from the endocardial surface of the right ventricle to the right septum (see Fig 6–9). Most commonly, the near-field resolution of the echocardiogram is too poor to demarcate the endocardial surface, and the end-diastolic right ventricular dimension is estimated by measuring the distance from the epicardial surface of the right ventricle to the right septum (see Fig 6–10) and subtracting 0.5 cm for the thickness of the right ventricular free wall. The normal range for this dimension is 0.7 to 2.7 cm. When possible, right ventricular cavity measurements should be made at end-expiration.

Left Ventricle.—The thickness of the interventricular septum and the posterior wall of the left ventricle are measured at end-diastole. This may be taken at the onset of the QRS (see Fig 6–9), at the time of maximum left ventricular diameter (see Fig 6–10), or immediately before the atrial kick. Measuring at the onset of the QRS offers more reproducible results and is preferred, particularly when comparisons between serial studies are anticipated. The interventricular septum is measured from the left to the right septal surfaces with care taken to avoid including the thickness of any right ventricular trabeculations. The posterior wall is measured from the leading edge of the endocardial surface to that of the epicardial surface. Care should be taken to exclude the thickness of overlying chordae tendineae from the endo-

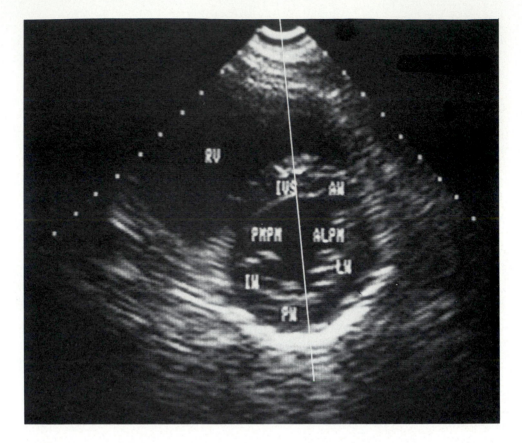

FIG 6–8.
Two-dimensional cross-sectional image of the left ventricle showing the position of the M-mode cursor (*solid line*) for measuring left ventricular wall thickness and cavity size. This position is identified by recognizing the chordae tendineae which originate from the posteromedial papillary muscle (*PMPM*) and the anterolateral papillary muscle (*ALPM*). The cursor is directed through the right ventricular cavity (*RV*), the interventricular septum (*IVS*), the left ventricular cavity, and the posterior wall of the left ventricle (*PW*). *AW* = anterior wall; *IW* = inferior wall; *LW* = lateral wall.

cardium, and the epicardium should be distinguished from the echodense pericardium. The most reliable estimates are obtained by measuring from the leading edge of each structure, identifying the border of the wall as the most rapidly moving continuous echo reflection. Normal values for left ventricular wall thickness range from 0.6 to 1.2 cm.

The left ventricular end-diastolic dimension is measured from the posterior wall endocardium to the left septum. Once again, this measurement is made at the onset of the QRS or at the maximum left ventricular diameter (see Figs 6–9 and 6–10). The normal range of the cavity dimension is 3.5 to 5.7 cm. The left ventricular end-systolic dimension is measured as the minimum distance separating the septum and posterior wall.

Left Ventricular Volume and Ejection Fraction.—The most commonly applied parameter for estimating left ventricular function is the ejection fraction. In ventricles that contract uniformly, that is, do not have segmental contraction abnormalities, M-mode echocardiography provides a reasonable estimate of left ventricular ejection

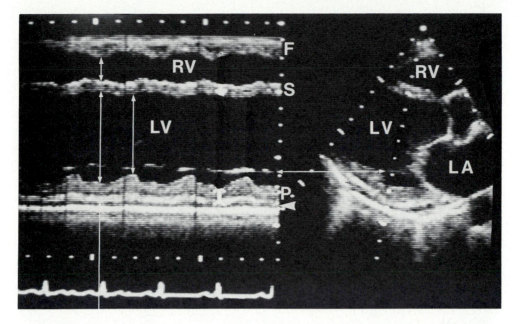

FIG 6–9.
Two-dimensional long-axis view of the left ventricle showing the position of the M-mode cursor (*dotted line*) at the level of the chordae tendineae (*horizontal arrow*). The M-mode beam traverses the free wall of the right ventricle (*F*), the right ventricular cavity (*RV*), the interventricular septum (*S*), the left ventricular cavity (*LV*), the posterior wall of the left ventricle (*P*), a small pericardial effusion (*arrowhead*), and the pericardium. The *vertical arrows* indicate the positions for measuring these structures. Diastolic measurements are shown at the onset of the QRS and systolic measurements are shown at the minimum dimension of the left ventricle. *LA* = left atrium.

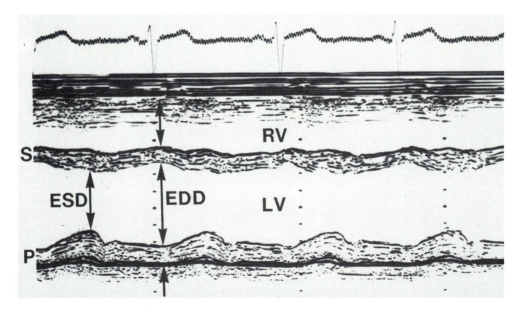

FIG 6–10.
M-mode tracing of the left ventricle showing the positions used to measure the dimension of the right ventricle (*RV*), the thickness of the septum (*S*) and posterior wall (*P*), and the end-diastolic dimension (*EDD*) and end-systolic dimension (*ESD*) of the left ventricle (*LV*). The measurements in this tracing are made at the time of the maximum and minimum dimensions of the left ventricle.

fraction. Ejection fraction is calculated as stroke volume divided by end-diastolic volume. Left ventricular stroke volume is determined as the difference between end-diastolic and end-systolic volume. These volumes are approximated using measurements of the left ventricular internal diameter at end-diastole and end-systole. The most widely applied formula for determining left ventricular ejection fraction

EJECTION FRACTION NOMOGRAM
M-MODE ECHOCARDIOGRAPHY

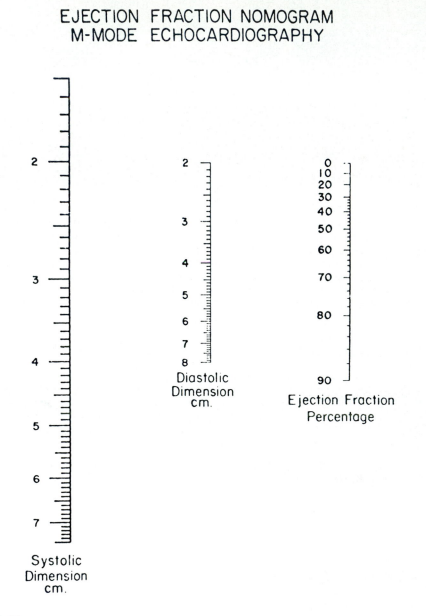

FIG 6–11.
Nomogram enabling calculation of the left ventricular ejection fraction from the end-diastolic and end-systolic dimensions measured from an M-mode echocardiogram. A line drawn from the end-systolic dimension on the left through the end-diastolic dimension in the middle crosses the right line enabling direct reading of the ejection fraction. (Courtesy of John M. Nicklas, M.D.)

by M-mode is the "cube formula." It assumes that the left ventricle has the shape of a spherical ellipse whose minor axis diameters are equal to one-half that of the major axis diameter. Using this geometry, left ventricular volume is equal to $\pi/3$ times the minor axis diameter cubed and therefore can be approximated as the cube of the internal (short-axis) dimension. The stroke volume is then estimated as the end-diastolic dimension (EDD) cubed minus the end-systolic dimension (ESD) cubed. The ejection fraction is estimated by dividing this by the cube of the end-diastolic dimension and can be simplified as the value $1 - (\text{ESD}/\text{EDD})^3$. Figure 6–11 shows a nomogram that enables the rapid determination of the ejection fraction from the end-diastolic and end-systolic dimensions of the left ventricle. The normal left ventricular ejection fraction is greater than 55%.

Another parameter reflecting left ventricular function is the percent fractional shortening. It is the percent reduction in left ventricular circumference from end-diastole to end-systole. Since the circumference is π times the ventricular diameter, this parameter can be calculated as $1 - \text{ESD}/\text{EDD}$. Normal fractional shortening exceeds 25%.

A less frequently used parameter of left ventricular function that can be estimated from M-mode echocardiography is the velocity of circumferential fiber shortening.[19] This is determined as the difference in end-diastolic and end-systolic circumference, normalized by dividing by the end-diastolic circumference, and divided by the time duration from end-diastole to end-systole. In practice it is obtained by dividing the fractional shortening expressed as a decimal fraction, by the time separating the end-diastolic and end-systolic measurements. The normal rate of contraction is greater than 0.85 per second.

If the M-mode tracing is digitized, rates of wall thickening, ventricular filling, and ventricular emptying can be calculated. Wall thickness and left ventricular cavity dimensions can be combined to generate other parameters such as left ventricular mass, regional ventricular function, and (with the addition of left ventricular systolic pressure) myocardial wall stress.

Although M-mode tracings of the tricuspid and pulmonic valves may be obtained using the left parasternal acoustic window, they are frequently difficult to image and are not routinely measured in clinical laboratories.

TWO-DIMENSIONAL ECHOCARDIOGRAPHY

By enabling the generation of tomographic images of the heart, two-dimensional echocardiography is well suited for measuring chamber and great vessel sizes.[20–22] The ability to image the heart in multiple planes makes the estimation of left ventricular volume less dependent on geometric assumptions, since the formulas that are applied do not require a symmetric, uniformly contracting ventricle. The most accurate estimates of chamber volume are generated on the basis of area and length measurements made from the two-dimensional images.[23] These require digitizing the endocardial borders of the cavity using a light pen, a video analyzer, or an off-line analysis system. While some authors have advocated the measurement of linear dimensions from the two-dimensional images, these require more stringent geometric assumptions in order to estimate volumes and ejection fractions. Although the most broadly applied echocardiographic measurements are the M-mode parameters described in the previous section, knowledge of two-dimensional measurements is

Abdomen

Chapter 7

Vascular Ultrasound Measurements

Wolfgang F. Dähnert, M.D.
Paul A. Dubbins, M.D.

The practice of radiology plays an important role in the workup of vascular disorders, including noncontrast radiography, angiography, nuclear medicine, and cross-sectional imaging with ultrasound, computed tomography (CT), and, most recently, magnetic resonance imaging (MRI). This chapter will focus on available morphologic data, that is, the measurement of vessel size in the normal individual. Vessel size may be determined across the center of the lumen from intima to intima or from serosa to serosa, including the wall thickness. The presented data refer to the caliber, that is, the inner diameter of a vessel.

VARIABLES AFFECTING DIAMETERS OF VESSELS

There is a wide variation of normal vessel size, as can be seen in the accompanying tables of this chapter. Some of the known factors responsible for these variations are related to intraindividual and interindividual factors as well as methodologic problems. These will be discussed in a general context in the following section.

Intraindividual Variables

Different diameters may be obtained within the same individual for the same vessel. The most obvious mistake may be related to the site where the measurement is taken. The normal gradual decrease in vessel caliber toward the periphery makes it necessary to identify a particular anatomic site. Once an anatomic landmark is established, it must be reproducible within the same individual for subsequent measurements and, also, transferable to another subject for comparison.

Developmental variants of vascular anatomy are common. As a result, the vessel under consideration may carry a larger or smaller flow volume which will affect the diameter of the vessel. Examples can be found in variations of the celiac trunk and renal vascular anatomy.

Vessel diameters may change during the period in which measurements are obtained. Arterial wall pulsations are initiated by the cardiac cycle[1] and dampened by the windkessel function of the aorta (*windkessel* refers to the elastic properties of the large arteries which transform a discontinuous into a continuous blood flow throughout the cardiac cycle). Pulsatory variations of arteries may be as large as 2.5 mm.[2] For example, a 5-mm fetal aorta may vary 20% in diameter between systole and diastole.[3] The diameter of the central and splanchnic veins is subject to changes with respiration. In veins, the problem can be minimized by measuring flow during light or suspended respiration. According to Gill's experience transient changes in venous flow last approximately 10 to 20 seconds before the normal average flow rate in the vein is reestablished.[4] A time-motion recorder can be used to measure the time-varying diameter of the vessel.[5]

Postural changes have an influence on the diameter of low-pressure vessels. Vessel diameters also adjust to demands on increased or decreased organ perfusion as occurs during physical activity, postprandial metabolism, or in the aging kidney. Vasoactive hormones and drugs[6, 7] will also influence measurements. Thus, a description of the exact conditions under which these measurements were obtained is required.

A vessel diameter measured in one plane may be an incorrect representation of the true lumen of the vessel. Cross sections of healthy arteries are usually circular secondary to the pressure gradient between intra- and perivascular compartments as well as their thick muscular walls. Most veins, however, show an elliptic cross section. In these cases, the minimal and maximal diameter have to be measured to arrive at the correct cross-sectional area. For example, a maximum diameter 30% larger than the minimum introduces an error of -24% or $+31\%$ if the calculation is based on the assumption that the vessel is circular.

Interindividual Variables

It appears sensible to expect vessels to adapt to the nutritional requirements of the perfused organ. The size of a vessel should then be related to size and activity of the organ supplied. It is immediately apparent that substitute measurements for organ activity and size, for instance, body height or weight, body surface area, bone size, age and sex of an individual must be inadequate and represent approximations at best. In addition, the aging process has an effect on the elastic properties of the arterial wall. For example, the aorta has been shown to become dilated and its wall thinned with age.[9]

Faced with the large biologic variation of vessel sizes, and in an effort to obtain meaningful results, absolute measurements have been adjusted to common denominators. The results of these adjusted measurements, however, are controversial. With regard to the aorta, all investigators agree that the aortic circumference increases with age (Fig 7–1). Cronenwett and Garrett[10] measured age, body surface area, height, weight, and bone size, correlating these data with aortic measurements. Although the body surface area showed the best correlation, overall correlation with the arterial diameter was poor. Corrections based on these variables were not helpful in defining small aortas in women and the authors suggested using absolute measurements instead. Correlating arteriographic with sonographic as well as postmortem studies, van Rinsum[11] demonstrated a significant variation of aortic diameter between sexes that could not be reduced by adjusting the diameter for body length. Similarly, Hoogendam et al.[12] were able to reduce the difference between male and female maximum aortic diameter only slightly when correcting it for body length (Fig 7–2). On the other hand, measurements of the thoracic aorta by CT showed a statistically

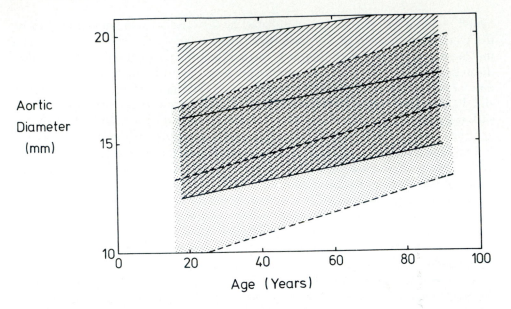

FIG 7–1.
Graph demonstrating the variation in aortic diameter with age for men (*hatched*) and women (*stippled*).
(Modified after Hoogendam J, Van Rinsum AC, Olystager J: *J Cardiovasc Surg* 1984; 25:408–413.)

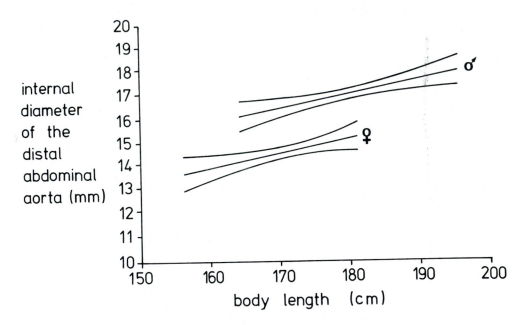

FIG 7–2.
Graph relating body length to the internal diameter of the distal abdominal aorta in females (♀) and
males (♂). Although both vary with body length, mean diameters for women are lower than those for
men. (After Van Rinsum AC: *Diameter of Normal and Pathological Aortic Bifurcations and the Development of Atherosclerosis.* Utrecht, Netherlands, BV Vitgeverij De Banier, 1984).

significant relationship to vertebral body width over and above the correlation due to age and sex.[13]

Branches of the aorta, however, appear to increase only to the fifth decade after which an increase of the outer diameter is secondary to thickening of the vessel wall.[14] This has not been confirmed in a study of 250 male and 250 female cadavers by Gulisano et al.[9] who determined the mean circumference of various arteries. All arteries increased with age, but the arterial circumferences increased further in the female than in the male, reducing male-female differences in the elderly population. Even though arteries were generally a little larger in the male than in the female population, and arteries of the right side somewhat larger than those on the left, these differences were statistically not significant. The only exception applies to the vertebral and coronary arteries, in which the left side is usually dominant.

CLINICAL IMPLICATION

Although vascular diseases may manifest as an increase or decrease in size of the affected vessel, it is only in certain selected instances that absolute measurements of vascular size are clinically useful. For example, conditions producing diffuse alterations of vessel dimension, such as arteriomegaly[15] as seen in ectatic atherosclerosis or peripheral arterial vasospastic disorders, may only be recognized if measurements fall outside the range of normal.

In order to judge a diseased stenotic or aneurysmal portion of a vessel, instead of using absolute measurements, direct comparison of an abnormal vascular segment with its adjacent normal part is common practice. In case of narrowing, the degree of stenosis may be expressed as a percentage of the adjacent normal caliber. However, two-dimensional representations of the arterial system, as in angiography, do not always permit assessment of the severity of a stenosis or the hemodynamic significance of a lesion. In fact, some hemodynamically significant stenoses may be missed completely on single-plane arteriography, and are detected only on oblique or lateral arteriograms. Cross-sectional imaging of a vessel lumen, on the other hand, displays the area reduction as opposed to merely the diameter of a stenosis. This difference may be quite striking so that, in general, Doppler wave-form analysis allows better quantitation of the hemodynamic significance of lumen reduction than angiography. Saccular or fusiform aneurysms are recognized by their shape and dissimilarity to the adjacent unaffected vessel. While the diagnosis depends on a comparison between abnormal and normal segment, the absolute size of the diameter bears prognostic relevance.[16, 17]

Judged by the few reports found in the literature, it appears that the complexity in obtaining reliable measurements, together with their limited clinical usefulness, have enticed few investigators to look into the topic of absolute measurements of vessel calibers.

METHODOLOGIC ERRORS

Imaging of vessels is possible due to contrast differences between the intraluminal components and the vessel wall or surrounding tissues. Only contrast differences of a sufficient magnitude will allow clear visualization of the lumen of the vessel. Contrast differences will diminish with decrease in vessel size. The inherent contrast of blood components can be detected by ultrasound and MRI. X-ray imaging, as in angiography and CT, requires injection of a dye to momentarily raise intravascular attenuation. Radionuclide imaging of individual vessels is marred by poor spatial resolution so that measurements of vessel calibers have not been attempted. Post-mortem figures of vessel caliber are commonly less than in vivo measurements, which is most likely from loss of the dilating effect of circulating blood.

Plain Radiography

Plain film radiography of vessel dimensions is ordinarily not feasible in healthy individuals. Vessel size may, however, be estimated in situations where the vessel wall is perceptibly different in x-ray transmission. Under pathologic conditions, radiographic contrast may be present as calcifications within the vessel wall. In a study of 283 patients with suspected aortic aneurysm, 55% had detectable calcifications of the aortic wall on plain abdominal radiographs, but in only 31.5% were the calcifications sufficient to adequately evaluate the aortic size.[18] Normal values for the size of abdominal vessels as assessed by plain radiography are, therefore, not available. Under normal conditions, vessel size may be measured within the chest where air-containing lung creates a natural contrast border. Few vessels, however, are totally or almost completely surrounded by air as in the case for the intrapulmonary course of the pulmonary veins and arteries. A small segment of the azygous vein and left superior intercostal vein can be measured. Crude estimates of vessel dimensions are obtained if soft tissue structures are applied to the vessel wall. In any case, the true lumen of the vessel cannot be assessed on plain film radiography. Posteroanterior (PA) and lateral radiographs of the chest do provide a means for estimates of aortic diameter. The transverse aortic diameter is a relatively insensitive measure, but the upper limit of 50 mm appears to have clinical usefulness.[19, 20]

Angiography

Practically every vascular province can be imaged with sophisticated angiographic techniques. The superb spatial resolution of x-ray images allows imaging of vessels down to precapillary levels with appropriate magnification. Angiographic determination of vessel diameters may be inaccurate secondary to catheter manipulation provoking spasm and secondary to pressure injection of an added contrast volume causing some degree of artificial dilatation. To avoid interference from instrumentation and added volume, Steinberg et al.[21] have chosen an intravenous method of contrast injection for measurement of the abdominal aorta. Of course, digital subtraction angiography with its improved contrast resolution eliminates these problems. Dependent on the duration of exposure, systolic and diastolic variations in the diameter may not be detectable.[21] In addition, the geometry of target-film distance must be considered to compensate for image magnification. Magnification can best be taken into account by using the diameter of the catheter for each plane as calibration.[22] Measurements are usually performed by ultrasound in the anteroposterior (AP) dimension because of the greater accuracy of axial measurements. Direct correlation with angiography can be achieved using the coronal approach. This plane of scan also allows more consistent visualization of the renal and iliac arteries (Fig 7–3).

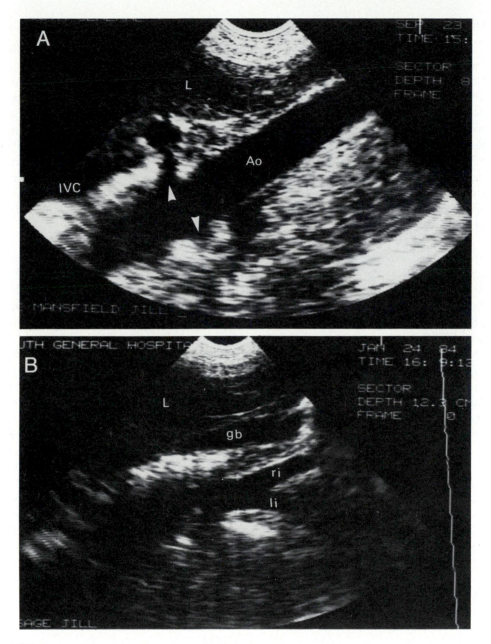

FIG 7–3.
A, coronal scan of normal aorta performed with the patient in the left lateral decubitus position demonstrates normal, regular aortic lumen (*Ao*). The origins of both renal arteries are also shown (*arrowheads*). *IVC* = inferior vena cava; *L* = right lobe of liver. **B,** coronal view of aortic bifurcation. Both right and left common iliac vessels are demonstrated (*ri;li*). Crosses identify the point of measurement at the level of bifurcation of the aorta. *L* = liver, *gb* = gallbladder.

Ultrasound

The initial limitations of vascular measurements by A-mode and bistable B-mode display have been overcome since the introduction of real-time gray-scale imaging. It is now possible to assess the diameter of a vessel instantaneously. In addition, M-mode ultrasound across the maximal diameter of a vessel registers caliber changes over time. The more recent introduction of combined Doppler and real-time ultrasound (duplex ultrasound) has added a powerful tool to identify and measure blood flow velocity and flow volume. The tremendous intra- and interobserver variability of flow measurements has directed attention to the most critical sources of errors, underlining the importance of correct sonographic measurements. Appropriate insonation of the vessel under investigation has to take into account the angle of approach and the direction of the imaging plane in relation to the long axis of the vessel.

A sound beam perpendicular to an interface will produce echoes of the shortest duration and greatest amplitude. The resultant strong echoes may generate image pixels larger than the true anatomic size. Measurement errors can be minimized by decreasing the overall gain which will result in smaller image pixels. Alternatively, the same is accomplished by systematically measuring from leading edge to leading edge or from maximal brightness to maximal brightness of the anterior and posterior wall (Fig 7–4).

The diameter will be accurately measured only if a plane perpendicular to the long axis of the vessel is used. Angle approaches of less than 90 degrees will either underestimate the diameter due to the effect of beam width, or overestimate the diameter if no correction is made for the angle of approach. Any error in estimating the angle of approach will effect the measurement of blood velocity and cross-sectional area. The accuracy of measurement is especially critical when relatively large angles are used, since the cosine of the angle varies more rapidly with large angles than with smaller ones. The imaging plane must be aligned with the axis of the vessel ensuring that the length of the vessel segment that is imaged is as long as possible. This will minimize underestimation of velocity (usually in the order of 3%–6%) since the apparent angle of approach is less than the true angle if the vessel is cutting through the scanning plane. Measurements of the laterolateral dimension, that is, perpendicular to the sound beam, are less accurate due to the poorer lateral resolution of the sound beam compared with the axial resolution.

The accuracy of measurement of the vessel diameter is most critical for calculations of flow within vessels since the area (A) depends on the square of the diameter (d^2) according to the formula

$$A = \pi \times d^2/4$$

A given percentage error in estimating d will result in an error of approximately twice that percentage in estimating flow. In the most favorable situation, variations of vessel diameter measurements of approximately 0.5 to 1.0 mm are obtained. Consequently, in vessel diameters between 10 and 14 mm, an error of 10% to 20% may be introduced. With smaller vessel diameters, as encountered in the fetus, the error will increase considerably. For example a 1-mm uncertainty in the measurement of a 6-mm vessel will produce a 33% variation in the flow calculation.

In diseased vessels, particularly those containing mural thrombus, the end points

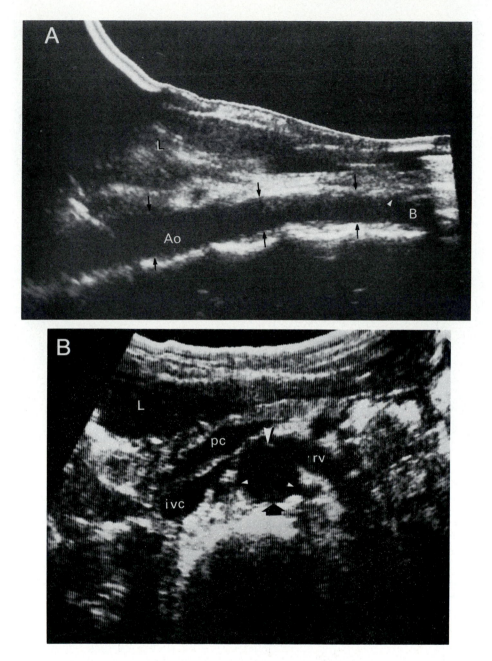

FIG 7–4.
A, long-axis scan of the abdominal aorta from the aortic hiatus (*Ao*) to the bifurcation (*B*). The *small arrowhead* indicates the origin of the superior rectal artery. The *arrows* indicate the points of measurement from anterior wall to posterior wall at the xiphoid, below the renal arteries and just above the bifurcation. *L* = liver. **B,** transverse scan at the level of the renal arteries, the origins of which are shown by the *small arrowheads.* The posterior point for aortic measurement is clearly shown by the *large arrow.* There is, however, slight confusion about the anterior point of measurement which is marked by the *large arrowhead.* The reason for this confusion is due to the left renal vein (*rv*) which courses over the anterior surface of the aorta and appears to be contiguous with the aortic wall. *pc* = portal venous confluence; *L* = liver; *IVC* = inferior vena cava.

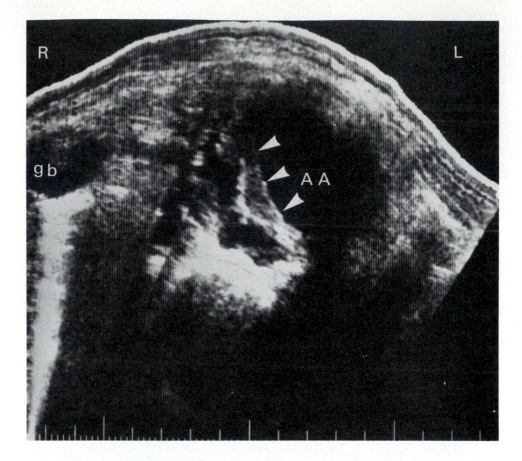

FIG 7–5.
Large abdominal aortic aneurysm (*AA*) in transverse section. The *arrowheads* indicate the large amount of mural clot in this patient which makes the assessment of end points for measurement somewhat difficult. In addition, sound reverberation in the anterior portion of the aneurysm, as a result of close proximity to the anterior abdominal wall, makes the anterior point of measurement also more difficult. *gb* = gallbladder; *R* = right; *L* = left.

of vascular measurements are more difficult to define. Findings at surgery in patients with aortic wall thrombus suggest that ultrasound usually underestimates the true contribution of the thrombus[23] (Fig 7–5).

Care must be taken not to exert too much pressure on a venous vessel during Doppler interrogation and during measurement of cross-sectional diameter. Pressure of a hand-held transducer can be minimized using an open water bag technique.[8]

MORPHOLOGIC VASCULAR MEASUREMENTS

In the following section, absolute measurements of vessel sizes are compiled as reported in the literature. Where applicable, reference is made to the technique of measurement, anatomic site of measurement, age, number, and sex of subjects, as well as to the conditions under which the examinations were performed. All of the measurements are given in diameters and converted into diameters where the authors have presented results in circumference or area. The results of measurements for individual vessels are listed in tables identified by source.

TABLE 7–1.
Measurements of Thoracic Aorta

Author (s)	Reference	Methodology	n	Age (yr)	Vessel Diameter (mm) (Average ±SD)	Range (mm)
Supravalvular						
Kani	14	Autopsy	19	9–58		13.7–25.8
Dotter & Steinberg	26	Arteriography	100	35.3 (5–65)	28.6*	16.0–38.0
Orlandini et al.	24	Autopsy	60 F	27–91	27.1 ±3.5	
			60 M	27–91	28.0 ±4.7	
Aronberg et al.	13	CT	102		36.2†	24.0–47.0
Aortic arch						
Kani	14	Autopsy	19	9–58		9.9–19.4
Dotter & Steinberg	26	Arteriography	44	35.3 (5–65)	24.8*	13.0–34.0
Goldberg	28	Ultrasound	21 M	34 (mean)	24.7 ±3.5	
			31 F	37 (mean)	21.7 ±3.8	
Aronberg et al.	13	CT	102		24.8†	16.0–37.0
Descending thoracic aorta						
Come	30	Ultrasound	50	56 (15–92)	20.0	13.0–27.0
Dotter & Steinberg	26	Arteriography	58	35.3 (5–65)	22.9*	12.0–32.0
Aronberg et al.	13	CT	102		24.8†	16.0–37.0
At level of diaphragm						
Kani	14	Autopsy	19	9–58		8.9–17.8
Dotter & Steinberg	26	Arteriography	54	35.3 (5–65)	19.7*	9.0–28.0
Aronberg et al.	13	CT	102		24.2†	14.0–33.0

*Not corrected for magnification.
†Outer diameter.

Arterial System

Thoracic Aorta (Table 7–1).—The aortic circumference increases with age and is larger in the male than in the female population. Kani[14] measured arterial walls and circumferences on 220 autopsy specimens of which only 19 qualified as normal standards according to medical history and cause of death. From wall thickness measurements he concluded that real growth occurs up to the age of 50 followed later by dilatation. The descending aorta showed an interesting constant relationship of 1.00 : 1.07 : 0.74 when measured at the diaphragm, distal to the arch, and above the bifurcation. These numbers were independent of age or sex. The ascending aorta, however, did not show such a strict relationship. Orlandini et al.[24] measured the circumference of the ascending aorta in an anatomic study of 120 fresh cadavers excluding "remarkable" pathologic vessel alterations. They noticed an increase in aortic circumference throughout the decades as well and a linear relationship between the circumference of the aorta and the pulmonary trunk. Increase in aortic diameter with aging may be partly related to the observation that aortic peak flow velocity decreases with age.[25]

Angiographically, the most satisfactory projection was established to be the left anterior oblique, which reveals the entire thoracic aorta. Left anterior oblique and left lateral measurements of the ascending aorta tended to be slightly greater (1–2 mm) than the corresponding frontal measurement, a fact partly accounted for by the phase at or after the R wave of the electrocardiogram, that is, between a and v waves of the venous pulse, considering only the minimal diameter. IVC diameter increased from the left lateral decubitus position to the supine position to the right lateral decubitus position. Correspondingly, the IVC changed from a slitlike or crescent shape into an oval and then into a round shape (Figs 7–6 A–C). The authors speculate that variable degrees of compression by the liver may be responsible for the positional changes or alteration in venous return. It was also noted that the IVC diameter did not correlate with the body surface area. Most importantly, an IVC diameter of over 10 mm in the left lateral decubitus position had a predictive accuracy of 95% (sensitivity 84%, specificity 96%) for the diagnosis of elevated right atrial pressure over 8 mm Hg.

In a study of 26 healthy persons with a mean age of 40.0 ± 15 years, Strohm et al.[6] observed a decrease in the diameter of the IVC by 22% within 5 minutes after administration of nitroglycerin.

Femoral Vein.—On CT examination, Junker et al.[58] observed an increase in the diameter of the femoral veins of approximately 33% during the Valsalva maneuver over 13 seconds, although two patients showed no change in size. The tomographic section was selected in the usual puncture area for transfemoral angiography. The mean diameter of the femoral veins increased from 12 mm during quiet respiration to 16 mm during the Valsalva maneuver.

Portal Venous System (see Table 7–6).—The main portal vein conveys blood from the viscera to the liver. In the normal situation the portal venous system in the adult is a low-pressure system and pathology affecting the portal venous system changes this normal pressure relationship. This might be expected to be reflected in a change in the size of the portal vein, and thus measurement of normal portal venous size should allow prediction of pathology of the portal system.

The site of measurement of the portal vein diameter may have a significant influence. Doehner et al.[59] found three configurations of the main portal vein. In 90% of cases, the portal vein diameter decreased along its course toward the liver hilum (Fig 7–7). In 4% the diameter remained the same, and in 4% it even increased in size approaching the hilum of the liver (Fig 7–8). An unusual variant, seen in one of 50 patients, was a fusiform portal vein having its largest diameter in the middle third. In the sonographic literature, the site of measurement is usually just distal to the union of the splenic and superior mesenteric veins[60] (Fig 7–9). Occasionally, the sample point is set at the midpoint between the confluence of the splenic and superior mesenteric veins and the portal bifurcation at the hepatic hilum, because it runs in a straight line with few branches and exhibits an almost round cross-sectional area.[61]

Test conditions for measurement of the portal vein must be standardized for comparison. Nevertheless, repeated measurements on subsequent days showed a coefficient of variation between 1.4% and 10.2%.[62, 63] Portal venous blood flow and pressure change with body position, physical activity, respiration, and state of fasting. Patients are usually positioned supine, but may have been examined in the right anterior oblique or left lateral decubitus position. Weinreb et al.[64] visualized the portal vein best and most readily in the right anterior oblique position. Ohnishi et al.[63] documented significant decreases in vessel diameter in the sitting position and with exercise. With inspiration, portal venous pressure increases while portal venous blood flow decreases secondary to compression of the liver parenchyma and its venous

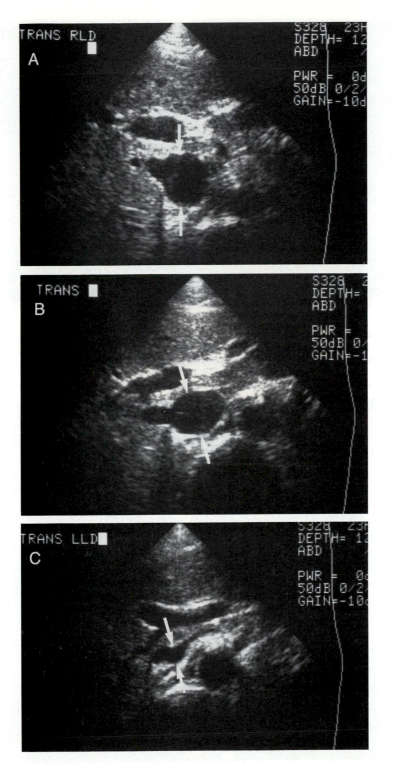

FIG 7–6.
Positional changes in shape and maximal diameter of the hepatic segment of the IVC during quiet respiration. Increasing compression of IVC from right lateral decubitus (**A**) over supine (**B**) into left lateral decubitus position (**C**) is depicted by a decrease in AP diameter of the vein (*arrows*).

between normals and cirrhotics. Bolondi et al.[66] reported that the portal vein was less than 13 mm in all normal patients, or greater in 47.8% of those with portal hypertension. The portal vein was best and most readily visualized in the right anterior oblique position. Kumari-Subaiva et al.[60] established the upper limit of normal of portal vein diameter as 12 mm.

In contrast, Moriyasu et al.[61] found a bimodal wide distribution of portal vein diameters in healthy volunteers secondary to sex differences. In cirrhotic patients the portal vein may be normal or even decreased in size after blood flow has been diverted into collateral vessels.[59, 67, 68] In an angiographic study of 64 biopsy-proven cirrhotics, Lafortune et al.[68] found no significant differences between the caliber of the portal vein in controls and those of cirrhotic patients. However, the caliber tended to diminish when collaterals developed.

Bolondi et al.[66] found a significant increase of 50% to 100% in the caliber of the splenic and superior mesenteric veins during inspiration. This respiratory response is diminished or absent depending on the severity of portal hypertension.

Lafortune et al.[68] could not find significant differences in measurements of the portal vein caliber on the direct portogram versus those obtained from the venous phase of the arteriogram in their cirrhotic patients. This observation, however, may not hold up in noncirrhotics.

REFERENCES

1. Gardin JM, Tobis JM, Dabestani A, et al: Superiority of two-dimensional measurement of aortic vessel diameter in Doppler echocardiographic estimates of left ventricular stroke volume. *J Am Coll Cardiol* 1985; 6:66–74.
2. Seitz K, Kubale R: *Duplexsonographie der abdominellen und retroperitonealen Gefässe.* Weinheim, West Germany, VCH Verlagsgesellschaft, 1988.
3. Eik-Nes SH, Marshal K, Kristofferson K: Methodology and basic problems related to blood flow studies in the human fetus. *Ultrasound Med Biol* 1984; 10:329–337.
4. Gill RW: Measurement of blood flow by ultrasound: accuracy and sources of error. *Ultrasound Med Biol* 1985; 11:625–641.
5. Godwin JD, Korobkin M: Acute disease of the aorta. Diagnosis by computed tomography and ultrasonography. *Radiol Clin North Am* 1983; 21:551–574.
6. Strohm WD, Rahn R, Cordes HJ, et al: Diameters of abdominal veins and arteries during nitrate therapy. *Z Kardiol* 1983; 72(suppl 3):56–61.
7. Fitzgerald DE, O'Shaughnessy AM: Cardiac and peripheral arterial responses to isoprenaline challenge. *Cardiovasc Res* 1984; 18:414–418.
8. Riley Jr. WA, Barnes RW, Schey HM: An approach to the noninvasive periodic assessment of arterial elasticity in the young. *Prev Med* 1984; 13:169–184.
9. Gulisano M, Zecchi S, Pacini P, et al: The behaviour of some human arteries as regards the corrected circumference: a statistical research. *Anat Anz* 1982; 152:341–357.
10. Cronenwett JL, Garrett HE: Arteriographic measurement of the abdominal aorta, iliac, and femoral arteries in women with atherosclerotic occlusive disease. *Radiology* 1983; 148:389–392.
11. Van Rinsum AC: *Diameter of Normal and Pathological Aortic Bifurcations and the Development of Atherosclerosis* Utrecht, Netherlands, BV Uitgeverij De Banier, 1984.
12. Hoogendam J, Van Rinsum AC, Olyslager J: The diameter of the distal abdominal aorta and the etiology of local atheroma. *J Cardiovasc Surg* 1984; 25:408–413.
13. Aronberg DJ, Glazer HS, Madson K, et al: Normal thoracic aortic diameters by computed tomography. *J Comput Assist Tomogr* 1984; 8:247–250.
14. Kani I: Systematische Lichtungs- und Dickenmessungen der grossen Arterien und ihre Bedeutung für die Pathologie der Gefässe. *Virchows Arch Pathol Anat* 1910; 201:45–78.
15. Callum KG, Gaunt JI, Thomas ML, et al: Physiologic studies in arteriomegaly. *Cardiovasc Res* 1974; 8:373–383.

16. Darling RC, Messina CR, Brewster DC: Autopsy study of unoperated abdominal aortic aneurysms. *Circulation* 1977; 56(suppl 2):161–164.
17. Fomon JJ, Kurzweg FT, Broadway RK: Aneurysms of the aorta: A review. *Ann Surg* 1967; 165:557–563.
18. Hardy DC, Lee JK, Weyman J, et al: Measurement of the abdominal aortic aneurysm, plain radiographic and ultrasonographic correlation. *Radiology* 1981; 141:821–823.
19. Ungerleider HE, Gubner R: Evaluation of heart size measurements. *Am Heart J* 1942; 24:494–510.
20. Sussman ML: Roentgen examination of the aorta and pulmonary artery. *Am J Roentgenol Radiother Nucl Med* 1939; 42:75–84.
21. Steinberg CR, Archer M, Steinberg I: Measurement of the abdominal aorta after intravenous aortography in health and arteriosclerotic peripheral vascular disease. *Am J Roentgenol* 1965; 95:703–708.
22. Marx GR, Goldberg SJ, Allen HD: Two methods for measurement of ascending aortic diameter by 2-D echocardiography as compared with cineangiography. *Am Heart J* 1986; 112:172–173.
23. Graeve AH, Carpenter CM, Wicks JD, et al: Discordance in the sizing of abdominal aortic aneurysm and its significance. *Am J Surg* 1982; 144:627–634.
24. Orlandini GE, Ruggiero C, Orlandini SZ: The corrected circumference of human pulmonary trunk and arteries in relation to the size of aorta and principal bronchi. *Anat Anz* 1986; 162:251–257.
25. Gardin JM, Davidson DM, Rohan MK, et al: Relationship between age, body size, gender, and blood pressure and Doppler flow measurements in the aorta and pulmonary artery. *Am Heart J* 1987; 113:101–109.
26. Dotter CT, Steinberg I: The angiocardiographic measurement of the normal great vessels. *Radiology* 1949; 52:353–358.
27. Goldberg BB, Ostrum BJ, Isard HJ: Ultrasonographic aortography. *JAMA* 1966; 198:353–358.
28. Goldberg BB: Suprasternal ultrasonography. *JAMA* 1971; 215:245–250.
29. Seward JB, Tajik AJ: Noninvasive visualization of the entire thoracic aorta: A new application of wide-angle two-dimensional sector echocardiographic technique (abstracted). *Am J Cardiol* 1979; 43:387.
30. Come PC: Improved cross-sectional echocardiographic techniques and visualization of the retrocardiac descending aorta in its long axis. *Am J Cardiol* 1983; 51:1029–1033.
31. George L, Deane Waldman J, Kirkpatrick SE, et al: Two dimensional echocardiographic visualization of the aortic arch by right parasternal scanning in neonates and infants. *Pediatr Cardiol* 1982; 2:277–280.
32. Reed KL, Anderson CF, Shenker L: Fetal pulmonary artery and aorta: two-dimensional Doppler echocardiography. *Obstet Gynecol* 1987; 69:175–178.
33. Fendel H, Fendel M, Warnking R: Fehlermöglichkeiten der gepulsten Dopplermethode zur Blutflussmessung am Feten. *Z Geburtshilfe Perinatol* 1983; 187:83–87.
34. Arnot RS, Louw JH: The anatomy of the posterior wall of the abdominal aorta. *S Afr Med J* 1973; 47:899–902.
35. Sato S. Ohnishi K, Sugita S, et al: Splenic artery and superior mesenteric artery blood flow: nonsurgical Doppler US measurement in healthy subjects and patients with chronic liver disease. *Radiology* 1987; 164:347–352.
36. Jäger K, Bollinger A, Valli C, et al: Measurement of mesenteric blood flow by duplex scanning. *J Vasc Surg* 1986; 3:462–469.
37. Qamar MI, Read AE, Skidmore R, et al: Transcutaneous Doppler ultrasound measurement of superior mesenteric artery blood flow in man. *Gut* 1986; 27:100–105.
38. Aldoori MI, Qamar MI, Read AE, et al: Increased flow in the superior mesenteric artery in dumping syndrome. *Br J Surg* 1985; 72:389–390.
39. Norryd C, Dencker H, Lunderquist A, et al: Superior mesenteric blood flow during digestion in man. *Acta Chir Scand* 1975; 141:197–202.
40. Buchardt-Hansen HJ, Engell HC, Ring-Larsen H, et al: Splanchnic blood flow in patients with abdominal angina before and after arterial reconstruction. *Ann Surg* 1977; 186:216–220.
41. Dubbins PA: Renal artery stenosis: duplex Doppler evaluation. *Br J Radiol* 1986; 59:225–229.
42. Avasthi PS, Voyles WF, Greene ER: Noninvasive diagnosis of renal artery stenosis by echo-Doppler velocimetry. *Kidney Int* 1984; 25:824–829.
43. Kohler TR, Zierler RE, Martin RL, et al: Noninvasive diagnosis of renal artery stenosis by ultrasonic duplex scanning. *J Vasc Surg* 1986; 4:450–456.
44. Rittgers SE, Norris CS, Barnes RW: Detection of renal artery stenosis: Experimental and clinical analysis of velocity waveforms. *Ultrasound Med Biol* 1985; 11:523–531.

TABLE 8–3.

Relationship of Body Type to Liver Morphotype*

	Body Type		
	Endomorph	Normotype	Ectomorph
Depth (cm)	14.7 ±1.6	12.1 ±1.3	11.4 ±1.0
Width (cm)	15.7 ±1.3	15.6 ±0.9	18.7 ±1.3
Length (cm)	15.0 ±1.2	18.5 ±1.8	15.6 ±1.3

*Adapted from Nimeh W: *Am J Gastroenterol* 1955; 23:147–156.

None of the above studies makes any allowance for the variations in hepatic anatomy. Variations in this anatomy have long been recognized, and a recent study[3] attempted to assess the relationship of body type to hepatic morphotype and the relationship of the latter to individual hepatic diameters. It should be noted that length was measured on a coronal image rather than the usual parasagittal image. This report, which evaluated only 74 subjects, found statistically significant differences in the length, width, and depth based on body morphology (ectomorph, endomorph, and normotype). The sizes reported are shown in Table 8–3.

No significant variation in volumetric index was found among the three body types in the study on hepatic morphotypes. A hepatic volumetric index is obtained by multiplying length times width times depth and dividing by 27. A normal falls within the range of 95 to 140 cc.[1]

CONCLUSION

There is some inconsistency in the many reports on hepatic size. Indirect signs are a useful means to quickly gauge liver size. The most widely used measurement is the length in the midclavicular line. If the liver exceeds 15 cm in length, hepatomegaly should be considered (Figs 8–1 and 8–2).

REFERENCES

1. Castell D, O'Brien KD, Nuench H, et al: Estimation of liver size by percussion in normal individuals. *Ann Intern Med* 1969; 70:1183–1189.
2. Naftalis J, Leevy C: Clinical estimation of liver size. *Am J Dig Dis* 1963; 8:236–243.
3. Nimeh W: New method for the determination of the size of the liver and spleen. *Am J Gastroenterol* 1955; 23:147–156.
4. International Commission On Radiological Protection. Task Group on Reference Man: *Report of the Task Group on Reference Man:* Prepared by the Task Group Committee no. 2, International Commission on Radiological Protection, Snyder WS (chairman). New York, Pergamon Press, 1975.
5. Riemenschneider P, Whalen J: The relative accuracy of estimation of enlargement of the liver and spleen by radiologic and clinical methods. *AJR* 1965; 94:462–468.
6. Pfahler GE: The measurement of the liver by means of roentgen rays based upon a study of 502 subjects. *AJR* 1926; 16:558–564.
7. Feldman M: Liver measurement. *Radiology* 1928; 10:496–499.
8. Halpern S, Coel M, Ashburn W, et al: Correlation of liver and spleen size. *Arch Intern Med* 1974; 134:123–124.

9. Rosenfield A, Schneider PB: Rapid evaluation of hepatic size on radioisotope scan. *J Nucl Med* 15:237–240.
10. Petri H, Boscaini M, Berthezene P, et al: Heptatic morphotypes. Their statistical individualization using ultrasonography. *J Ultrasound Med* 1988; 7:189–196.
11. Igidbashian VN, Liu S, Goldberg BB: Hepatic ultrasound. *Semin Liver Dis* 1989; 9:16–31.
12. Kane R: Ultrasonographic anatomy of the liver and biliary tree. *Semin Ultrasound* 1980; 1:87–95.
13. Kane R: Sonographic anatomy of the liver. *Semin Ultrasound* 1981; 2:190–197.
14. Sapira JD, Williams DL: How big is the normal liver? *Arch Intern Med* 1979; 139:971–973.
15. Gosink BB, Leymaster CE: Ultrasonic determination of hepatomegaly. *J Clin Ultrasound* 1981; 9:37–41.
16. Niederau C, Sonnenber A, Miller JE, et al: Sonographic measurement of the normal liver, spleen, pancreas and portal vein. *Radiology* 1983; 149:537–540.

Chapter 9

Common Bile Duct Measurements

Alan H. Wolson, M.D.

Ultrasound has played a role in evaluation of surgical vs. nonsurgical jaundice for several years. Earlier equipment could not regularly visualize extrahepatic ducts, and it was necessary to rely on visualization of dilated intrahepatic ducts to distinguish obstructive from nonobstructive jaundice. However, with mild and/or early obstruction, evaluation of intrahepatic ducts is difficult and inaccurate and only extrahepatic dilatation may be present.[3, 7]

The advent of high-resolution ultrasound equipment, especially real-time systems, has made it possible to visualize the normal extrahepatic ducts in almost all patients. It is therefore essential to know the size of the normal common duct to recognize minimal degrees of dilatation.[3, 7]

ANATOMY OF EXTRAHEPATIC DUCTS

Considerable variability exists in the reported size of the ducts. Sources of data include both autopsy and surgical studies. The difficulty in applying these data to clinical work is the nonphysiologic state of the duct at the time of measurement. Dowdy et al.,[8] in a detailed autopsy study, found the extrahepatic ducts varied from "prominent to almost undiscernible." The common hepatic duct (CHD) measured as follows: length 0.8 to 5.2 cm, average 2 cm; diameter 0.4 to 2.5 cm, average 0.8 cm. The common bile duct (CBD) measured: length 1.5 to 9 cm, average 5 cm; diameter 0.4 to 1.3 cm, average 0.66 cm. The diameters refer to external diameters.

Mahour et al.[19] studied the CBD in autopsy specimens and reported outside diameters ranging from 4 to 12 mm, with an average of 7.39 mm. The diameter increased with age but there was no correlation with body weight or length.

Kune[15] measured casts of the CBD made by injecting the duct at physiologic pressures. The diameters decreased from proximal to distal from 8 mm to 7 mm at the three sites chosen for measurements.

Two surgical studies show considerable discrepancy in the reported results. Ferris and Vibert[10] found the external diameter in apparently normal CBDs to be 8.87 mm (range 4–17 mm). Leslie[17] found the average external diameter without disease was 12 mm (range 5–17 mm); in diseased ducts the average external diameter was 21 mm (range 9–58 mm). Another surgical study[6] found the external diameter was a much less accurate predictor of CBD disease than internal diameters measured on intravenous (IV) cholangiograms. The error was believed to be related to variable thickness of the wall. Consequently, external diameters do not reflect luminal size.

RADIOGRAPHY

Radiographic studies, with the exception of computed tomography (CT), suffer from a common source of error in evaluation of the extrahepatic bile ducts, that is, the nonphysiologic state of the ducts. Intravenous cholangiography contrast material produces a choleretic effect, while endoscopic retrograde cholangiopancreatography (ERCP) introduces injection pressure as a source of error[16]. In addition, there is an element of magnification which is variable with patient size and different radiographic units.

Anderson[1] reported the average diameter of the CBD was 7.8 mm (range 7–9 mm) on a series of IV cholangiograms. He also reported the right and left hepatic ducts to be half the diameter of the CBD. Wise et al.[29] in a study of partial obstruction of the CBD, used 5.6 mm as the normal size with a range of 2 to 20 mm.

Computed tomography visualizes the extrahepatic ducts in a physiologic manner unless cholangiographic dye is administered. Foley et al.[11] reported that normal CHDs and CBDs could be visualized with optimal technique in 30% of patients. The diameters ranged from 4 to 6 mm. A more recent report[2] found 53% of patients with gallbladders had visible common ducts (mean diameter 5.3 mm) while 87% of postcholecystectomy patients had visible ducts (mean diameter 8.2 mm).

ULTRASOUND

The normal extrahepatic bile ducts are identified with high regularity with current equipment. Using a right posterior oblique position, Dewbury[7] reported 94% visualization with gray-scale B-scanners and Cooperberg[3] reported 98% visualization with a mechanical sector scanner. Because the cystic duct cannot be identified it is not possible to distinguish between the CHD and CBD. Many simply refer to the extrahepatic duct as the common duct. To standardize results several authors used the point at which common duct passes anterior to the right portal vein, often with the hepatic artery seen in cross section between the duct and the vein (Fig 9–1). It is important to measure the widest longitudinal section of the duct rather than a tangential section, which decreases the measurement. Only the lumen is measured inside the bright echoes of the anterior and posterior walls and the measurement should be perpendicular to the walls. Several reports have indicated that 4 mm is the upper limit for the normal common duct.[3, 4, 22, 23, 25, 27] Niederau et al.[22] found 95% were less than or equal to 4 mm. Sample et al.,[25] using non-real-time equipment, reported 5 mm as the upper limit of normal. Dewbury[7] reported a range of 2 to 5 mm, also using static imaging. Cooperberg et al.[4] and Sauerbrei et al.[26] both used 5 mm as a gray zone with any duct larger requiring further evaluation. Cooperberg et al.[4] reported 99% sensitivity and 87% specificity using these criteria to evaluate extrahepatic ducts as a cause of obstructive jaundice (Fig 9–2).

Measurement of the common ducts after a fatty meal has been utilized to detect

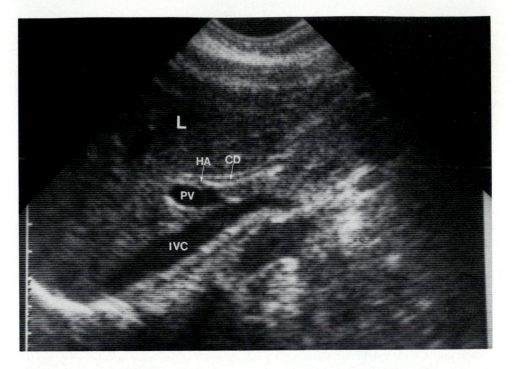

FIG 9–1.
Longitudinal image of a normal common duct. *L* = liver; *CD* = common duct; *HA* = hepatic artery;
PV = portal vein; *IVC* = inferior vena cava.

the presence of partial common duct obstruction.[5, 27, 28] One report used different
criteria for those with and without gallbladder and with a normal or dilated duct.[27]
In this study, if the duct was 6 mm or less, the result was positive only if the duct
increased by 1 mm or more. If the duct size initially was greater than 6 mm the
result was positive with either no change or an increase in diameter. However, two
more recent studies[5, 28] found that lack of change after a fatty meal is normal in a
dilated duct. Two recent studies noted normal intermeasurement variations of 1
mm,[5, 24] presumably due to normal temporal variations or errors in measurement.
Consequently, Darweesh et al.[5] concluded that high sensitivity and specificity would
be achieved in all patients if a test were considered positive only with an increase
in duct diameter equal to or greater than 2 mm.

Controversy persists regarding duct size following cholecystectomy. Some have
proposed that the common duct dilates following cholecystectomy and functions as
a reservoir.[5, 14, 20, 21, 22] Others,[1, 9, 12, 13, 18, 21, 30] however, contend that the duct does
not enlarge as a result of cholecystectomy, and dilatation greater than 6 mm suggests
partial obstruction or loss of elasticity due to preexisting obstruction. Darweesh et
al.[5] suggest that both etiologies most probably exist, and our experience confirms
this. We have examined a group of asymptomatic patients following cholecystectomy
in whom the common duct was dilated despite a normal-caliber duct prior to surgery.
Therefore, duct dilatation may not be indicative of obstruction after cholecystectomy.

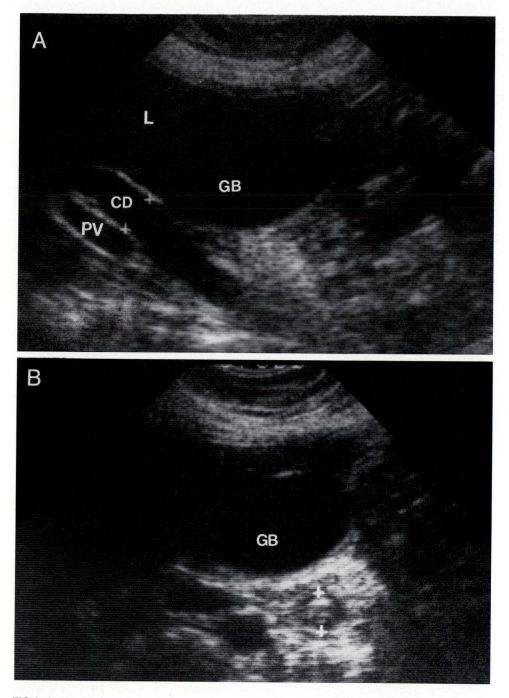

FIG 9–2.
A, longitudinal section of a dilated common bile duct (*CD*). *L* = liver; *GB* = gallbladder; *CD* = common duct; *PV* = portal vein. **B,** transverse section of dilated duct (*crosses*) with echogenic stone within the duct. *GB* = gallbladder.

CONCLUSION

The normal extrahepatic ducts are easily visualized with ultrasound, especially real-time high-resolution scanners. There is some discrepancy in the size of the normal duct as reported in radiographic and ultrasound studies. Numerous reasons are cited for these discrepancies. Among these are magnification, choleresis (IV cholangiography), and injection pressure (ERCP) on radiographic studies[4, 20, 26] and underestimation of duct size due to "blooming" of wall echoes on ultrasound.[7, 26] In addition, there are discrepancies in site of measurement between ultrasound and radiographic studies, that is, CHD on ultrasound versus CBD on IV cholangiography and ERCP. Finally, Mueller et al.[20] found that marked distensibility of the extrahepatic ducts resulted in rapid change in size.

The normal common duct should be measured as it crosses the right portal vein. Up to 5 mm is normal. A gray zone exists between 5 mm and 6 mm, but over 6 mm is abnormal, and warrants further investigation.

REFERENCES

1. Anderson F: The biliary tract in the normal and cholecystectomized patient. *AJR* 1957; 78:623–630.
2. Co CS, Shea WJ, Goldberg HI: Evaluation of common bile duct diameter using high resolution computed tomography. *J Comput Assist Tomogr* 1986; 10:424–427.
3. Cooperberg PL: High-resolution real-time ultrasound in the evaluation of the normal and obstructed biliary tract. *Radiology* 1978; 129:477–480.
4. Cooperberg PL, Li D, Wong P, Cohen MM, et al: Accuracy of common hepatic duct size in the evaluation of extrahepatic biliary obstruction. *Radiology* 1980; 135:141–144.
5. Darweesh RM, Dodds WJ, Hogan WJ, et al: Fatty meal sonography for evaluating patients with suspected partial common duct obstruction. *AJR* 1988; 151:63–68.
6. Deitch E: In vivo measurements of the internal and external diameters of the common bile duct in man. *Surg Gynecol Obstet* 1981; 152:642–644.
7. Dewbury KC: Visualization of normal biliary ducts with ultrasound. *Br J Radiol* 1980; 53:774–780.
8. Dowdy GS, Waldron GW, Brown WG: Surgical anatomy of the pancreatobiliary ductal system. *Arch Surg* 1962; 94:229–246.
9. Edmunds R, Rucker C, Finby N: Intravenous cholangiography. *Arch Surg* 1965; 90:73–75.
10. Ferris DO, Vibert JC: The common bile duct. *Ann Surg* 1959; 149:249–251.
11. Foley WD, Wilson CR, Quiroz FA, et al: Demonstration of the normal extrahepatic biliary tract with computed tomography. *J Comput Assist Tomogr* 1980; 4:48–52.
12. Graham MF, Cooperberg PL, Cohen MM, et al: Ultrasonic screening of the common hepatic duct in symptomatic patients after cholecystectomy. *Radiology* 1981; 138:137–139.
13. Graham MF, Cooperberg PL, Cohen MM, et al: The size of the normal common hepatic duct following cholecystectomy: An ultrasonographic sign. *Radiology* 1980; 135:137–139.
14. Hughes J, LoCurcio SB, Edmunds R, et al: The common bile duct after cholecystectomy. *JAMA* 1966; 197:247–249.
15. Kune GA: Surgical anatomy of common bile duct. *Arch Surg* 1964; 89:995–1004.
16. Lasser RB, Silvis SE, Vennes JA: The normal cholangiogram. *Dig Dis* 1978; 23:586–590.
17. Leslie D: The width of the common bile duct. *Surg Gynecol Obstet* 1968; 126:761–763.
18. Longo MF, Hodgson JR, Ferris DO: Size of the common bile duct follwoing cholecystectomy. *Ann Surg* 1967; 165:250–253.
19. Mahour GH, Wakin KG, Ferris DO: The common bile duct in man: Its diameter and circumference. *Ann Surg* 1967; 165:415–419.
20. Mueller PR, Ferrucci JT, Simeone JF, et al: Observations on the distensibility of the common duct. *Radiology* 1982; 142:467–472.
21. Mueller PR, Ferrucci JT, Simeone JF, et al: Post-cholecystectomy bile duct dilatation: Myth or reality. *Radiology* 1981; 136:355–358.

22. Niederau C, Muller J, Sonnenberg A, et al: Extrahepatic bile ducts in healthy subjects, in patients with cholelithiasis, and in postcholecystectomy patients: A prospective ultrasonic study. *J Clin Ultrasound* 1983; 11:23–27.

23. Parulekar SG: Ultrasound evaluation of common bile duct size. *Radiology* 1979; 133:703–707.

24. Raptopoulos V, Smith EH, Karellas A, et al: Daytime constancy of bile duct diameter. *AJR* 1987; 148:557–558.

25. Sample WF, Sarte DA, Goldstein LI, et al: Gray-scale ultrasonography of the jaundiced patient. *Radiology* 1978; 128:719–725.

26. Sauerbrei EE, Cooperberg PL, Gordon P, et al: The discrepancy between radiographic and sonographic bile duct measurements. *Radiology* 1980; 137:751–755.

27. Simeone JF, Butch RJ, Mueller PR, et al: The bile ducts after a fatty meal: Further sonographic observations. *Radiology* 1985; 154:763–768.

28. Willson SA, Gosink BB, van Sonnenberg E: Unchanged size of a dilated common bile duct after a fatty meal: Results and significance. *Radiology* 1986; 160:29–31.

29. Wise RE, Johnston DE, Salzman FA: The intravenous cholangiographic diagnosis of partial obstruction of the common bile duct. *Radiology* 1957; 68:507–525.

Chapter 10

Ultrasound Measurements of the Gallbladder

Alan H. Wolson, M.D.

A discussion of measurements of the gallbladder must include measurements of size of the gallbladder and measurements of gallbladder wall thickness. The latter measurement has become a factor only since the advent of high-resolution ultrasound and computed tomography (CT).

While there are reports that give standards for the size of the gallbladder, it is important to recognize that considerable variability exists. The gallbladder size varies both with body habitus and, to some extent, with the type of mesentery. In addition, a very distended gallbladder that contracts normally with a fatty meal or cholecystokinin is of no significance. Absence of contractility also may not be significant. In contrast, a small or normal-sized gallbladder may be unable to distend due to chronic fibrotic changes.[1]

Dowdy et al.,[3] in a report of surgical anatomy, found the average gallbladder length was 8.5 cm with a range of 4 to 14 cm. The report of the Task Group on Reference Man[11] gives both newborn and adult sizes. Volumes are also presented. They are as follows:

Size
Newborn
  Length 30–32 mm
  Width 1/3 of length
Adult
  Length 10 cm (range 8–12 cm)
  Width 4–5 cm

Volume
1–3 months 3.2 mL
3–10 years 8.5 mL
6–9 years 33.6 mL
Adult 50–65 mL

RADIOLOGY

The size of the gallbladder as seen on oral cholecystography seems well established,[9] generally reported as being approximately 7 to 10 cm in length. A recent article[10] also confirms this size, reporting 97% of normals had length less than 11 cm and width less than 4 cm.

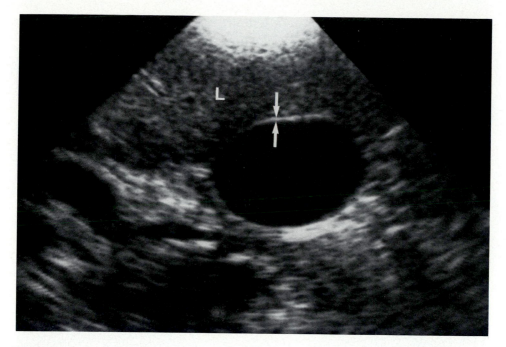

FIG 10–1.
Normal gallbladder wall (*arrows*) thickness. *L* = liver.

ULTRASOUND

The size of the normal gallbladder as reported in the ultrasound literature correlates well with the radiology measurements. One study[17] found the gallbladder was less than 4 cm in diameter in 96% of asymptomatic fasting patients. Diameters greater than 4 cm are seen in a high percentage of patients with acute cholecystitis, but can be seen in a variety of other conditions as well. Kane[14] reported the normal gallbladder measures 8 to 10 cm in length and 5 cm in diameter. Weissberg and Gosink[26] found normal gallbladders usually were approximately 8 cm in length, but could be up to 13 cm. We have used a diameter of up to 4 cm as normal.

Relatively little attention has been given to volume measurements, perhaps because of the difficulty in performing them. However, one report[2] found that a rather simple formula [Volume = 0.52 (length × width × height)] compared very favorably with the more complex sum-of-the-cylinders method. Two studies[5, 10] dealing with volumes reported widely disparate values for fasting volunteers. In one[10] the volume was 27 cc while in the other[5] it was 16.7 cc.

The wall of the gallbladder measures 1 to 2 mm on pathologic specimens.[8, 24] It can swell dramatically (up to ten times normal) with inflammation due to infiltration of fluid.

Numerous ultrasound studies have reported both normal and abnormal wall measurements in a variety of conditions. Many disorders besides cholecystitis produce thickening due to edema and the wall is not always abnormal in cholecystitis.[1, 4, 6, 7, 8, 13, 16, 18, 19, 21, 22]

Considerable variation exists in the reported normal thickness of the gallbladder wall measured by ultrasound. Some of this inconsistency arises from confusion over

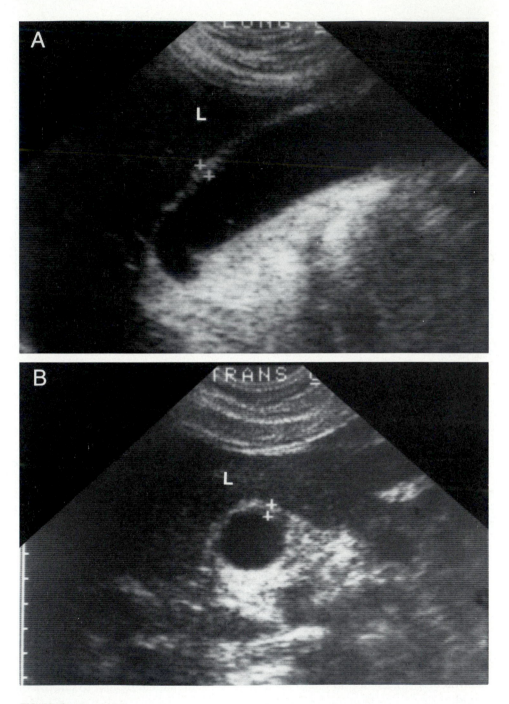

FIG 10–2.
A and B, longitudinal and transverse sections showing a thickened gallbladder wall (6 mm) (*crosses*).
L = liver.

what constitutes the wall echoes. Most reports use the bright echodense line as the wall echo while one[8] measures only the low-level echoes inside the bright line. Sanders[21] compared the results of measuring the bright line only versus including the bright line and inner soft echoes.

Many reports[6, 18, 20-22] use 2 mm as the normal wall thickness, while others[1, 4, 12, 18, 20, 25] use 3 mm as normal. Raghavendra[18] reported that 70% of normals were 2 mm and 96% were 3 mm. Ralls et al.[20] evaluated 25 normal volunteers. In the fasting state the wall measured 1 to 2 mm with a median of 1.5 mm. After a fatty meal the wall did not exceed 3 mm. Sanders[21] found 2 mm was the normal thickness using only the bright echodense line, whereas the wall was 5 mm thick if both bright line and soft inner echoes were included. Only two reports[6, 16] used 5 mm as the upper limit of normal but one[6] found the wall to be 2 mm or less in 97%. Two reports of wall thickness measured by CT[15, 23] also found 2 mm to be normal. We have found the majority of normals are 2 mm but accept up to 3 mm as normal (Figs 10–1 and 10–2).

CONCLUSION

The gallbladder is frequently and easily assessed with ultrasound. Normal values are fairly well established. The gallbladder may be up to 13 cm in length and 4 cm in diameter. The wall typically measures about 2 mm but up to 3 mm is normal.

REFERENCES

1. Croce F, Montali G, Solbrati L, et al: Ultrasonography in acute cholecystitis. *Br J Radiol* 1981; 54:927–931.
2. Dodds WJ, Groh WJ, Daweesh RMA, et al: Sonographic measurement of GB volume. *AJR* 1985; 145:1009–1011.
3. Dowdy GS, Waldron GW, Brown WG: Surgical anatomy of the pancreatobiliary ductal system. *Arch Surg* 1962; 84:229–246.
4. Engel JM, Deitch EA, Sikkena W: Gallbladder wall thickness: Sonographic accuracy and relation to disease. *AJR* 1980; 134:907–909.
5. Everson GT, Braverman DZ, Johnson ML, et al: A critical evaluation of real time ultrasonography for the study of gallbladder volume and contraction. *Gastroenterology* 1980; 79:40–46.
6. Finberg H, Bernholz J: Ultrasound evaluation of the gallbladder wall. *Radiology* 1979; 133:693–698.
7. Fiske CE, Laing F, Brown TW: Ultrasonographic evidence of gallbladder wall thickening in association with hypoalbuminemia. *Radiology* 1980; 135:713–716.
8. Handler SJ: Ultrasound of gallbladder wall thickening and its relation to cholecystitis. *AJR* 1979; 132:581–585.
9. Hatfield PM, Wise RE: Anatomic variation in the gallbladder and bile ducts. *Semin Roentgenol* 1976; 10:157–167.
10. Hopman WPM, Rosenbusch G, Jansen JBMJ, et al: Gallbladder contraction: Effect of fatty meals and cholecystokinin. *Radiology* 1985; 157:37–39.
11. International Committee on Radiological Protection. Task Group on Reference Man: *Report of the Task Group on Reference Man.* Prepared by the Task Group Committee no. 2, International Committee on Radiological Protection, Snyder WS (chairman). New York, Pergamon Press, 1975.
12. Juttner H-U, Ralls PW, Quinn MF, et al: Thickening of the gallbladder wall in acute hepatitis: Ultrasound demonstration. *Radiology* 1982; 142:465–466.
13. Kaftori JK, Pery M, Green J, et al: Thickness of the gallbladder wall in patients with hypoalbuminemia: A sonographic study of patients on peritoneal dialysis. *AJR* 1987; 148:1117.
14. Kane RA: Ultrasonic evaluation of the gallbladder. *CRC Crit Rev Diagn Imaging* 1982; 17:107–159.

15. Koehler RE, Stanley RJ: Computed tomography of the gallbladder and bile ducts, in Berk RN, Ferrucci JT, Leopold GR (eds): *Radiology of the Gallbladder and Bile Ducts: Diagnosis and Intervention.* Philadelphia, WB Saunders Co, 1983, pp 239–260.

16. Mindell HJ, Ring BA: Gallbladder wall thickening: Ultrasonic findings. *Radiology* 1979; 132:699–701.

17. Nathan NJ, Newman A, Murray DJ: Normal findings in oral and cholecystokinin cholecystography. *JAMA* 1978; 240:2271–2272.

18. Raghavendra NB, Feiner HD, Subramangam BR, et al: Acute cholecystitis: Sonographic pathologic analysis. *AJR* 1981; 137:327–332.

19. Raghavendra BN, Subramanyam BR, Balthazar EJ, et al: Sonography of adenomyomatosis of the gallbladder: Radiologic pathologic correlation. *Radiology* 1983; 146:747–752.

20. Ralls PW, Quinn MF, Juttner HU, et al: Gallbladder wall thickening: Patients without intrinsic gallbladder disease. *AJR* 1981; 137:65–68.

21. Samuels BI, Freitas JE, Bree RL, et al: A comparison of radionuclide hepatobiliary imaging and real-time ultrasound for the detection of acute cholecystitis. *Radiology* 1983; 147:207–210.

22. Sanders RC: The significance of sonographic gallbladder wall thickening. *J Clin Ultrasound* 1980; 8:143–146.

23. Shlaer WJ, Leopold GR, Scheible FW: Sonography of the thickened gallbladder wall: A nonspecific finding. *AJR* 1981; 136:337–339.

24. Stanley RJ: Liver and biliary tract, in Lee JKT, Sagel S, Stanley RJ (eds): *Computed Body Tomography.* New York, Raven Press, 1983, pp 167–211.

25. Tsujimoto F, Miyamoto Y, Tada S: Differentiation of benign from malignant ascites by sonographic evaluation of gallbladder wall. *Radiology* 1985; 157:503–504.

26. Weissberg DL, Gosink BB: Grayscale evaluation of the gallbladder. *Appl Radiol* 1978; 7:113–120.

Chapter 11

Ultrasound Measurements of the Pancreas

Gordon S. Perlmutter, M.D.

PANCREAS

Prior to the advent of sophisticated cross-sectional imaging modalities, such as ultrasound and computed tomography (CT), detailed evaluation of the pancreas was possible only intraoperatively or on postmortem specimens. From autopsy data, the weight of the pancreas for the normal reference male is determined to be 100 g; and for the normal reference female, 85 g. The pancreas gradually enlarges in size and weight as a function of age, reaching full growth after 20 years of age. The transverse diameter (or length) of the adult pancreas measures 14 to 18 cm, the anteroposterior (AP) diameter (or width) is 3 to 9 cm, and the vertical diameter (or thickness) is 2 to 3 cm.[1] These measurements were further refined into anatomic areas of the pancreas in autopsy results obtained by Kreel et al.,[2] where the normal AP diameters for the pancreatic head are 24 mm; for the neck, 17 mm; for the body, 20 mm; and for the tail, 15 mm. The normal craniocaudad diameters for the pancreatic head are 44 mm; for the neck 34 mm; for the body, 35 mm; and for the tail, 30 mm (Table 11–1).[2]

Attention has also been given to measurements of the pancreatic duct and these will be considered in a separate section of this chapter.

Computed Tomography

CT imaging of the pancreas is the most recent and, probably, the most precise method for visualizing the pancreas due to a relative lack of artifacts compared to ultrasound imaging modalities where bowel gas artifacts have proved to be a serious limiting factor in imaging the pancreas in a small percentage of patients. From CT data, Kreel et al.[2] determined that the measurements for the head of the pancreas are 23 ± 3.0 mm; for the neck of the pancreas, 19 ± 2.5 mm; for the body, 20 ± 3.0 mm; and for the tail, 15 ± 2.5 mm. Maximal normal measurements are 3 cm for the head of the pancreas, 2.5 cm for the neck and body of the pancreas, and 2 cm for the tail of the pancreas. All measurements were obtained perpendicular to the anterior border of the pancreas and are, consequently, at varying degrees of angulation to the AP axis of the patient, particularly in the region of the head of the

TABLE 11–1.
Normal Pancreas Measurements (cm)*

	Head	Neck/Isthmus	Body	Tail
Autopsy				
Kreel et al.[2]				
AP	2.4	1.7	2.0	1.5
CC	4.4	3.4	3.5	3.0
Computed Tomography				
Kreel et al.[2]				
AP	2.3 ± 0.3	1.9 ± 0.25	2 ± 0.3	1.5 ± 0.25
Max nl	3.0	2.5	2.5	2
Ultrasound				
Doust and Pearce[6]				
AP			0.8	
Max nl			1.5	
Haber et al.[7]				
AP		2.7 ± 0.7	2.2 ± 0.7	2.4 ± 0.4
CC		3.6 ± 1.2	3.0 ± 0.6	2.9 ± 0.4
Weill et al.[8]	1.1–3.0	0.4–2.1		0.7–2.8
Max nl	3.0			
de Graaff[9]				
AP	2.08 ± 0.4	0.95 ± 0.26	1.16 ± 0.29	
CC	2.01 ± 0.39	1.00 ± 0.30	1.18 ± 0.36	
96th percentile	2.8			
Arger et al.[10] AP	<2.5		<2	<2
Coleman et al.[11] (pediatric)				
0–18 yr AP	1.0–2.0		0.4–1.0	0.8–1.8
0–6 yr AP	1.6 (1.0–1.9)		0.7 (0.4–1.0)	1.2 (0.8–1.6)
7–12 yr AP	1.9 (1.7–2.0)		0.9 (0.6–1.0)	1.4 (1.3–1.6)
13–18 yr AP	2.0 (1.8–2.2)		1.0 (0.7–1.0)	1.6 (1.3–1.8)
Niederau et al.[12]	2.2 ± 0.3		1.8 ± 0.3	
AP	2.6		2.2	
95th percentile				
Shawker et al.[13]			1.18 (0.8–2.0)	

*AP = anteroposterior; CC = craniocaudad; Max nl = maximum normal.

pancreas.[2] Other articles by Sheedy et al.[2] and Haaga et al.[4] relate pancreatic measurements to the transverse diameter of the L2 vertebral body with the normal pancreatic head being no greater than the transverse diameter of the vertebral body, and the body and tail regions of the pancreas being no greater than two-thirds of the transverse diameter of L2. Since there is an approximate 2:1 ratio between the craniocaudad and AP diameters of the pancreas, it is felt that any scanning method using an angled gantry, such as that employed by Haaga et al.,[4] probably results in an overestimation of the size of the true AP diameter of the pancreas.[2] Also, in determining the CT measurements of the pancreas, care must be taken to opacify adjacent surrounding structures such as bowel and vessels in order not to include them as part of the pancreas (see Table 11–1).

Ultrasound

Numerous studies are available in the literature reporting normal ultrasound parameters of the pancreas. In several instances, direct comparison is not possible due to differences in equipment and the technique of measurement. One of the earliest attempts at measuring the normal pancreas was made by Doust in 1975 wherein he determined that the pancreas is significantly enlarged when the AP diameter of the pancreas overlying the aorta exceeds 2 cm.[5] Additional studies by Doust and Pearce[6] determined the maximum AP diameter in normal patients to be 15 mm with an average AP diameter of 8 mm. It was further determined that measurements equal to, or in excess of, 12 mm in diameter should be considered to be significantly enlarged. These data indicate that there is an overlap between the large normal and the pathologically enlarged pancreas.[6] Haber et al.[7] further refined measurements of the pancreas into three anatomic regions both in the AP and craniocaudad planes. Normal AP measurements for the head, body, and tail of the pancreas are 2.7 ±0.7 cm, 2.2 ±0.7 cm, and 2.4 ±0.4 cm, respectively. Craniocaudad measurements for the same anatomic areas are 3.6 ±1.2 cm, 3.0 ±0.6 cm, and 2.9 ±0.4 cm, respectively.[7] The larger craniocaudad dimensions of the pancreas concur with the anatomic and CT findings reported by Kreel et al.[2] Approximately 1 year later, and almost coincident in time with the article on CT measurements of the pancreas by Kreel et al., an article was published by Weill et al.[8] using ultrasonic measurement techniques virtually identical to those of Kreel et al. (i.e., measuring pancreatic thickness perpendicular to the anterior border of the pancreas). The normal range of measurements for the head, the isthmus, and the tail of the pancreas are given by Weill et al. as 11 to 30 mm, 4 to 21 mm, and 7 to 28 mm, respectively. Pancreatic head thickness in excess of 30 mm is considered to be significantly enlarged.[8]

In 1978, de Graaff et al. published measurements for the normal pancreas in the AP and craniocaudad dimensions. AP dimensions for the head, neck, and body of the pancreas are 2.08 ±0.4 cm, 0.95 ±0.26 cm, and 1.16 ±0.29 cm, respectively. Craniocaudad dimensions for the same anatomic areas are 2.01 ±0.39 cm, 1.00 ±0.30 cm, and 1.18 ±0.36 cm. In this article it was found that a maximum dimension of 2.8 cm embraces approximately 96% of the normal population.[9] In comparison to the earlier article of Haber et al., it can be seen that the data of de Graaff et al. indicate smaller normal dimensions in all planes of measurement. This probably was a result of improvement in instrumentation in the 2-year period between the two studies. In 1979 Arger et al.,[10] in comparing normal to enlarged pancreata in pancreatitis, determined that 100% of normal patients had pancreatic heads less than 2.5 cm, 94% of normal patients had pancreatic bodies less than 2 cm, and 97% of patients had pancreatic tails less than 2 cm. In a subsequent article by Coleman et al.[11] in 1983, these measurements were further refined for the pediatric age group. The normal range for the head of the pancreas is given as 1.0 to 2.2 cm; for the body of the pancreas, 0.04 to 1.0 cm; and for the tail of the pancreas, 0.8 to 1.8 cm. In their series, patients with pancreatic enlargement due to pancreatitis had dimensions of the head, body, and tail of the pancreas of 2.2 to 4.0 cm, 0.8 to 2.0 cm, and 1.4 to 3.5 cm, respectively. In this study, there was a further breakdown of the size of the normal pancreas by age group as shown in Table 11–2.

In a recent series, Niederau et al. reported the AP diameter of the pancreatic head to be 2.2 ±0.3 cm, with the 95th percentile at 2.6 cm, and the body of the pancreas to be 1.8 ±0.3 cm, with the 95th percentile at 2.2 cm.[12] Shawker et al. found the AP diameter of the body of the pancreas to be 1.18 cm (range 0.8 –2.0 cm) with a pancreatic-vertebral ratio of 0.25 ±0.04 (see Table 11–1).[13]

DISCUSSION

It can be seen from the foregoing that there are definite differences in measurement of the pancreas depending on the method employed, whether it be at autopsy or from in vivo images produced with CT or ultrasound (see Table 11–1). There is also a significant variation in measurements reported by various studies using ultrasound as the imaging modality. A general trend toward smaller dimensions of normal is seen relative to how recently the study was published, which may indicate that newer instrumentation with higher resolution has resulted in more closely defined parameters for the normal pancreas. It would also appear, therefore, that the most recent studies are probably the most accurate, with the data of Arger et al.,[10] Coleman et al.,[11] and Niederau et al.,[12] being the best in this regard.

For purposes of comparison it appears from these articles that most ultrasound measurements of the pancreas were performed in the AP diameter with the exception of the study by Weill et al.[8] that employed a diameter perpendicular to the anterior wall of the pancreas corresponding to the technique used by Kreel et al.[2] in evaluating CT images of the pancreas. It also appears that measurements for the tail of the pancreas in the article of Coleman et al. were performed perpendicular to the long axis of the pancreas rather than in a true AP diameter. It should be noted that measurements given for the body of the pancreas by Haber et al.,[7] Arger et al., Coleman et al., Niederau et al., and de Graaff et al.[9] were obtained anterior to the superior mesenteric artery conforming to the dimension given as the neck of the pancreas by Kreel et al. Dimensions given for the tail of the pancreas by Haber et al., Weill et al., Arger et al., and Coleman et al. correspond to the diameter for the tail of the pancreas given by Kreel et al. using CT measurements. Doust[5] and Doust and Pearce[6] do not specify the site of measurement.

All ultrasound dimensions are similar to but significantly smaller than those given for CT. This may be on a technical basis due to gain settings on ultrasound, window and center settings and gantry angulation on CT, and partial volume effect with both modalities.

In summary, it is recommended that measurements for the head and body of the pancreas be obtained in the AP diameter whereas measurements for the tail of the pancreas be obtained in a diameter perpendicular to the anterior wall of the pancreas (i.e., in the anatomic ventral-dorsal axis of the gland) according to the method described by Coleman et al. (Figs 11–1 to 11–3). The normal pancreas should measure

TABLE 11–2.
Size of the Normal Pancreas by Age Group*

Age Group (yr)	Head	Body	Tail
0–6	1.6 (1.0–1.9) cm	0.7 (0.4–1.0) cm	1.2 (0.8–1.6) cm
7–12	1.9 (1.7–2.0) cm	0.9 (0.6–1.0) cm	1.4 (1.3–1.6) cm
13–18	2.0 (1.8–2.2) cm	1.0 (0.7–1.0) cm	1.6 (1.3–1.8) cm

*Data from Coleman BG, Arger PH, Rosenberg HK, et al: *Radiology* 1983; 146:145.

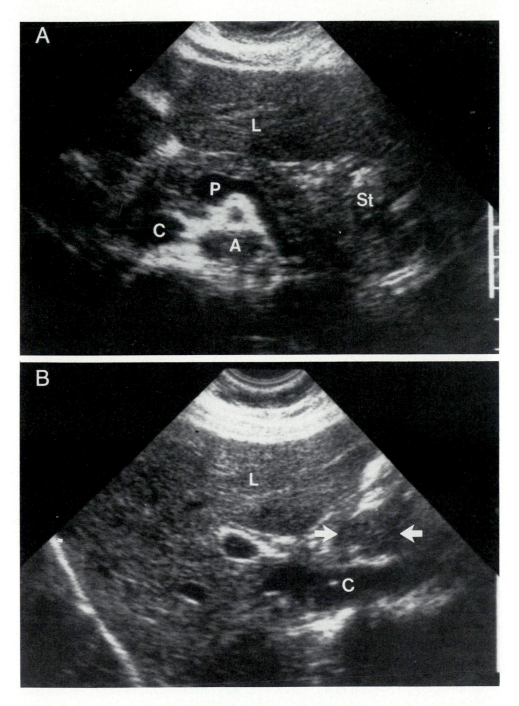

FIG 11–1.
A, transverse section of the upper abdomen at the level of the pancreas. *L* = liver; *St* = stomach; *A* = aorta; *C* = inferior vena cava; *P* = portal vein. **B,** sagittal section of pancreas (*arrows*) at the level of the vena cava (*C*). *L* = liver.

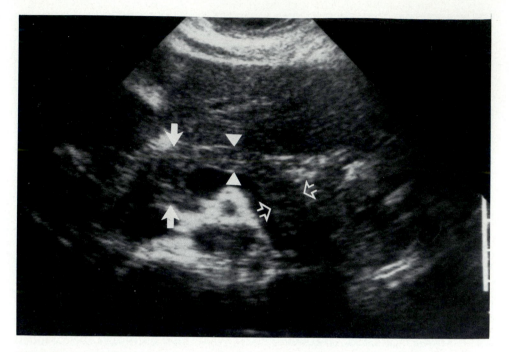

FIG 11–2.
Transverse section of the pancreas. The head of the pancreas (*closed arrows*) measures 1.8 cm, the body of the pancreas (*arrowheads*) measures 1.2 cm, and the tail of the pancreas (*open arrows*) measures 1.6 cm. Note that measurements of the pancreatic tail are performed in an AP axis relative to the anterior wall of the pancreas rather than relative to the patient.

less than 2.5 cm in the head region, less than 2 cm in the body, and less than 2 cm in the tail. In the pediatric age group these dimensions are somewhat smaller with the normal pancreas measuring less than 2.2 cm in the head region, less than 1.0 cm in the body, and less than 1.8 cm in the tail.

PANCREATIC DUCT

With the advent of higher-resolution ultrasound and CT scanners, as well as the development of endoscopic retrograde cholangiopancreatography (ERCP), it became possible to directly image the pancreatic duct, or duct of Wirsung. In a large autopsy study, Millbourn[14] reported the mean maximal diameter of the pancreatic duct to be 3.3 mm (range 3.0–4.0 mm) in the 16- to 20-year age group, increasing to a mean maximal diameter of 6.0 mm (range 3.5–10.0 mm) in the 81- to 92-year age group. Composite figures for the age groups of 16 to 92 years are a mean maximal diameter of 4.4 mm (range 2.0–11.0 mm).[14] Data were also obtained in this study on the size of pancreatic ducts as measured on intraoperative cholangiography with a mean maximal diameter of 2.2 mm (range 1–3 mm) in the 21- to 30-year age group, increasing to a mean maximum of 3.4 mm (range 2–4 mm) in the 61- to 70-year age group for an overall mean maximal diameter of 3.1 mm (range 1–7 mm) for the 20- to 65-year age groups combined.[14] It is clear from these data that there is a definite age discrepancy in the upper end of the range of normalcy but no significant age effect at the lower end of the normal range.

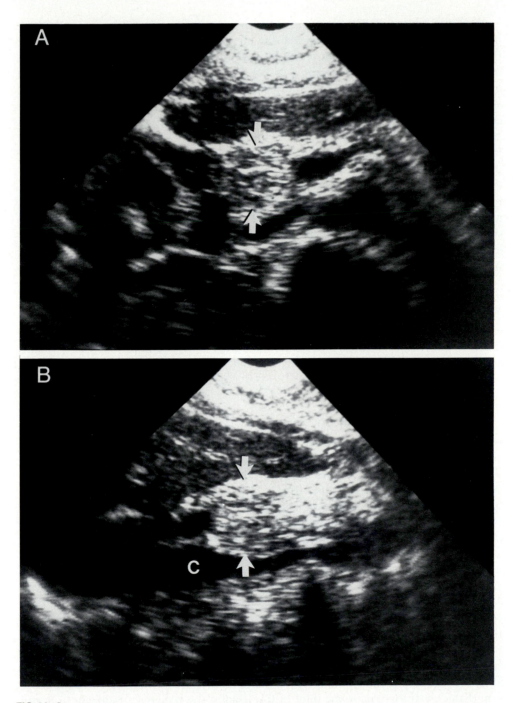

FIG 11–3.
A, the large solid mass (*arrows*) in the head of the pancreas proved to be a pancreatic carcinoma. **B,** the mass (*arrows*) in the sagittal section compresses the inferior vena cava (*C*).

With the advent of ERCP, direct measurement of the opacified pancreatic duct became feasible. The range of normal for measurements of the pancreatic duct in the head of the pancreas is 2.6 to 3.5 mm; in the body of the pancreas, 2.0 to 2.7 mm; and in the tail of the pancreas, 1.0 to 1.7 mm, with a mean maximum diameter of 3.5 ±0.9 mm, as reported in a study by Kasugai et al. in 1972.[15] Pancreatic duct size did not appear to be sex-dependent and there was only a slightly positive correlation of pancreatic size with age in this study. In a more recent study, Ferrucci observed that dimensions of the pancreatic duct at ERCP ranged from 3 to 4 mm in the head of the pancreas, tapering gradually to 1 to 2 mm in the tail of the pancreas.[16] Varley et al.,[17] in a more extensive evaluation of the pancreatic duct at ERCP, reported that the normal duct diameter in the pancreatic head is 3.1 ±0.9 mm (range 1.5–6.9 mm); in the body of the pancreas, 2.0 ±0.7 mm (range 1.3–3.6 mm); and in the tail of the pancreas, 0.9 ±0.4 mm (range 0.6–2.3 mm). In this same study, the overall length of the pancreatic duct was reported to be 169 ±27 mm (range 107–223 mm).[17] Cotton, using pooled data from ERCP studies performed at several centers, reported average actual duct measurements in the head of the pancreas of 4 mm (range 2–6 mm); in the body, 3 mm (range 2–4 mm); and in the tail, 2 mm (range 1–3 mm).[18] Didier et al.,[19] in a more recent series, found the dimensions of the pancreatic duct at ERCP to be 3.4 ±0.9 mm (1.5–5.0 mm) in the head, 2.6 ±0.7 mm (1.5–4.0 mm) in the body, and 1.6 ±0.5 mm (1.5–2.5 mm) in the tail. Ducts were diagnosed as being dilated when the diameter exceeded 5 mm, 4 mm, and 2.5 mm in the head, body, and tail, respectively (Table 11–3).[19]

Computed Tomography

Fishman et al.[20] reported that dilatation of the pancreatic duct could be imaged on CT scans. Although no normal measurements were given for duct size on CT scans, the author did reference an earlier work by MacCarty indicating the normal duct size at ERCP to be 3.3 mm in the 30- to 50-year age group and 4.6 mm in the 70- to 90-year age group.[20] Callen et al.[21] noted that ducts that are dilated may not be visible with 10-mm collimation, but may be seen with narrower 5-mm sections. No normal measurement for duct size were given on the basis of CT but these authors cited data at ERCP by Ohto indicating an average normal duct size of 3.9 mm with a range of 2.0 to 6.5 mm.[21] Hauser et al.[22] reported being able to image dilated ducts in the 4 to 20-mm range, but again did not cite any CT parameters for normal duct size. They did, however, reference ERCP data giving a normal duct size as 3.3 to 3.4 mm, but also noted that the duct size at ERCP tends to be 1 mm larger than corresponding anatomic sections due to radiologic magnification and distention of the duct due to the injection pressure.[22] Berland et al.[23] reported normal duct size with thin-section CT to be 5 mm in the pancreatic head, tapering to 2 mm in the tail of the pancreas. Using a correction factor of 15% for magnification of duct size at ERCP, this report indicated close correlation between ERCP data indicating a 7-mm diameter of the pancreatic duct in the head of the pancreas, tapering to 3 mm in the tail of the pancreas.[23] Lawson noted that the normal pancreatic duct, as identified by CT, is usually less than 4 mm in diameter with the abnormal duct being greater than 4 mm in diameter in the pancreatic head and 2 mm in diameter in the body of the pancreas (see Table 11–3).[24]

TABLE 11–3.
Normal Pancreatic Duct Measurements (mm)*

Autopsy	
Millbourn[14]	4.4 mean max (2.0–11.0)
or Cholangiography	
Millbourn[14]	3.1 mean max (1–7)
ERCP	
Kasugai et al.[15]	3.5 ±0.9 mean max
	Head 2.6–3.5
	Body 2.0–2.7
	Tail 1.0–1.7
Ferrucci[16]	3–4 head tapering to 1–2 tail
Varley et al.[17]	Head 3.1 ±0.9 (1.5–6.9)
	Body 2.0 ±0.7 (1.3–3.6)
	Tail 0.9 ±0.4 (0.6–2.3)
	Length 169 ±27 (107–223)
Cotton[18]	Head 4 max av (2–6)
	Body 3 max av (2–4)
	Tail 2 max av (1–3)
Didier et al.[19]	Head 3.4 ±0.9 (1.5–5.0)
	Body 2.6 ±0.7 (1.5–4.0)
	Tail 1.6 ±0.5 (1.5–2.5)
Computed Tomography	
Berland et al.[23]	5 head tapering to 2 tail
Lawson[24]	4 head tapering to 2 tail
Ultrasound	
Weinstein and Weinstein[26]	Body 1–2, >2 abnormal
Eisenscher and Weill[28]	Body 3, >3 abnormal
Parulekar[29]	Body 1.3 (0.6–2.6); >2 abnormal
Lawson et al.[30]	Body 1.3 (1.0–2.0); >2 abnormal
Hadadi[31]	Head/neck 3 (2.8–3.3)
	Body (SMA) 2.1 (2.0–2.4)
	Body 1.6 (1.0–1.7)
Didier et al.[19]	Body 2.6, >2.6 abnormal

*ERCP = endoscopic retrograde cholangiopancreatography; SMA = superior mesenteric artery.

Ultrasound

In an early article on the subject published in 1978, Gosink and Leopold[25] reported being able to demonstrate dilated pancreatic ducts in the size range of 5 to 12 mm with the average measurement being 8 mm. Presumably, the pancreatic duct in the normal state could not be visualized by these authors and, as a consequence, no normal measurements for the pancreatic duct were given.[25] Weinstein and Weinstein[26] reported the threshold of visualization of the pancreatic duct in the body of the pancreas to be 2 mm, corresponding to magnification-corrected normal values at ERCP. Visualization of the pancreatic duct, therefore, was concluded to be indicative of pathologic dilatation.[26] In an article published 1 year later, Weinstein and Weinstein observed that with newer high-resolution equipment it was possible to identify pancreatic ducts in the 1- to 2-mm size range, with 2 mm being the upper limit of normal diameter.[27] Eisenscher and Weill reported dilated pancreatic ducts as being greater than 3 mm in diameter.[28] Presumably, the measurements reported by Weinstein and Weinstein and Eisenscher and Weill were obtained in the region of the body of the pancreas. In a more detailed study, Parulekar[29] reported the mean normal diameter of the pancreatic duct in the body of the pancreas at the level of the superior mesenteric artery to be 1.3 mm (range 0.6–2.6 mm). Ducts greater than 2 mm in diameter were considered to be pathologically dilated. The minimum detectability threshold of duct diameter by ultrasound was 0.6 mm.[29] Lawson et al.[30] reported the normal pancreatic duct to be 1.3 mm (range 1–2 mm) with normal ducts being less than 2 mm in diameter with parallel walls. Abnormally enlarged ducts were reported as being greater than or equal to 2 mm with nonparallelism of the walls. In this series, abnormally dilated ducts had a mean diameter of 5 mm (range 2–18 mm).[30] More recently, Hadadi reported the normal pancreatic duct in the head and neck of the pancreas to be 3 mm (range 2.8–3.3 mm), in the body of the pancreas overlying the superior mesenteric artery to be 2.1 mm (range 2.0–2.4 mm), and more distally in the body of the pancreas to be 1.6 mm (range 1.0–1.7 mm).[31] Didier et al.,[19] using ERCP and ultrasound results in the same patients, classified normal ducts as being less than 2.6 mm by ultrasound measurement with dilated ducts being greater than 2.6 mm. Reported results yielded a high specificity (0.96) but with a large number of false-negatives (sensitivity 0.65) (see Table 11–3).[19]

DISCUSSION

It would appear from the foregoing that the normal pancreatic duct can be imaged reliably with modern high-resolution ultrasound equipment. The duct can be imaged more consistently in the region of the body of the pancreas and less reliably in the head of the pancreas due to the dorsoventral course of the pancreatic duct in the pancreatic head. In the tail of the pancreas, it is difficult to visualize the pancreatic duct due to overlying loops of gas-containing bowel and also due to the normal caliber of the pancreatic duct at this site approximating the threshold of visualization with ultrasound. The size of the normal pancreatic duct determined by ultrasound is dependent on technique and equipment, with pancreatic ducts of normal caliber not visible on older scanning units. Appropriately focused high-frequency transducers and low gain settings are essential for obtaining maximal luminal diameter measurements. These technical factors may account for variations in measurements reported for the normal pancreatic duct (see Table 11–3). In addition, it appears that there is a significant overlap between the upper range of normal and the lower range of abnormally dilated pancreatic ducts.

It is recommended that the pancreatic duct be measured in the body of the pancreas since this is the region most readily imaged and that the diameter of the normal pancreatic duct not exceed 2 mm at this site (Figs 11–4, 11–5).

Ultrasonic measurements of the pancreatic duct are significantly smaller than those reported at ERCP. This probably is due to a combination of geometric magnification and pressure distention of the duct at ERCP as opposed to the tendency for minification of the size of the pancreatic duct by less than optimal technique at ultrasound. Assuming an average maximal diameter of the pancreatic duct in the body of the pancreas at ERCP to be approximately 3 mm, this appears to correlate reasonably well with the top normal measurement of 2 mm at ultrasound when all factors are

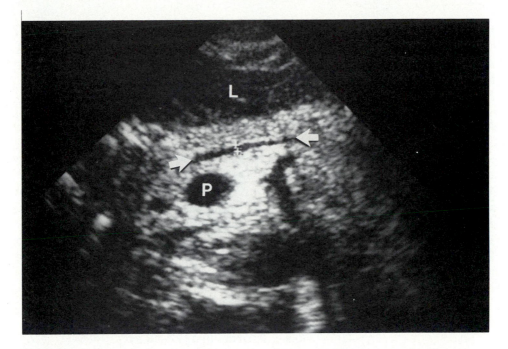

FIG 11–4.
Transverse scan demonstrates a normal pancreatic duct (*arrows*) in the body of the pancreas measuring 2 mm in diameter. Due to the advanced age of the patient, note the increased echogenicity of the pancreas. *L* = liver; *P* = portal vien.

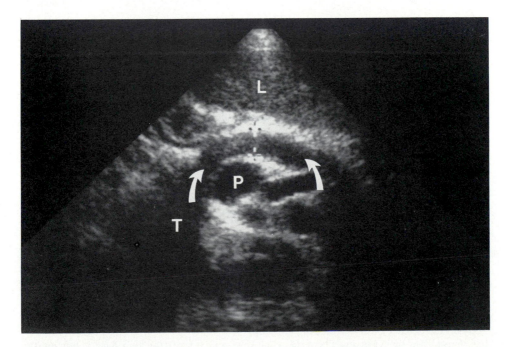

FIG 11–5.
Transverse section demonstrates a pathologically dilated pancreatic duct (*arrows*) measuring 16 mm in maximal diameter due to an obstructing tumor (*T*) in the head of the pancreas. *P* = portal vein; *L* = liver.

taken into consideration. There is also close correlation between the mean maximal diameter of the pancreatic duct at intraoperative cholangiography and at ERCP. CT measurements correlate closely with ultrasound in the body and tail regions but are significantly larger in the head of the pancreas for some unexplained reason.

MISCELLANEOUS MEASUREMENTS

Measurements are also available for the vessels surrounding the pancreas. The normal diameter of the splenic vein on CT scans is given as 9 mm by Kreel et al.[2] Using ultrasound scans, Doust and Pearce reported the average normal diameter of the splenic vein to be 6 mm and that of the portal vein to be 10 mm, with maximal AP diameters of 10 mm for the splenic vein and 15 mm for the portal vein.[6] Niederau et al. cite the mean maximal diameter of the portal vein as being 1.2 ±0.2 cm with the 95th percentile at 1.4 cm.[12] Weinreb et al. determined that the size of the portal vein is age-dependent with measurements as follows:[32]

Age (yr)	Measurement	
0–10	8.5 ± 2.7 mm	(range 5–12 mm)
11–20	10.0 ± 2.0 mm	(range 7–13 mm)
21–30	11.0 ± 2.0 mm	(range 6–15 mm)
31–40	11.0 ± 2.0 mm	(range 6–15 mm)
Mean	11.0 ± 2.0 mm	(range 6–15 mm)

REFERENCES

1. International Commission on Radiological Protection. Task Group on Reference Man: *Report of the Task Group on Reference Man.* Report of the Task Group Committee no. 2, International Commission on Radiological Protection, Snyder WS (chairman). New York, Pergamon Press, 1975, pp 149–151.
2. Kreel L, Haertel M, Katz D: Computed tomography of the normal pancreas. *J Comput Assist Tomogr* 1977; 1:290.
3. Sheedy PF, Stephens DH, Hattery RR, et al: Computed tomography in the evaluation of patients with suspected carcinoma of the pancreas. *Radiology* 1977; 124:731.
4. Haaga JR, Alfidi RJ, Havrilla TR, et al: Definitive role of CT scanning of the pancreas. *Radiology* 1977; 124:723.
5. Doust BD: Ultrasonic examination of the pancreas. *Radiol Clin North Am* 1975; 13:467.
6. Doust BD, Pearce JD: Gray-scale ultrasonic properties of the normal and inflamed pancreas. *Radiology* 1976; 120:653.
7. Haber K, Freimanis AK, Asher WM: Demonstration and dimensional analysis of normal pancreas with gray-scale echography. *AJR* 1976; 126:624.
8. Weill F, Schraub A, Eisenscher A, et al: Ultrasonography of the normal pancreas. *Radiology* 1977; 123:417.
9. de Graaff CS, Taylor KJW, Simonds BD, et al: Gray-scale echography of the pancreas. *Radiology* 1978; 129:157.
10. Arger PH, Mulhern CB, Bonavita JA, et al: An analysis of pancreatic sonography in suspected pancreatic disease. *J Clin Ultrasound* 1979; 7:91.
11. Coleman BG, Arger PH, Rosenberg HK, et al: Gray-scale sonographic assessment of pancreatitis in children. *Radiology* 1983; 146:145.
12. Niederau C, Sonnenberg A, Muller JE, et al: Sonographic measurement on the normal liver, spleen, pancreas, and portal vein. *Radiology* 1983; 149:537.

13. Shawker TH, Linzer M, Hubbard VS: Chronic pancreatitis: the diagnostic significance of pancreatic size and echo amplitude. *J Ultrasound Med* 1984; 3:267.
14. Millbourn E: Calibre and appearance of the pancreatic ducts and relevant clinical problems. *Acta Chir Scand* 1960; 118:286.
15. Kasugai T, Kuno N, Kobayashi S, et al: Endoscopic pancreatocholangiography. I. The normal endoscopic pancreatocholangiogram. *Gastroenterology* 1972; 63:217.
16. Ferrucci JT: Radiology of the pancreas, 1976. Sonography and ductography. *Radiol Clin North Am* 1976; 14:543.
17. Varley PF, Rohrmann CA, Silvis SE, et al: The normal endoscopic pancreatogram. *Radiology* 1976; 118:295.
18. Cotton PB: The normal endoscopic pancreatogram. *Endoscopy* 1974; 6:65.
19. Didier D, Deschamps JP, Rohmer P, et al: Evaluation of the pancreatic duct: a reappraisal based on a retrospective correlative study by sonography and pancreatography in 117 normal and pathologic subjects. *Ultrasound Med Biol* 1983; 9:509.
20. Fishman A, Isikoff MB, Barkin JS, et al: Significance of a dilated pancreatic duct on CT examination. *AJR* 1979; 133:255.
21. Callen PW, London SS, Moss AA: Computed tomographic evaluation of the dilated pancreatic duct. *Radiology* 1980; 134:253.
22. Hauser H, Battikha JG, Wettstein P: Computed tomography of the dilated main pancreatic duct. *J Comput Assist Tomogr* 1980; 4:53.
23. Berland LL, Lawson TL, Foley WD et al: Computed tomography of the normal and abnormal pancreatic duct: correlation with pancreatic ductography. *Radiology* 1981; 141:715.
24. Lawson TL: CT evaluation of pancreatic inflammation and complications. Presented at the Sixth Annual Course in Computed Body Tomography, San Diego, February, 1983.
25. Gosink BB, Leopold GL: The dilated pancreatic duct: ultrasonic evaluation. *Radiology* 1978; 126:475.
26. Weinstein DP, Weinstein BJ: Ultrasonic demonstration of the pancreatic duct: an analysis of 41 cases. *Radiology* 1979; 130:729.
27. Weinstein BJ, Weinstein DP: Sonographic anatomy of the pancreas. *Semin Ultrasound* 1980; 1:156.
28. Eisenscher A, Weill F: Ultrasonic visualization of Wirsung's duct: dream or reality? *J Clin Ultrasound* 1979; 7:41.
29. Parulekar SG: Ultrasonic evaluation of the pancreatic duct. *J Clin Ultrasound* 1980; 8:457.
30. Lawson TL, Berland LL, Foley WD, et al: Ultrasonic visualization of the pancreatic duct. *Radiology* 1982; 144:865.
31. Hadadi A: Pancreatic duct diameter: Sonographic measurement in normal subjects. *J Clin Ultrasound* 1983; 11:17.
32. Weinreb J, Kamuri S, Phillips G, et al: Portal vein measurements by real-time sonography. *AJR* 1982; 139:497.

Chapter 12

Ultrasound Measurements of the Spleen

Gordon S. Perlmutter, M.D.

The spleen is the largest lymphoid-containing organ in the body, as well as the largest structure in the reticuloendothelial system. As such, it has been the subject of measurements using virtually every modality available for assessing the size of this organ, from the simplest—palpation of the tip of the spleen—to highly sophisticated volumetric determinations using complex imaging modalities. In the normal state, the spleen is a rather variable organ in size and shape with wide ranges of normal limits. Using autopsy specimens, Krumbhaar and Lippincott have found the spleen to weigh approximately 170 g in the 16- to 20-year age group, decreasing to 155 to 160 g in the 26- to 65-year age group, and further decreasing to approximately 100 g in weight above the age of 65.[1] Spleens are usually larger in whites than in blacks and in males than in females.[1, 2] Deland, using autopsy material, found a poor correlation of splenic weight with patient body habitus but did observe that the spleen tended to decrease in size with age and increase in size with weight, height, and surface area.[3] The report of the Task Group on Reference Man lists the reference male spleen at 180 g and the reference female spleen at 150 g and gives a formula relating splenic weight to body weight (Table 12–1).[4]

In an extensive review of the subject, Aito found that palpation and radiographic estimates of splenic size were best, with nuclear medicine giving additional information when necessary.[5] Ultrasound was determined to be the least accurate of the modalities he investigated. This article, however, was published in 1974, prior to the era of computed tomography (CT) and modern high-resolution ultrasound equipment.

RADIOGRAPHY

Riemenschneider and Whalen estimated splenic weight (Wt) using the height and the width of the spleen 7 cm above the tip at right angles to the length using the formula: $Wt = (W/2)^2 \times L$, where W is the width and L is the length of the spleen.[6] Other authors have reported an average length of the spleen, radiographically, of 12.9 cm (range 7–16 cm) and an average width of 6 cm (range 3.5–10 cm).[7] Whitley et al. reported that 98% of spleens greater than 200 g in weight had a length in

TABLE 12–1.
Normal Spleen Measurements—Autopsy

Krumbhaar & Lippincott[1]	
Age (yr)	Weight
16–20	170 g
26–65	155–160 g
>65	100 g
Task Group on Reference Man[4]	
Male	180 g
Female	150 g

*Formula relating splenic weight to body weight: log s = log c + q log w where c = 3.5×10^{-8}, q = 0.97, w = total body weight in kg, and s = weight of spleen in grams.

excess of 13.6 cm corrected for magnification and a length multiplied by width measurement greater than 75 cm².[8] Other authors have used a width measurement 2 cm above the splenic tip with an average measurement of 3.4 to 3.5 cm and a range of 2.0 to 4.6 cm.[9, 10] Hopfan et al., using radiographs at angiography, determined the average splenic length to be 9.5 cm (range 7–13 cm) and width to be 6.0 cm (range 4–8 cm).[11] Using splenic area determined on anteroposterior (AP) views of the abdomen taken during angiography, Itzchak and Glickman determined that the normal splenic area is less than 80 cm² (Table 12–2).[12] This correlates well with earlier autopsy studies by Blendis et al. who found the mean splenic weight to be 198 ±61 g and the mean splenic area on AP radiographs to be 75 ±17 cm² corrected for magnification (see Table 12–2).[13]

TABLE 12–2.
Normal Spleen Measurements—Radiography

Riemenschneider & Whalen[6]

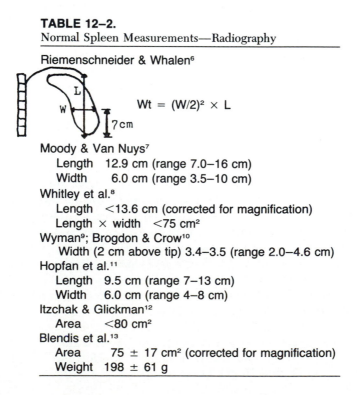

$$Wt = (W/2)^2 \times L$$

Moody & Van Nuys[7]
    Length   12.9 cm (range 7.0–16 cm)
    Width   6.0 cm (range 3.5–10 cm)
Whitley et al.[8]
    Length <13.6 cm (corrected for magnification)
    Length × width <75 cm²
Wyman[9]; Brogdon & Crow[10]
    Width (2 cm above tip) 3.4–3.5 (range 2.0–4.6 cm)
Hopfan et al.[11]
    Length 9.5 cm (range 7–13 cm)
    Width   6.0 cm (range 4–8 cm)
Itzchak & Glickman[12]
    Area   <80 cm²
Blendis et al.[13]
    Area   75 ± 17 cm² (corrected for magnification)
    Weight 198 ± 61 g

TABLE 12–3.
Normal Spleen Measurements—Nuclear Scans

Sigel et al.[14]
 Length 10.6 ±1.5 cm; 95th percentile—14 cm
Larson et al.[15]

	Posterior	Lateral
Length	10.0 ± 1.5 cm	10.0 ± 1.5 cm
Width	6.5 ± 1.0 cm	7.1 ± 1.6 cm
Circumference	27.7 ± 3.7 cm	27.5 ± 3.8 cm
Area	52.8 ± 14.6 cm²	56.2 ± 18.9 cm²

Length; 95th percentile—13 cm
Wt = 71.0 × L—537; r^2 = .960

RADIONUCLIDE IMAGING

Using nuclear imaging techniques, Sigel et al. determined the normal splenic height (or length) on posterior views to be 10.6 ±1.5 cm with 95% of normal spleens being less than 14 cm.[14] Spleens measuring 6 to 14 cm in length were within normal limits, those between 15 and 18 cm were enlarged, and spleens 19 cm and greater were diagnosed as being markedly enlarged. Larson et al., using multiple radionuclide measurements on both posterior and lateral views, determined that 95% of normal spleens were less than 13 cm in posterior length, with the normal weight of the spleen measuring between 150 and 200 g using the formula: Wt = 71.0 × L − 537, where L equals the posterior length of the spleen, with correlation of .96.[15] Similar to previously reported autopsy data, Larson et al. found no significant correlation between splenic weight and body weight, height, or surface area (Table 12–3). Ingeberg et al., using two different measurement techniques for determining splenic weight, found excellent correlation between each method and actual weight, but also found equal accuracy with "eyeball" evaluation by experienced examiners.[16]

COMPUTED TOMOGRAPHY

CT has been used extensively in evaluating the spleen. Methods have varied from eyeball assessment of splenic size to estimating volume from summation of cross-sectional areas. Henderson et al. have reported a mean splenic volume of 209 ±76 cm² using summation of cross-sectional areas on CT scans.[17] Other authors have determined that this summation-of-areas technique for splenic volume determination is very accurate with errors in the range of 3% to 5% (Table 12–4).[18] Using linear measurements of maximal width (W), thickness (T) (perpendicular to midwidth), and length (L), Cools et al. were able to derive volume (V) by the equation: V = 0.776 × L × W × T + 10.97, and closely correlate it with the more cumbersome direct volumetric methods (r = .991) (see Table 12–4).[19]

L = 7.56 ±3.32 cm (range 3.2–17.8 cm)
W = 9.95 ±2.55 cm (range 3.2–18.2 cm)
T = 3.26 ±1.14 cm (range 1.8–6.4 cm)

Another similar approach was published by Strijk et al.[20] using the Lackner splenic index (SI) where SI = length × maximal width × thickness at the hilum. They found a 91% accuracy for detecting splenomegaly when the SI exceeded 480 and that splenic weight (Wt) could be estimated from the splenic index by the formula Wt = SI × 0.55 (see Table 12–4).[20]

ULTRASOUND

Ultrasonic techniques have also been used to evaluate splenic size. Scanning techniques vary from author to author with views including transverse sections of the spleen with the patient either supine or in the right lateral decubitus position, longitudinal scans in the coronal plane, and oblique scans paralleling the left rib cage usually between the eighth and 11th rib interspaces. Carlsen reports the normal spleen to approximate 12 cm in length and 7 cm in diameter on images obtained paralleling the rib cage at the tenth to 11th intercostal space.[21] Koga and Morikawa, using scanning techniques paralleling the rib cage at the eighth to ninth intercostal space, determined the maximal normal splenic area to be 20 cm² using the formula: Area = K × L × W, where K = 0.8 in normal patients, and 0.9 in patients with liver disease.[22] They found no correlation with cross-sectional area and the patient's weight, height, or surface area. Using the same technique, Koga subsequently found that splenic volume could be determined as a function of cross-sectional area with the formula: Volume = 7.5 (area) − 77.5, with a correlation of .956.[23] Rasmussen et al.,[24] using Simpson's formula for summation of cross-sectional area, were able to calculate splenic volume with ±1 SD of 125 mL. They reported a normal splenic volume to be 300 mL with spleens greater than 2 SD above normal, or in excess of 550 mL, being definitely enlarged.[24] Niederau et al. evaluated spleen size using the section affording the maximal cross-sectional area of the spleen in the coronal plane with the patient in the right lateral decubitus position and in deep inspiration.[25]

TABLE 12–4.
Normal Spleen Measurements—Computed Tomography

Henderson et al.[17]
  Volume 209 ± 76 cm²
Cools et al.[19]

Volume = 0.776 × L × W × T + 10.97

L = 7.56 ± 3.32 cm (range 3.2–17.8 cm)
W = 9.95 ± 2.55 cm (range 3.2–18.2 cm)
T = 3.26 ± 1.14 cm (range 1.8–6.4 cm)

Strijk et al.[20]

Splenic index (SI) = L × W × T
SI = 120–480
Wt = SI × 0.55 (normal 65–265 g)

Transverse (T), longitudinal (L), and diagonal (D) measurements were obtained as follows:

$$T = 5.5 \pm 1.4 \text{ cm with a 95th percentile} = 7.8 \text{ cm}$$
$$L = 5.8 \pm 1.8 \text{ cm with a 95th percentile} = 8.7 \text{ cm}$$
$$D = 3.7 \pm 1.0 \text{ cm with a 95th percentile} = 5.4 \text{ cm}$$

The area (A) of the spleen was also determined by the formula: $A = (D \times \sqrt{T^2 + L^2})/2$. All measurements correlated well with each other, with diagonal and area measurements found to add no significant additional information compared to the longitudinal and transverse measurements in assessing splenic size. Splenic size was seen to decrease with age and increase with weight and body surface area in this series. Aito[5] found the best estimate for splenic volume using ultrasound techniques was given by the formula: $V = 1.6 \times L \times W$ for splenic volumes in the range of 15 to 535 cc. He used longitudinal (coronal) sections with the patient in the right lateral decubitus position with measurements performed on the scan in which the dimensions and area of the spleen were maximal.[5] In this study, splenic volume relates the splenic weight by the specific gravity of 1.14 g/cc. Another estimation of splenic size employs transverse sections with the patient either supine or in the right lateral decubitus position. The section demonstrating maximal area is used for measurement. Maximal long- and short-axis measurements are obtained and the area determined by the formula: Area $= L \times W$. Normal area is less than or equal to 55 cm^2, borderline enlargement is equal to 65 cm^2, and splenomegaly is equal to or greater than 75 cm^2 (Table 12–5).[26]

Pietri and Boscaini,[27] using an articulated arm scanner, measured height (H) (length), breadth (B) (maximal transverse diameter), and thickness (T) (maximal AP diameter) and derived a splenic volume index (SVI) where SVI $= H \times B \times T/27$. Ninety-five percent of normals had an SVI between 8 and 34. Other measurements are as follows (see also Table 12–5)[27]:

$$\text{SVI} = 21.5 \pm 6.4 \text{ (range 9–35)}$$
$$\text{Height} = 9.0 \pm 1.7 \text{ cm (range 5.5–14 cm)}$$
$$\text{Breadth} = 8.0 \pm 1.2 \text{ cm (range 6–12 cm)}$$
$$\text{Thickness} = 8.0 \pm 1.7 \text{ cm (range 5–12 cm)}$$

One additional parameter unique to the ultrasound method is determining the echogenicity of the normal spleen. Mittelstaedt and Partain[28] found that the echogenicity of the normal spleen is approximately the same as that of the liver. Rosenfield et al.[29] found that the spleen is slightly more echogenic than the adjacent left renal cortex.

DISCUSSION

Inherent variation in the size and shape of the normal spleen, as well as the multiple ultrasound approaches used in measuring the spleen, render it difficult to establish one best method for determining splenic size. Because of the difficulties in obtaining ultrasonic images of the spleen due to air in the lung on the superior aspect of the spleen, interfering ribs along the periphery of the spleen, and bowel

TABLE 12–5.
Normal Spleen Measurements—Ultrasound

Carlsen[21] (oblique views at 10–11th intercostal space)
  Length   12 cm
  Width   7 cm
Koga & Moritama[22]; Koga[23] (oblique views at 8–9th intercostal space)

Area = K × L × W
        K = 0.8 normal patients
        k = 0.9 liver diseases

Area <20 cm²
Volume = area × 7.5 − 77.5; r^2 = .956
Aito[5] (coronal sections)

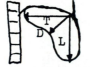

Volume = 1.6 × L × W

Volume = 166.4 ± 72.4 cm²
Wt = 1.14 × volume
Niederau et al.[25] (coronal sections)

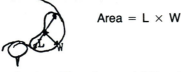

T = 5.5 ±1.4 cm; 95th percentile = 7.8 cm
L = 5.8 ±1.8 cm; 95th percentile = 8.7 cm
D = 3.7 ±1.0 cm; 95th percentile = 5.4 cm

Area = (D × $\sqrt{T^2 + L^2}$)/2
Perlmutter[26] (transverse sections)

Area = L × W

Area = 55 cm² normal (65 cm² borderline; 75 cm² enlarged)

Rasmussen et al.[24] (summation technique)
  Volume = 300 ± 125 mL (550 mL definitely enlarged)
Pietri & Boscaini[27]

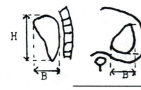

SVI = H × B × T/27
SVI = 21.5 ± 6.4 (range 9–35)
  H = 9 ± 1.7 cm (range 5.5–14 cm)
  B = 8 ± 1.2 cm (range 6–12 cm)
  T = 8 ± 1.7 cm (range 5–12 cm)

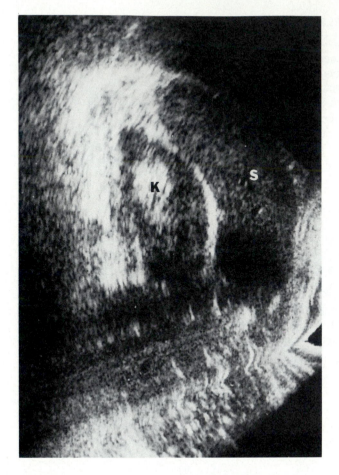

FIG 12–1.
Coronal section of the left upper quadrant. *S* = spleen; *K* = kidney.

gas artifact along the medial aspect of the spleen, it would appear that the best measurements should be those most easily obtained. To this extent, the transverse and longitudinal measurements of Niederau et al.,[25] the volume measurements of Aito,[5] and the cross-sectional area measurements of Perlmutter[26] would seem the most appropriate in estimating splenic size (Figs 12–1 through 12–6). Koga's method for measuring the cross-sectional area and volume of the spleen using the eighth to ninth intercostal space also would appear to be satisfactory. It should be noted,

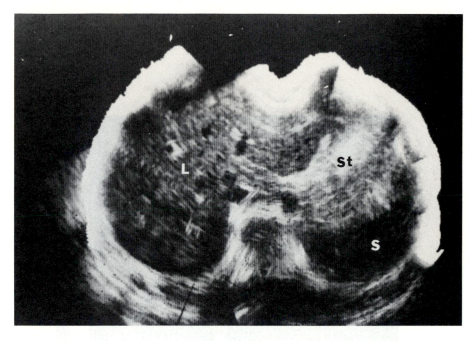

FIG 12–2.
Transverse section of the upper abdomen in the plane of the spleen. *S* = spleen; *L* = liver; *St* = stomach.

however, that Koga's data were derived from Japanese populations and that his data for maximal normal splenic area of 20 cm² and his formula for volume would result in a top normal volume of 72.5 cc. Assuming the specific gravity of the spleen at 1.14 g/cm,[5] this would result in a top normal splenic weight of 82.6 g, which would be considerably less than estimated weights for normal whites. For this reason, Koga's data may have limited applicability in non-Asian populations. On the other hand, Aito's formula for determination of splenic volume is easy to use and probably more appropriate to Western populations. The estimation for splenic volume of Rasmussen et al.,[24] which uses cross-sectional areas and Simpson's formula, is the most difficult of the methods available and probably not applicable to routine ultrasound practice.

Summarizing measurements from all modalities, it would appear that splenic weight in excess of 200 g and volume in excess of 175 to 200 cc, determined by any of the methods discussed, can be considered to be abnormal. It would also appear that splenic length in excess of 14 cm and maximal width in excess of 8 cm, irrespective of the measurement, would indicate the presence of splenomegaly.

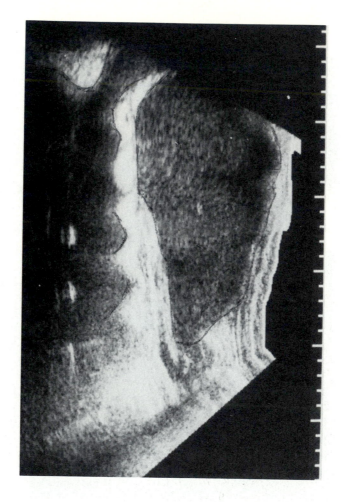

FIG 12–5.
Coronal section of an enlarged spleen. A = 9.2 cm; B = 14.5 cm; C = 17.3 cm; D = 9.2 cm. Volume = 254.6 cc; weight = 290.3 g. Diameters are defined on Fig 12–3.

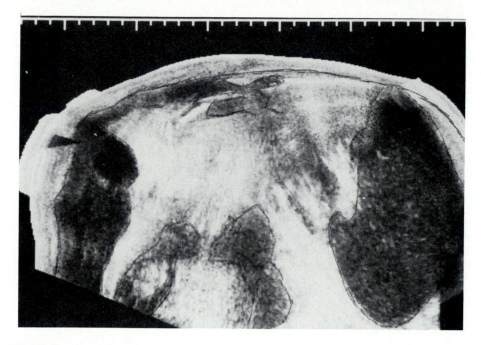

FIG 12–6.
Transverse section of an enlarged spleen. E = 15.7 cm; F = 7.8 cm. Area = 122.5 cm². Diameters are defined on Fig 12–4.

REFERENCES

1. Krumbhaar EB, Lippincott SW: The postmortem weight of the "normal" human spleen at different ages. *Am J Med Sci* 1939; 197:344–359.
2. McCormick WF, Kashgarian M: The weight of the adult human spleen. *Am J Clin Pathol* 1965; 43:332–333.
3. DeLand FH: Normal spleen size. *Radiology* 1970; 97:589–592.
4. International Commission on Radiological Protection. Task Group on Reference Man: *Report of the Task Group on Reference Man*. Prepared by the Task Group Committee no. 2, International Commission on Radiological Protection, Snyder WS (chairman). New York, Pergamon Press, 1975.
5. Aito H: The estimation of the size of the spleen by radiological methods. *Ann Clin Res* 1974; (suppl) 15:1–54.
6. Riemenschneider PA, Whalen JP: The relative accuracy of estimation of enlargement of the liver and spleen by radiologic and clinical methods. *Am J Roentgenol* 1965; 94:462–468.
7. Moody RO, Van Nuys RG: Some results of study of roentgenograms of the abdominal viscera. *Am J Roentgenol* 1928; 20:348.
8. Whitley JE, Maynard DD, Rhyne AL: A computer approach to the prediction of spleen weight from routine films. *Radiology* 1966; 86:73.
9. Wyman AC: Traumatic rupture of the spleen. *Am J Roentgenol* 1954; 72:51.
10. Brogden BG, Crow NE: Observations on the "normal" spleen. *Radiology* 1959; 72:412.
11. Hopfan S, Watson R, Benua R: Splenic irradiation portals. *Radiology* 1974; 112:417–420.
12. Itzchak Y, Glickman MG: Splenic vein thrombosis in patients with a normal size spleen. *Invest Radiol* 1977; 12:158–163.
13. Blendis IM, Williams R, Kreel L: Radiological determination of spleen size. *Gut* 1969; 10:433–435.
14. Sigel RM, Becker DV, Hurley JR: Evaluation of splenic size during routine liver imaging with 99m Tc and the scintillation camera. *J Nucl Med* 1970; 11:689–692.
15. Larson SM, Tuell SH, Moores KD, et al: Dimensions of the normal adult spleen scan and prediction of spleen weight. *J Nucl Med* 1971; 12:123–126.
16. Ingeberg S. Stockel M, Sorensen PJ: Prediction of spleen size by routine radioisotope scintigriphy. *Acta Haematol* 1983; 69:243–248.

17. Henderson JM, Heymsfield SB, Horowitz J, et al: Measurement of liver and spleen volume by computed tomography. *Radiology* 1981; 141:525–527.

18. Brieman RS, Beck JW, Korobkin M, et al: Volume determinations using computed tomography. *Am J Roentgenol* 1982; 138:329–333.

19. Cools L, Osteaux M, Divano L, et al: Prediction of splenic volume by a simple CT measurement: a statistical study. *J Comput Assist Tomogr* 1983; 7:426–430.

20. Strijk SP, Wagener DJ, Bogman MJJT, et al: The spleen in Hodgkin disease: diagnostic value of CT. *Radiology* 1985; 154:753–757.

21. Carlsen EN: Liver, gallbladder, and spleen. *Radiol Clin North Am* 1975; 13:543–555.

22. Koga T, Morikawa Y: Ultrasonic determination of the splenic size and its clinical usefulness in various liver diseases. *Radiology* 1975; 115:157–161.

23. Koga T: Correlation between sectional area of the spleen by ultrasonic tomography and actual volume of the removed spleen. *J Clin Ultrasound* 1979; 7:119–120.

24. Rasmussen SN, Christensen BE, Holm HH, et al: Spleen volume determination by ultrasonic scanning. *Scand J Haematol* 1973; 10:298–304.

25. Niederau C, Sonnenberg A, Muller JE, et al: Sonographic measurement of the normal liver, spleen, pancreas and portal vein. *Radiology* 1983; 149:537–540.

26. Perlmutter GS: Unpublished personal experience.

27. Pietri H, Boscaini M: Determination of splenic volume index by ultrasonic scanning. *J Ultrasound Med* 1984; 3:19–23.

28. Mittelstaedt CA, Partain CL: Ultrasonic-pathologic classification of splenic abnormalities. Grey-scale patterns. *Radiology* 1980; 134:697–705.

29. Rosenfield AT, Taylor KJW, Jaffe CC: Clinical applications of ultrasound tissue characterization. *Radiol Clin North Am* 1980; 18:31–58.

Chapter 13

Ultrasound Measurements of the Bowel

Laurence Needleman, M.D.

Sonographic measurements of the gastrointestinal tract usually consist of measurement of the bowel wall. The bowel has several layers sonographically: the inner echogenic layer corresponding to the bowel contents, mucus, and the mucosa; the outer echogenic serosa; and the echo-poor wall. Using high-resolution equipment the specific layers of the bowel, such as the submucosa and the muscularis propria, can be separated, but their identification is not necessary in the routine measurement of the bowel.

The ultrasonic thickness of the stomach, small intestine, or colon wall is the thickness of the echo-poor layer. The measurement is made from the inner edge of the mucosal layer, or intraluminal mucus or gas, to the echogenic layer representing the serosa (Fig 13–1).

The measurement is best made on transverse images of the bowel since oblique images may falsely increase the measurement. When possible, the nondependent portion of the wall should be measured since this will be the most distended portion of the bowel. This will not always be possible since some bowel pathology will thicken bowel loops nonuniformly.

STOMACH

The thickness of the stomach was best evaluated in two studies.[1, 2] Fleischer et al.[1] found the range of normal nondistended stomach to be 2 to 6 mm and the distended stomach to be slightly smaller, 2 to 4 mm. Kuroiwa et al.[2] found the range to be 1 to 7 mm. There was no significant difference in wall thickness due to sex, body habitus, or age. The mean wall thickness was 2.5 mm and the standard deviation was 1.0 mm. The upper normal limit of gastric wall thickness is considered to be 5.0 mm.

SMALL AND LARGE BOWEL

Measurements of the small and large intestines were reported in one study of a

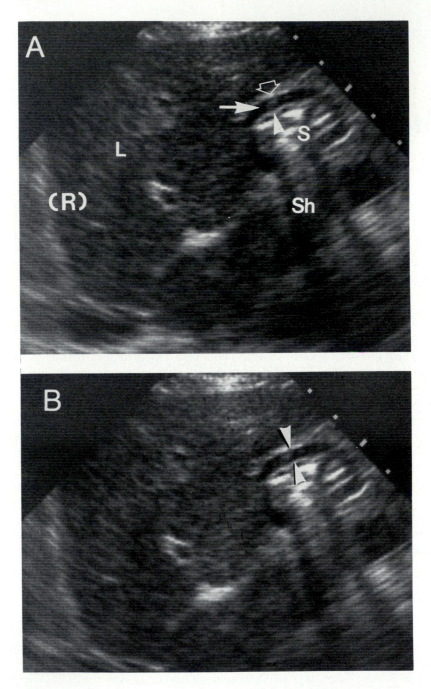

FIG 13–1.
Sonographic measurement of bowel wall thickness. **A,** longitudinal sonogram of the stomach (*S*) and left lober of the liver (*L*). The echo-poor bowel wall (*longer arrow*) is separable from the echogenic mucosal lining (*arrowhead*) and echogenic serosa (*short open arrow*). The stomach contains mucus and gas. The gas produces bright intraluminal echoes and shadowing (*Sh*). (*R*) = toward patient's head. **B,** bowel wall thickness is defined as the width of the echo-poor layer (*arrowheads*). The nondependent portion is usually used as it is the most distended. Five millimeters is considered the upper normal limit of the stomach, small bowel, or colonic wall thickness.

small number of patients. Fleischer et al.[1] found the small bowel to average 3 mm, with a range of 2 to 3 mm in 11 patients. There was no difference between nondistended and distended loops.

The same group[1] studied the large bowel in seven normals and found the mean to be 6 mm in the nondistended colon and 3 mm in the distended state. The measurement of 9 mm was found in the nondistended transverse colon of one patient. Excluding this unusual case, colonic thickening is considered when the bowel thickness is greater than 5 mm. In practice, a wall thickness of 5 mm is a good discriminator of bowel wall thickening, especially when there is other evidence of pathology such as abnormal compressibility or absent peristaltic activity.

TABLE 13–1.
Range of Measurements of the Infantile Pylorus

	Pyloric Diameter (mm)	Pyloric Muscle Thickness (mm)	Canal Length (mm)
Normal	6–13[5–7, 10]	1–4[5–7, 9, 10]	5–16[5, 7, 10]
HPS*	9–20[4–7]	2–7[4–7, 9]	16–28[5, 7]

*HPS = hypertrophic pyloric stenosis.

INFANTILE HYPERTROPHIC PYLORIC STENOSIS

Since the initial report by Teele and Smith[3] of the usefulness of sonography to diagnose infantile hypertrophic pyloric stenosis (HPS), many investigations have been performed. The diagnosis is made on the basis of both measurements of the pylorus and sonographic signs identifying the abnormal morphology and physiology of this region.[4–8]

High-resolution equipment (at least 5 MHz) is utilized and the pylorus is identified below the xiphoid and just to the right of the midline. Long-axis (Fig 13–2) and transverse (Fig 13–3) views of the pylorus are used for measurements. In long-axis measurements the echogenic line of the mucosa delineates the pyloric canal length (see Fig 13–2). The pyloric diameter is obtained from transverse (short-axis) planes. This is the anteroposterior (AP) diameter of the pylorus from the outer anterior edge of pyloric muscle to the outer posterior edge of pyloric muscle (see Fig 13–3). The pyloric muscle thickness is measured in either view and is measured from the edge of the mucosa (inner edge of pyloric muscle) to the outer edge of pyloric muscle (see Figs 13–2 and 13–3).

TABLE 13–2.
Measurement Criteria for Infantile
Hypertrophic Pyloric Stenosis*

Canal length	≥ 18 mm
Pyloric diameter	≥ 15 mm
Pyloric muscle thickness	≥ 4 mm

*Adapted from Haller JO, Cohen HL: *Radiology* 1986; 161:335–339.

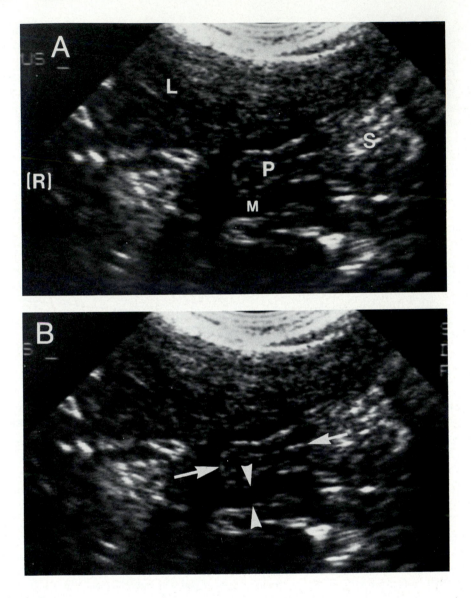

FIG 13–2.
Sonographic measurement of the infant pylorus. **A,** long-axis sonogram of the pylorus showing the closed pylorus (*P*), echo-poor pyloric muscle (*M*), and material within the stomach (*S*). The echogenic line indicating the mucosa must be visualized to make this measurement. (*R*) = toward patient's right; *L* = liver. **B,** canal length and muscle thickness measurements: The canal length measurement is made from one end of the echogenic line of the mucosa to the other (*between arrows*). The pyloric muscle thickness is obtained from the edge of the echogenic mucosa to the outer edge of the pyloric muscle (*between arrowheads*). It may be measured in either long-axis or in transverse planes (see Fig 13–3).

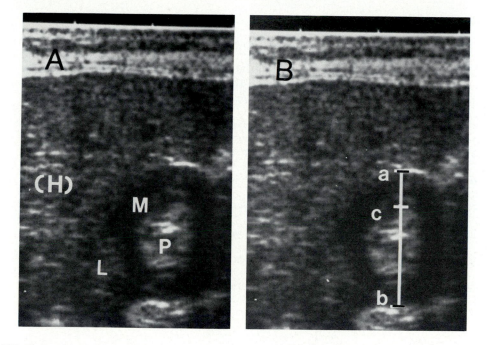

FIG 13–3.
Sonographic measurement of the infant pylorus (same patient as in Fig 13–2). **A,** transverse (short-axis) sonogram of the pylorus showing the echogenic mucosa and bowel contents (*P*) and pyloric muscle (*M*). *L* = liver; (*H*) = toward patient's head. **B,** pyloric diameter and muscle thickness measurements: The AP diameter of the pylorus (*line* from *a* to *b*) is obtained from the anterior edge of the pyloric muscle to the posterior edge of the pyloric muscle. The pyloric muscle thickness is obtained from the edge of the echogenic mucosa to the outer edge of pyloric muscle (*line* from *a* to *c*).

Three measurements are usually regarded as standard: canal length, pyloric diameter, and pyloric muscle thickness. Graif et al.[5] measured 24 normal infants and found the mean pyloric canal length and standard deviation was 12.0 ±3.7 mm. Pyloric diameter was 7.5 ±2.2 mm, and pyloric muscle thickness was 2.3 ±0.7 mm.

In HPS these three measurements are increased. Since overdiagnosing HPS can lead to unnecessary surgery, it is important to set the upper limit of normal high enough to minimize false-positive diagnoses. Table 13–1 examines the range of these measurements in normal infants and infants with HPS. Based on this evaluation the criteria for abnormal pyloric measurements are summarized in Table 13–2.

The pyloric canal length is the most accurate measurement. In two reported series using this measurement[5, 7] only one of the 128 patients with HPS had a canal shorter than 18 mm. No normal patient (0/145) had a length longer than 16 mm. An upper limit of 18 mm for the pyloric canal length yields a sensitivity of 99.2% and a specificity of 100%.

The most overlap of normal and abnormal measurements occurs in the pyloric diameter and pyloric muscle thickness. Therefore, so the sensitivity of these measurements is correspondingly lower.[5–7] The specificity of the measurements is excellent, however, being 100% for pyloric diameter and 99.1% for muscle thickness.[4–6] These measurements are useful, therefore, if they are abnormal, but cannot completely exclude the diagnosis if normal.

REFERENCES

1. Fleischer AC, Muhletaler CA, James AE Jr: Sonographic assessment of the bowel wall. *AJR* 1981; 136:887–891.
2. Kuwoiwa T, Hirata H, Yasumori K, et al: Ultrasonographic measurements of the normal gastric wall. *Nippon Igaku Hoshasen Gakkai Zasshi* 1983; 43:1273.
3. Teele RL, Smith EH: Ultrasound in the diagnosis of idiopathic hypertrophic pyloric stenosis. *N Engl J Med* 1977; 296:1149.
4. Ball TI, Atkinson GO Jr, Gay BB Jr: Ultrasound diagnosis of hypertrophic pyloric stenosis: Real-time application and the demonstration of a new sonographic sign. *Radiology* 1983; 147:499–502.
5. Graif M, Itzchak Y, Avigad I, et al: The pylorus in infancy: Overall sonographic assessment. *Pediatr Radiol* 1984; 14:14–17.
6. Wilson DA, Vanhoutte JJ: The reliable sonographic diagnosis of hypertrophic pyloric stenosis. *J Clin Ultrasound* 1984; 12:201–204.
7. Stunden RJ, LeQuesne GW, Little KET: The improved ultrasound diagnosis of hypertrophic pyloric stenosis. *Pediatr Radiol* 1986; 16:200–205.
8. Haller JO, Cohen HL: Hypertrophic pyloric stenosis: Diagnosis using US. *Radiology* 1986; 161:335–339.
9. Blumhagen JD, Noble HGS: Muscle thickness in hypertrophic pyloric stenosis: Sonographic determination. *AJR* 1983; 140:221–223.
10. Sauerbrei EE, Paloschi GGB: The ultrasonic features of hypertrophic pyloric stenosis, with emphasis on the postoperative appearance. *Radiology* 1983; 147:503–506.

PART IV

Genitourinary

Normal Renal Ultrasound Measurements

Steven L. Edell, D.O.

Alfred B. Kurtz, M.D.

Matthew D. Rifkin, M.D.

The kidneys are the primary structures of the urinary system and are responsible for removing toxic waste products from the body. They are paired, coffee bean–shaped organs located in the retroperitoneum on either side of the vertebral column surrounded by retroperitoneal fat and areolar tissue.[1, 2] The kidneys extend from the cranial margin of the 12th thoracic vertebral body to the caudal aspect of the third lumbar vertebral body with the right kidney commonly located 1 to 2 cm lower than the left[2] (Fig 14–1). The renal axes follow the course of the psoas muscles so that their inferior poles are directed inferiorly and laterally. In the adult, the kidneys average 11.25 cm in length, 5 to 7.5 cm in transverse (width) dimension, and 2.5 cm in thickness (anteroposterior [AP] dimension) with the left kidney often longer and narrower than the right.[2] The average kidney weighs 125 to 170 g in the adult male and 115 to 155 g in the adult female.[2] Because the kidneys are not fixed to the abdominal wall or other retroperitoneal structures, they move caphalad and caudad during inspiration and expiration.

Grossly, the kidney can be divided into two major portions, the renal sinus and the renal parenchyma[1, 2] (see Fig 14–1). The renal sinus, the center of the kidney, contains the major branches of the renal artery and the renal vein, and the major and minor calcyces of the renal collecting system. Adipose tissue is dispersed throughout. The renal sinus is surrounded by the renal parenchyma, which consists of the central medulla and the peripheral cortex. Surrounding the cortex is the renal capsule.

Since Voelcker and Litchtenberg[3] first reported contrast studies of the urinary tract in 1906, there has been a need for standardization of normal renal measurements to compare the varying change in the size of the kidneys in diagnosing and managing renal disorders. Radiographic measurements of the kidneys derived from conventional supine abdominal radiographs as well as intravenous (IV) urography had been considered the gold standard for obtaining renal measurements. However, there have been various errors from these techniques which have necessitated the need for a more accurate imaging modality. The magnification effect during conventional

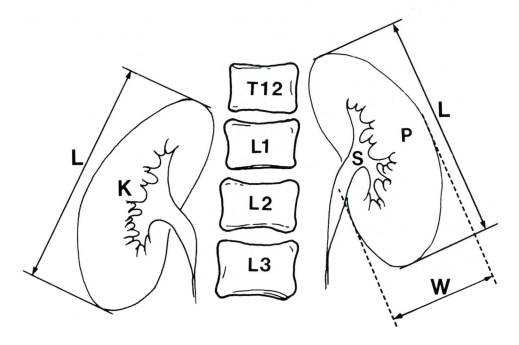

FIG 14–1.
Diagram of kidneys (*K*) in their normal axis parallel to the psoas muscles. The renal parenchyma (*P*) and sinus (*S*) are shown. *L* = length and *W* = width measurements. The 12th thoracic (T12) to third lumbar (L3) vertebral bodies are shown.

supine abdominal radiographs has resulted in increased renal size of approximately 17.5% and has been the major source of error in obtaining adequate measurements.[4] This magnification factor, along with the osmotic diuresis during IV infusion of contrast agents, has artifactually increased the longitudinal renal measurements approximately 1 to 1.5 cm. Conversely, foreshortening of the renal length has been caused by renal inclination and malrotation. Dure-Smith and McArdle[5] reported a mean angle of 16 ± 5.8 degrees (1 SD) between the longitudinal axis of the kidney and the horizontal plane. Griffiths et al.[6] reported that this angle ranged from 8 to 20 degrees in cadavers (mean 12 to 15 degrees on the right, 10 degrees on the left). Rotation of the kidney from 0 to 20 degrees about its transverse axis reduced its length by 1 cm, causing considerable shortening of the kidney.

Sonographic measurements, on the other hand, offer a more accurate determination of renal size and calculated renal volumes. Because this modality is a more anatomic type of examination, able to clearly define the renal borders without the theoretical detrimental side effects of radiation and problems with radiation magnification, this imaging study has gained considerable acceptance in recent years. The ability of ultrasound to evaluate patients in either renal failure or with contrast allergies is well known and has further helped to establish renal sonography as the procedure of choice in assessing kidney size.

However, ultrasound is not without its sources of error. (1) A significant renal malrotation, either primary or caused secondarily by a spinal curvature, adjacent organ enlargement, or mass, may lead to failure to fully evaluate renal size, especially length. When spinal curvature is considered a source of inaccurate renal measurements, comparison to conventional radiographs of the thoracolumbar spine may be of help to determine the correct scanning plane. (2) Lack of adequate renal and perirenal fat has been shown to be a significant source of error in obtaining adequate sonographic visualization of the renal borders, causing renal measurement inaccuracies especially in newborns and in very cachectic patients.[7] (3) Distortion of the renal contour from renal scarring may also make accurate measurements difficult. (4) Involuntary movements commonly occur when the patient is in extreme pain, febrile, or unable to suspend respiration and have tended to blur the ultrasound image, making the renal borders indistinct and occasionally exaggerating the longitudinal measurements. Paravertebral muscle contractions may also produce movement artifacts which can affect both longitudinal and transverse measurements. These movement artifacts have to a large extent been eliminated by the use of dynamic real-time scanners. (5) Inadequate visualization of the upper renal pole is often caused by the overlying ribs, making it difficult to adequately assess the superior portion of the kidney and obtain precise measurements. Since this difficulty is more prevalent on the left, this may account for the greater variation in the measurements of the left kidney. Normally the left kidney is approximately 1 cm longer than the right kidney. Obtaining images in multiple projections and using real-time small-headed sector transducers has led to obtaining more satisfactory visualization of the superior pole of the left kidney and hence more satisfactory longitudinal renal measurements.

These problems notwithstanding, optimum renal measurements can be obtained in most cases, commonly produced with the patient in the supine or decubitus position utilizing the liver as an acoustic window for the right kidney and the spleen as an acoustic window for the left kidney. Having the patient suspend respiration during the time of scanning will help to remove any blurring of the image caused by breathing that may develop during the course of the procedure. Three renal measurements are obtained: length, AP, and width dimensions. The longitudinal (length) measurement is obtained from the sagittal scan, by scanning the kidney from the superior to the inferior pole obliquely along its longest axis following the course of the psoas muscle margins (Figs 14–1 and 14–2). The maximum AP dimension is measured from this same sagittal image measured perpendicular to the long axis (Fig 14–2, A and B). The width is measured from a transaxial renal image, at its greatest thickness perpendicular to the length of the kidney, usually at the renal hilum or immediately above or below the hilum (Fig 14–2, C and D).

Although the supine position is usually optimal for obtaining renal measurements, it is sometimes necessary to utilize a more lateral (coronal) and rarely a prone approach to define renal dimensions. If the long-axis measurement is taken from a coronal image, it may be difficult to measure the AP dimension. When this occurs, the transaxial image can be used instead, provided the image is obtained exactly perpendicular to the renal length at its largest width. In addition, regardless of how the transaxial image is obtained, that is, sagittal, coronal, or prone, the width measurement should be taken from the lateral margin of the kidney through the renal hilum (see Fig 14–2, D).

Because of the higher position of the left kidney, the overlying costal margins may produce shadowing artifact and distortion of the left upper quadrant, making it difficult to adequately determine the most superior aspect of the left kidney. The earlier articles defining renal measurements were performed with the static articulated arm scanners and utilized the prone position exclusively. With the advent of the more sophisticated real-time sector scanners, the prone position has been almost entirely replaced by the supine or decubitus position. When the upper pole is difficult to image, placing the patient in the decubitus position with a towel under the lower flank and the upper arm extended over the head can be a useful technique. It raises the costochondral margins, opens up the rib spaces, and frequently allows better images of the upper pole either subcostally or intercostally. In infants, some examiners still prefer the prone position in evaluating infants with a rolled-up pillow placed under the costal margin allowing better penetration and optimal delineation for evaluating the entire outline of each kidney. This technique may also prove helpful in evaluating obese adults or those with scoliotic or kyphotic deformities of the thoracolumbar spine.

Echogenicity of the kidneys does not, per se, enter into renal measurements. However, to accurately identify the kidneys and to know where to measure and analyze for abnormalities, echogenicity is important. In the child and adult, the echo patterns are relatively constant for the parenchyma and the renal sinus. The paren-

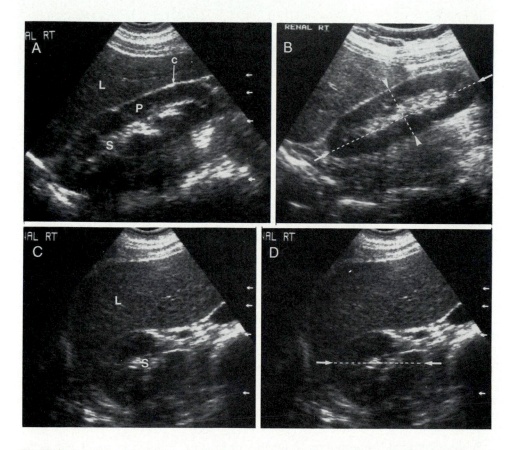

FIG 14–2.
Adult kidney. **A** and **B** are longitudinal ultrasound images of the right kidney. **A** shows hypoechoic renal parenchyma (*P*) surrounding the hyperechoic renal sinus (*S*). Note the bright thin capsule (*C*). *L* = liver.**B,** measurements of long axis (*arrows* and *dotted lines*) and the perpendicular AP dimension (*arrowheads* and *dotted lines*). **C** and **D** are transaxial ultrasound images of the right kidney at the level of the renal sinus (*S*). Measurement of width is shown in **D** by *arrows* and *dotted line*. *L* = liver.

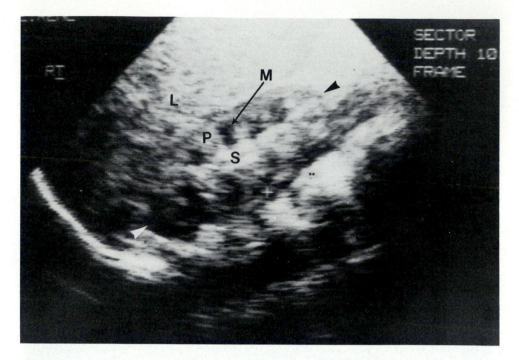

FIG 14–3.
Neonatal kidney (denoted by *arrowheads*). Long-axis ultrasound image of right kidney shows a hyperechoic renal parenchyma (*P*) blending with the adjacent liver (*L*). Note the hypoechoic medullary pyramids (*M*) and less pronounced renal sinus (*S*).

chymal cortex has a uniformly low-level echogenicity, less than the adjacent liver and spleen (see Fig 14–2, A and C). The thin hyperechoic renal capsule can be clearly identified. In approximately 20% of cases, the almost anechoic medullary pyramids can be identified lining the outer edge of the renal sinus. The sinus has variable echogenicity, but due to the multiple structures within it, is usually hyperechoic.

The neonatal kidney echogenicity appears differently.[7] The renal cortex has an overall increased echogenicity, equal to that of the adjacent liver and spleen (Fig 14–3). Due to the increased echogenicity, the (anechoic) medullary pyramids are almost always identified and the hyperechoic capsule is difficult to define. In addition, the sinus is less hyperechoic and usually has a similar echogenicity to the cortex. This cortical pattern is identified in the newborn period, with all cases reverting to the normally less hyperechoic child and adult pattern by 1 to 1.5 years of age.

NEWBORN RENAL MEASUREMENT

Schlesinger et al.[8] reported on 52 healthy premature infants examined within the first 72 hours of life. Normal renal lengths measured sonographically were compared with four parameters: body weight, body length, body surface area, and gestational age. Their data indicated that kidney length correlated better with body weight than with body length. The authors hypothesized that the poor correlation between the lengths of the kidney and body might be caused by difficulty in obtaining adequate body length measurements since infants in the neonatal period are frequently in the flexed position. Body weight, on the other hand, is a more accurate and reproducible measurement. Their table comparing renal length to body weight ranging from 600 to 3,000 g is recommended (Table 14–1).

Further evaluation of newborn full-term infant kidneys under the age of 1 year was reported by Blane et al.[9] who obtained an average from three sonographic images of each kidney and correlated this measurement with the infant weight (kg) and length (cm). There was no significant difference between males and females. Although their sample included only 34 patients (68 kidneys), the measurements were statistically significant to develop a morphometric nomogram for full-term infant kidneys (Fig 14–4). Using the infant's weight and length, the average renal length with a 2-SD range is shown in graph form.

TABLE 14–1.

Premature Infant Renal Measurements: Normal Standards for Body Weight Versus Renal Length*

Body Weight (g)	Kidney Length (mm)	
	Lower Limit	Upper Limit
	(at 95% Confidence Limits)	
600	26.4	35.7
700	27.2	36.5
800	27.9	37.2
900	28.7	38.0
1000	29.4	38.7
1100	30.1	39.5
1200	30.9	40.2
1300	31.6	41.0
1400	32.4	41.7
1500	33.1	42.5
1600	33.9	43.2
1700	34.6	43.9
1800	35.4	44.7
1900	36.1	45.4
2000	36.9	46.2
2100	37.6	46.9
2200	38.4	47.7
2300	39.1	48.4
2400	39.9	49.2
2500	40.6	49.9
2600	41.3	50.7
2700	42.1	51.4
2800	42.8	52.2
2900	43.6	52.9
3000	44.3	53.7

*From Schlesinger AE, Hedlund GL, Pierson WP, et al: *Radiology* 1987; 164:127–129. Used by permission.

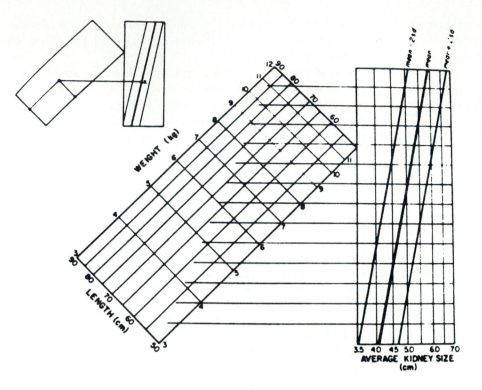

FIG 14–4.
Nomogram for the determination of normal infant kidney length. The infant's weight and length determine two oblique lines on the left side of the plot. The horizontal lines should be extended from left to right to where they intersect the heavy, nearly vertical, line on the right graph. The right graph predicts the mean kidney length indicated on the x-axis at the bottom with the fainter parallel lines delineating the 95% confidence limits (2 SD). (From Blane CE, Bookstein FL, DiPietro MA, et al: *AJR* 1985; 145:1289–1291. Used by permission.)

CHILDHOOD RENAL MEASUREMENTS

Sonographic measurements for children have been calculated for normal kidneys. Renal length was found in numerous reports to be the most accurate and usually the most easily obtainable renal measurement and could be related to the patient's age. Rosenbaum et al.[10] compared 203 patients ranging in age from several hours to 19 years, utilizing the regression equation of length (cm) = 4.98 + 0.155 × age (months) (SD = 0.69). For the subpopulation, aged 1 year and older, length (cm) = 6.79 + 0.22 × age (years) (SD = 0.79), with the average left kidney only 1.9 mm longer than the right (of no statistical significance). Their measurements are recommended (Table 14–2). Despite these findings, other investigators still feel that the renal length measurement obtained radiographically is the most practical and can be easily related to the patient's age or to a segment of lumbar spine on the radiographs.[10, 11]

Han and Babcock[12] studied 122 normal children from newborn to 17 years of age, measuring all 244 kidneys sonographically. They compared renal length and volume measurements to age, body weight, height, and total body surface at the predicted means and 95% prediction intervals. They also compared the renal parenchyma and sinus echogenicity in the neonate and its change from the neonatal to the adult kidney. Han and Babcock[12] felt that the increased neonatal cortical echogenicity was caused by a greater number of glomeruli occupying a greater cortical volume during the first 2 months of life (18%) (when compared to 8.6% in the adult) and a greater volume of cellular components of the glomerular tuft. They compared the maximum renal length to age, height, weight, and total body surface and renal volume to the same parameters only in graph form, and these are recommended (Figs 14–5 and 14–6).

Other investigators have also compared renal to body parameters and have obtained similar results.[13–15] While these results are therefore not recommended, the following description summarizes their works. Dremsek et al.[13] studied children from 4 weeks of age through 16 years, measuring renal length, width, depth, parenchymal areas, and a volume calculated by the equation for a prolate ellipsoid (described in the next paragraph). These were compared to the body weight, body length, length of the trunk and upper and lower limbs, width of the thorax and pelvis, head circumference, maximum cranial length, and maximum cranial breadth. The closest correlations were found between kidney parameters and the pelvic width, arm, and leg length, between the renal length and the body length, and between the renal volume and the body length and weight. Christophe et al.[14] studied children from newborn to 15 years, measuring renal length, thickness, width, volume, and largest

TABLE 14–2.
Childhood Renal Measurements: Summary of Grouped Observations—Mean Renal Length*

Average Age[†]	Mean Renal Interval[†]	Length (mm)	SD
0 mo	0–1 wk	44.8	3.1
2 mo	1 wk–4 mo	52.8	6.6
6 mo	4–8 mo	61.5	6.7
10 mo	8 mo–1 yr	62.3	6.3
1.5	1–2	66.5	5.4
2.5	2–3	73.6	5.4
3.5	3–4	73.6	6.4
4.5	4–5	78.7	5.0
5.5	5–6	80.9	5.4
6.5	6–7	78.3	7.2
7.5	7–8	83.3	5.1
8.5	8–9	89.0	8.8
9.5	9–10	92.0	9.0
10.5	10–11	91.7	8.2
11.5	11–12	96.0	6.4
12.5	12–13	104.2	8.7
13.5	13–14	97.9	7.5
14.5	14–15	100.5	6.2
15.5	15–16	109.3	7.6
16.5	16–17	100.4	8.6
17.5	17–18	105.3	2.9
18.5	18–19	108.1	11.3

*From Rosenbaum DM, Korngold E, Littlewood-Teele R: *AJR* 1984; 142:467–469. Used by permission.
[†]Years unless specified otherwise.

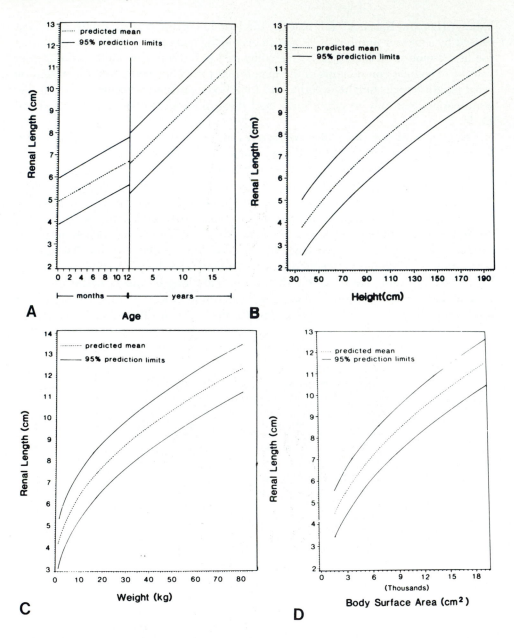

FIG 14–5.
Graphs of maximum renal length in children versus (*A*) age, (*B*) height, (*C*) weight, and (*D*) total body surface. The predicted mean and 95% confidence limits are shown. (From Han BK, Babcock DS: *AJR* 1985; 145:611–616. Used by permission.)

sagittal and transverse surface areas and plotted them against the children's height and body surface. They found similar close correlations with the same parameters.

Renal volume has also been evaluated in two articles but is not recommended in the childhood period. Dinkel et al.[15] reported on the sonographic measurements of 325 children without renal pathology, calculating the kidney volume by the formula for a prolate ellipsoid.

A satisfactory correlation was obtained between renal volume and body weight; no correlation was present between renal volume and body surface area. Moskowitz et al.[16] also measured the renal volume in 11 children with concurrent IV urography. They reported that the sonographic renal volume correlated well with the urographic renal volume, better than a comparison of their lengths. Henderstrom and Forsberg,[17] however, confirmed renal length measurements to be accurate and a reliable alternative to urographic assessment of renal size and growth. Nevertheless, Mos-

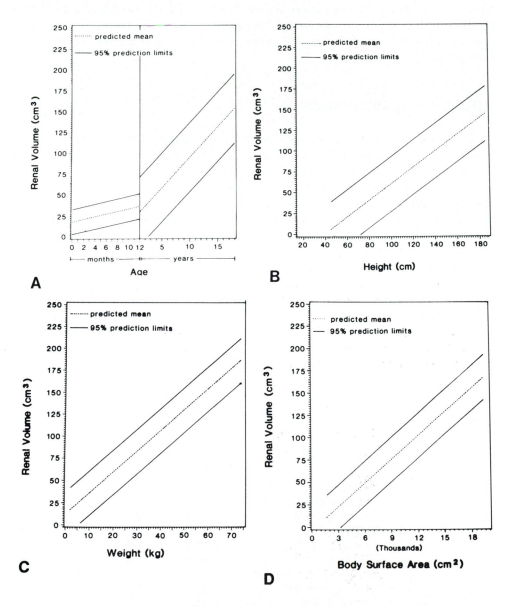

FIG 14–6.
Graphs of renal volume in children versus (*A*) age, (*B*) height, (*C*) weight, and (*D*) total body surface. The predicted mean and 95% confidence limits are shown. (From Han BK, Babcock DS: *AJR* 1985; 145:611–616.

kowitz et al.[16] did suggest that the sonographic measurement of renal length did not involve the inherent inaccuracies related to the angle of inclination found during IV urography and that sonography was therefore a more accurate measurement of true renal length.

The accuracy of renal volume, calculated by ultrasound, has even been proposed in children with urinary tract infections as an alternative and possible replacement for glomerular filtration rate and effective renal plasma flow. Troell et al.[18] compared renal parenchymal sonographic volume and renal parenchymal urographic area with glomerular filtration rate and renal plasma flow in children and found a good correlation. While this is a good concept because it attempts to compare an anatomic measurement to renal function, the work is confusing and further evaluation is warranted.

ADULT RENAL MEASUREMENTS

There is a need to standardize the adult kidney sonographic measurements, especially in evaluating renal allografts, various renal disorders, and in assessing patients following unilateral nephrectomy. Brandt et al.[19] reported a retrospective study of 52 patients performed with a commercially available articulated B-scanner for obtaining length, width, and depth measurements. Their study included images obtained in both the supine and prone position. They encountered difficulty in obtaining adequate true supine measurements, presumably because the static B-scanner did not have as much flexibility as more sophisticated real-time units in obtaining these measurements. Tables 14–3 and 14–4 demonstrate the renal dimensions of the right and left kidney, respectively, utilizing the three measured renal parameters of length, width, and AP dimension (depth). Although radiologic studies have demonstrated renal lengths averaging 12.5 to 13.5 cm with the average width 6 cm, the ultrasound findings are approximately 1.0 to 1.5 cm smaller due to a more physiologic type of examination not subject to either geometric magnification or osmotic diuresis from iodinated contrast material during IV urography.

TABLE 14–3.
Adult Renal Measurements: Right Renal Dimensions in Sample Groups of Patients Examined Retrospectively*

	Mean (mm)	SD
Length		
Oblique (n = 52)	106.5	13.5
Prone (n = 51)	107.4	13.5
Width†		
Oblique (n = 35)	49.2	6.4
Prone (n = 32)	50.5	7.6
Anteroposterior (depth)†		
Oblique (n = 19)	39.5	8.1
Prone (n = 9)	41.7	5.1

*From Brandt TD, Neiman HL, Dragowski MJ, et al: *J Ultrasound Med* 1982; 1:49–52. Used by permission.
†Approximate values.

TABLE 14–4.
Adult Renal Measurements: Left Renal
Dimensions in Sample Groups of Patients
Examined Retrospectively*

	Mean (mm)	SD
Length		
Oblique (n = 50)	101.3	11.7
Prone (n = 50)	111.0	11.5
Width[†]		
Oblique (n = 36)	53.0	7.4
Prone (n = 31)	53.0	8.0
Anteroposterior (depth)[†]		
Oblique (n = 18)	35.8	9.1
Prone (n = 10)	41.4	8.4

*From Brandt TD, Neiman HL, Dragowski MJ, et al: *J Ultra-sound Med* 1982; 1:49–52. Used by permission.
[†]Approximate values.

Renal volumes have been reported to be the most specific measurement for evaluating renal pathology since the volume correlates more accurately with renal mass. Hricak and Lieto[20] calculated the renal volume of three canine and 34 human kidneys, correlating the two variables within 24 hours after nephrectomy in humans and 1 hour after nephrectomy in dogs. The sonographic images were performed with both static and real-time scanners; the volumes (V) calculated according to the equation for an ellipsoid (prolated ellipsoid): $V = 0.523 \times L \times W \times AP$ were correlated with renal mass. The average ratio of the two was 0.99. The kidneys were also correlated with the amount of water displacement to the ultrasound volume with a ratio of 0.94. Based on this water displacement measurement, the ellipsoid equation was modified to: $V = 0.49 \times L \times W \times AP$. This equation provided more accuracy for calculating renal volume. Jones et al.[21] obtained volumes and surface areas son-ographically in vivo before autopsy and in water-bath phantom after autopsy by means of ellipsoid and stepped section methods. They too found that the ellipsoid method was also the simplest and provided sufficient accuracy for clinical use. Renal volume correlated with renal mass with a coefficient of .93.

Surface area was also calculated[21] and was found to vary as the two-thirds power of volume; thus, an effective renal surface area (SA) was defined as follows: $SA = \pi (L \times W \times T)^{2/3}$ where L, W, and T were the greatest dimensions of renal length, width, and thickness (AP dimension) in three orthogonal planes. Regression analysis was performed to obtain the best method to compute renal mass (M), resulting in the following formula: $M = -0.326V + 1.916SA - 63.21$

Surface area, while interesting, does not appear to have well-defined clinical value. Renal volume, on the other hand, does. Therefore, in addition to renal length, renal volume is also recommended using the modified formula of a prolate ellipsoid by Hricak and Lieto[20]: $V = 0.49 \times L \times W \times AP$ (Table 14–5). Since there are no well-defined normal limits for renal mass, absolute values and tables of renal volume are not available. When a patient has a renal abnormality, however, a change in size from one study to the next (relative value) may be helpful in determining the severity of disease.

TABLE 14–5.
Renal Volume Calculated From Modified Prolate
Ellipsoid Formula*

V = 0.49 × L × W × AP
where V = volume (cc)
L = renal length (cm)
W = renal width (cm)
AP = renal anteroposterior dimension (cm)

*From Hricak H, Lieto RP: *Radiology* 1983; 148:311–312. Used
by permission.

THE RENAL TRANSPLANT

The renal transplant sizes are the same as the donor kidney, whether a child or
an adult (see Tables 14–2, 14–3, 14–4). To complicate this, however, the transplant
undergoes approximately a 20% increase in size (hypertrophy) within the first 3
months following transplantation. Since one of the first signs in transplant rejection
is a change in the size of the transplanted kidney, any change of greater than 20%
during the first 3 months, or continued increase after 3 months, should be viewed
with suspicion. Ultrasound offers an excellent imaging modality for evaluating the
transplanted kidney undergoing rejection, especially when renal failure has made it
difficult to image the kidney with other imaging techniques. The calculation of
sonographic renal measurements, especially length and volume, and the appearance
of the renal echogenicity has been significant in investigating transplant rejection.
However, all the results are not uniform. Babcock et al.[22] reported no significant
association between renal volume and renal function in children with chronic transplant rejection, while Absy et al.[23] found that the transplant volume increased in
acute rejection and reversed toward normal following medical treatment. They also
demonstrated that the transplant volume seemed to stabilize after 6 months and
correlated positively with the renal transplant function.

The medullary pyramid size has also proved helpful in evaluating acute renal
transplant rejection (Fig 14–7,A). Paling and Black[24] proposed a revised measurement, termed the medullary renal ratio (MRR), calculated by the formula: MRR =
1/2 pyramid width × pyramid height/cortical AP dimension × renal length. They
compared their formula to the previous medullary pyramid index (MPI)[25] where MPI
= 1/2 pyramid length × pyramid width/cortical thickness. Paling and Black[24] felt
that the initial MPI formula should be changed because it only took into account the
length change during rejection. The authors postulated that with rejection there is
an inverse relationship between renal length and width.[24] As one dimension gets
bigger, the other gets smaller and vice versa. The older MPI was derived by dividing
a two-dimensional measurement by a one-dimensional thickness, making the MPI
directly proportional only to renal length. Because the newer MRR divided area by
area, it remained constant and independent of renal size and shape and hence would
be a more accurate measurement. Although there was no series of cases with their
article, the mathematical concept seems reasonable, and their MRR concept is
recommended[24] (Fig 14–7,B).

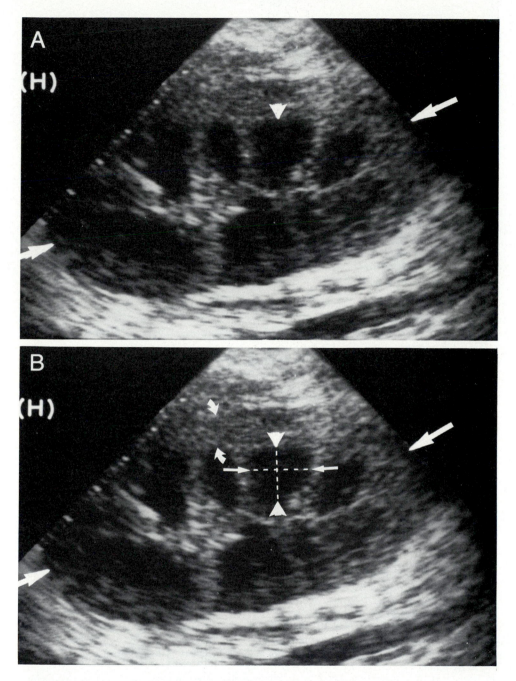

FIG 14–7.
Long-axis ultrasound image of a renal transplant (*large arrows*) in acute rejection. **A,** note the enlarged medullary pyramids (one denoted by an *arrowhead*). **B,** for the medullary renal ratio, the medullary pyramid width (*arrows* and *dotted lines*) and height (*arrowheads* and *dotted lines*) are shown. The cortical thickness is identified between the *two curved arrows.* (*H*) = toward patient's head.

REFERENCES

1. Netter FH: *Kidneys. Ureters and Urinary Bladder, in The CIBA Collection of Medical Illustrations,* vol 6. Summit, NJ, Ciba-Geigy Corp, 1973.
2. Goss CM (ed): *Gray's Anatomy of the Human Body,* ed Philadelphia, Lea & Febiger, 1959.
3. Voelcker F, von Lichtenberg: *Pyelographie* (Rontgenographie des Nierenbackens nach Kollargöfüllung). MMW 53:105, 1906.
4. Moell H: Kidney size and its deviation from normal in acute renal failure. *Reta Radiol (Suppl)* 1961; 206:1–74.
5. Dure-Smith P, McArdle GH: Tomography during excretory urography. Technical aspects *Br J Radiol* 1972; 45:896–901.
6. Griffiths GJ, Cartwright G, McLachlan MSF: Estimation of renal size from radiographs: Is the effect worthwhile? *Clin Radiol* 1974; 26:249–256.
7. Hricak H, Slovis TL, Callen CW, et al: Neonatal kidneys: Sonographic anatomic correlation. *Radiology* 1983; 147:699–702.
8. Schlesinger AE, Hedlund GL, Pierson WP, et al: Normal standards for kidney length in premature infants: Determination with US. *Radiology* 1987; 164:127–129.
9. Blane CE, Bookstein FL, DiPietro MA, et al: Sonographic standards for normal infant kidney length. *AJR* 1985; 145:1289–1291.
10. Rosenbaum DM, Korngold E, Littlewood-Teele R: Sonographic assessment of renal length in normal children. *AJR* 1984; 142:467–469.
11. Currarino G: Roentgenographic estimation of kidney size in normal individuals with emphasis on children. *AJR* 1985; 93:464–466.
12. Han BK, Babcock DS: Sonographic measurements and appearance of normal kidneys in children. *AJR* 1985; 145:611–616.
13. Dremsek PA, Kirtscher H, Bohm G, et al: Kidney dimensions in ultrasound compared to somatometric parameters in normal children. *Pediatr Radiol* 1987; 17:285–290.
14. Christophe C, Cantraine F, Bogaert C, et al: Ultrasound: A method for kidney size monitoring in children. *Euro J Pediatr* 1986; 145:532–538.
15. Dinkel E, Ertel M, Dittrich M, et al: Kidney size in childhood sonographical growth charts for kidney length and volume. *Pediatr Radiol* 1985; 15:38–43.
16. Moskowitz PS, Carroll BA, McCoy JM: Ultrasonic renal volumetry in children. *Radiology* 1980; 134:61–64.
17. Henderstrom E, Forsberg L: Accuracy of repeated kidney size estimation by ultrasonography and urography in children. *Acta Radiol [Diagn] (Stockh)* 1985; 26:603–607.
18. Troell S, Berg U, Johansson B, et al: Comparison between renal parenchyma sonographic volume, renal parenchyma urographic area, glomerular filtration rate and plasma flow in children. *Scand J Urol Nephrol* 1988; 22:207–214.
19. Brandt TD, Neiman HL, Dragowski MJ, et al: Ultrasound assessment of normal renal dimension. *J Ultrasound Med* 1982; 1:49–52.
20. Hricak H, Lieto RP: *Sonographic determination of renal volume. Radiology* 1983; 148:311–312.
21. Jones TB, Riddick LR, Harpen, et al: Ultrasonographic determination of renal mass and renal volume. *J Ultrasound Med* 1983; 2:151–154.
22. Babcock DS, Slovis TL, Han BK, et al: Renal transplants in children: Long-term follow-up using sonography. *Radiology* 1985; 156:165–167.
23. Asby M, Metreweli C, Matthews DCR, et al: Changes in transplanted kidney volume measured by ultrasound. *Br J Radiol* 1987; 60:525–529.
24. Paling MR, Black WC: Quantitation of the prominent medullary pyramid: A reappraisal. *J Can Assoc Radiol* 1986; 37:90–93.
25. Fried AM, Woodring JH, Loh FK, et al: The medullary pyramid index: An objective assessment of prominence in renal transplant rejection. *Radiology* 1983; 149:787–791.

Measurements of the Normal Adrenal Gland

Matthew D. Rifkin, M.D.

The adrenal glands are small structures measuring approximately 4 cm in cephalo-caudad length with a maximum of 2 cm in width, but are only approximately 3 to 6 mm in thickness. Thus, because of the thickness of the gland and because both the right and the left adrenals are often wing-shaped, visualization of the normal adrenals may be incomplete.

While the adrenals have been called suprarenal glands, only the right is, in fact, suprarenal in position, being slightly superior and medial to the right kidney. It is usually situated just lateral and posterior to the inferior vena cava. The left adrenal gland is slightly more variable in position and is situated, oftentimes, at the same level as the upper pole. There may be variable positions of the left adrenal gland, some being superior to the left kidney and others situated as low as the renal hilum. The left gland is posterolateral to the aorta.

The kidneys are quite movable during inspiration. The adrenal glands, however, are fixed to the apical portion of Gerota's fascia. Therefore, they do not move with respiration to the same degree as the kidneys.

Prior to the advent of cross-sectional imaging, identification of the small normal adrenal glands was difficult.[1] However, because they are surrounded by fat, they are ideally suited to identification by computed tomography (CT) and magnetic resonance imaging (MRI).[2–4] Identification of the kidneys by ultrasound is best obtained by scanning through the liver, either anteriorly or from the lateral aspect to identify the right kidney and through the spleen or from the back to identify the left kidney.[5–11] Because of the thinness of the kidneys, and because of their high position, complete visualization of both wings is infrequent and only partial identification may be possible. Some studies have suggested up to a 98% success rate in identification of the normal gland.[8, 9] Others have been less successful, with greater ability to identify the right adrenal than the left.[6–9]

Our personal experience has been similar in that identification of the normal right gland is possible but visualization of the normal left adrenal is quite difficult. However, a new technique for evaluation of the left adrenal gland has been suggested.[11] Scanning through the liver, inferior vena cava, and aorta may improve visualization of the left side.

TABLE 15–1.

Total Weight of Both Adrenal Glands in Male and Female as a Function of Postnatal Age*

	Male			Female		
Age	n	Mean Weight (g)	SD	n	Mean Weight (g)	SD
Newborn–1 mo	81	6.22	2.37	147	5.23	2.12
2–12 mo	30	3.35	1.51	102	3.15	1.0
1–5 yr	27	4.6	1.51	109	4.2	1.48
6–10 yr	15	6.6	1.7	43	6.01	1.81
11–15 yr	6	8.63	1.58	30	7.99	2.1
16–20 yr	63	12.95	2.95	46	11.00	3.15
21–30 yr	166	13.71	2.78	97	12.97	3.03
31–40 yr	111	13.91	2.78	91	13.02	2.9
41–50 yr	51	13.84	2.95	89	12.00	2.77
51–60 yr	26	13.36	3.2	84	11.65	2.74
61–70 yr	14	13.00	2.52	87	12.14	3.02
>70 yr	11	12.16	1.82	57	11.72	3.03

*From International Commission on Radiological Protection. Task Group on Reference Man: *Report of the Task Group on Reference Man*. Prepared for the Task Group Committee no. 2, International Commission on Radiological Protection, Snyder WS (chairman). New York, Pergamon Press, 1975, pp 203–205.

The adrenals are generally a subtly hypoechoic structure, surrounded by echogenic periadrenal fat; there may be subtle hyperechoic internal areas of the gland, the adrenal medulla surrounded by the more hypoechoic cortex.

The normal adrenal gland decreases markedly in weight (Table 15–1) and size (Table 15–2)[12, 13] in the first 3 postnatal months.

Adrenals that appear rounded or greater than 1.5 cm in anteroposterior (AP) or transverse dimension should be highly suspicious for mass and/or enlargement.

The normal adrenal glands have distinctly different echogenic layers. There is a hypoechoic outer layer and a more echogenic center. The outer, hypoechoic layer is the adrenal cortex. The inner, more hyperechoic area is the adrenal medulla. A third layer, actually exterior to the adrenals, is the hyperechoic fat surrounding the suprarenal glands.

To measure the adrenal, the length and width of the limbs can be calculated[14] (Figs 15–1 through 15–3). While this will obtain measurements of size, because of the difficulty in evaluating the entire adrenal, calculating the adrenal volume is quite difficult because of the marked irregularity of the shape of the glands.

TABLE 15–2.

Dimensions of the Adrenal Glands*

Age	Transverse Diameter (cm)	Vertical Diameter (cm)	AP Diameter (cm)
Newborn	3.3–3.5	2.3–2.8	1.2–1.3
Adult	3.0–7.0	2.0–3.5	0.3–0.8

*From International Commission of Radiological Protection. Task Group on Reference Man: *Report of the Task Group on Reference Man*. Prepared by the Task Group Committee no. 2, International Commission on Radiological Protection, Snyder WS (chairman). New York, Pergamon Press, 1975, pp 203–205.

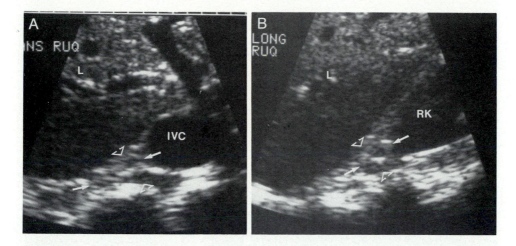

FIG 15–1.
Right adrenal. A transverse (**A**) and longitudinal (**B**) scan of the right upper quadrant demonstrates portions of the liver (*L*), the inferior vena cava (*IVC*), and the right kidney (*RK*). The adrenal gland can be measured by its cephalocaudad dimension (*arrows* in **B**) and transverse dimensions (*arrows* in **A**). The AP dimension (*arrowheads*) can be measured by either view. The adrenal gland is identified as a structure with a highly echogenic center with a surrounding low-level echogenic cortex. Periadrenal fat is seen as an echogenic border.

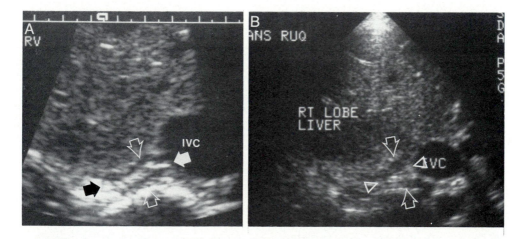

FIG 15–2.
Right adrenal. The right adrenal gland in this patient is adjacent to the inferior vena cava (*IVC*) in both the transverse (**A**) and longitudinal (**B**) image. The cephalocaudad (*closed arrows*), transverse (*arrowheads*), and AP (*open arrows*) dimensions can be measured.

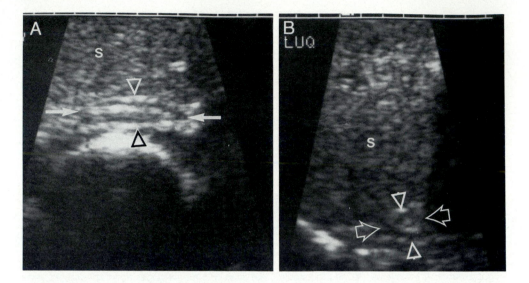

FIG 15–3.
Left adrenal gland. A longitudinal (**A**) and transverse (**B**) image of the left adrenal gland through the spleen (*S*) demonstrates the highly echogenic center, surrounding hypoechoic cortex, and the periadrenal fat as an echogenic periphery. The longitudinal dimension (*arrows*) is identified on the longitudinal scan. The transverse dimension (*open arrows*) is seen on the transverse image, and the AP dimension (*arrowheads*) can be measured on either view.

REFERENCES

1. Krebs CA, Eisenberg RL, Ratcliff S, et al: Cava-suprarenal line: New position for sonographic imaging of left adrenal gland. *J Clin Ultrasound* 1986; 14:535–539.
2. Reinig JW, Doppman JL, Dwyer AJ, et al: Adrenal masses differentiated by MR. *Radiology* 1986; 158:81–84.
3. Bernardino ME: Management of the asymptomatic patient with a unilateral adrenal mass. *Radiology* 1988; 166:121–123.
4. Glazer GM, Woolsey EJ, Borrello J, et al: Adrenal tissue characterization using MR imaging. *Radiology* 1986; 158:73–79.
5. Yeh H: Ultrasonography of the adrenal gland, in Resnick MI, Sanders RC (eds): *Ultrasound in Urology*, ed 2. Baltimore, Williams & Wilkins Co, 1984, pp 285–306.
6. Yeh H: Somography of the adrenal glands: Normal glands and small masses. *AJR* 1980; 135:1167–1177.
7. Sample WF: A new technique for the evaluation of the adrenal gland with gray scale ultrasonography. *Radiology* 1977; 124:463–469.
8. Gunther RW, Kelbel C, Lenner V: Real-time ultrasound of normal adrenal glands and small tumors. *J Clin Ultrasound* 1984; 12:211–217.
9. Zappasodi F, Derchi LE, Rizzatto G: Ultrasonography of the normal adrenal glands: Study using linear array real-time equipment. *Br J Radiol* 1986; 59:759.
10. Marchal G, Gelin J, Verbeken E, et al: High resolution real-time sonography of the adrenal glands: A routine examination? *J Ultrasound Med* 1986; 5:65–68.
11. Yeh H: Adrenal gland and non-renal retroperitoneum. *Urol Radiol* 1987; 9:127–140.
12. International Commission on Radiological Protection. Task Group on Reference Man. *Report of the Task Group on Reference Man.* Prepared by the Task Group Committee no. 2, International Commission on Radiological Protection, Snyder WS (chairman). New York, Pergamon Press, 1975, pp 203–205.
13. Kangerloo H, Diament MJ, Gold RH, et al: Sonography of adrenal glands in neonates and children: Changes in appearance with age. *J Clin Ultrasound* 1986; 14:43–47.
14. Oppenheimer DA, Carroll BA, Yousem S: Sonography of the normal neonatal adrenal gland. *Radiology* 1983; 146:157–160.

Chapter 16

Urinary Bladder Measurements
Matthew D. Rifkin, M.D.

The urinary bladder, when distended, occupies much of the pelvis. The peritoneum-covered dome or superior aspect of the urinary bladder separates the potential peritoneal-covered spaces, the anterior paravesical space, and the posterior cul-de-sac. The urinary bladder is in direct contact with the pubic bones anteriorly, the anterior peritoneal reflection superiorly, and the prostate (in the male) inferiorly. In the female, the inferior margin is the urogenital diaphragm. The rectum is the posterior margin of the urinary bladder.

There are various anatomic positions and orientations of the pelvic structures in the female. Thus, there is inconstant position of these structures.

The determination of bladder size and fluid content (urine) volume is difficult to calculate, regardless of the techniques for measurements. This is because the size, shape, and position of the bladder vary, not only from patient to patient but within an individual patient in the same area of the bladder because of changes in the distention and, thus, in the shape of the bladder (Fig 16–1). Not all bladders, and not even the same bladder, assumes a constant shape in a single space in time. For this reason, determination of accurate volume has always been difficult. Inaccuracies generally result because of an invalid assumption that the bladder is a single specific shape.

The importance of bladder volume determination is also variable. Absolute total bladder volume is not necessarily important. The most important clinical evaluation of bladder volume is in measuring the residual volume. This is a measurement following voiding to see if the postvoid residua is clinically significant (usually greater than 50–100 mL).

Regardless of the difficulties, there have been a number of formulas that have been applied to the determination of bladder volume. The simplest[1] measures only the transverse diameter (see Fig 16–1) of the bladder and compares the results to a chart (Table 16–1). All others require measurements of the height (the cephalocaudad or superior-inferior dimension), the depth (the anteroposterior [AP] dimension, or width), and the transverse (lateral) dimensions of the fluid-filled urinary bladder. The following are formulas that have been developed and utilized.

4. Orgaz RE, Gomez AZ, Ramirez CT, et al: Applications of bladder ultrasonography. I. Bladder content and residue. *J Urol* 1981; 125:174–176.

5. Ravichandran G, Fellows GJ: The accuracy of a hand-held real time ultrasound scanner for estimating bladder volume. *J Urol* 1983; 55:25–27.

6. Harrison NW, Parks C, Sherwood T: Ultrasound assessment of residual urine in children. *Br J Urol* 1976; 47:805–814.

7. McLean GK, Edell SL: Determination of bladder volumes by gray scale ultrasonography. *Radiology* 1978; 128:181–182.

8. van Erpecum KJ, Koch CW, Jones B, et al: Bladder content and residual urine in renal transplant patients: Measurement using ultrasonography and relevance to urinary tract infection. *World J Urol* 1986; 4:228–230.

9. Rodriguez E, Holzer J, Trivino X, et al: Capacidad vesical, edad, peso, talla y superficie corporal an ninos. *Rev Chil Pediatr* 1985; 56:81–83.

10. Holmes JH: Ultrasonic studies of the bladder. *J Urol* 1987; 97:654–663.

11. Pedersen JF, Bartrum RJ Jr, Grytter C: Residual urine determination by ultrasonic scanning. *AJR* 1975; 125:474–478.

12. Doust BD, Baum JK, Maklad NF, et al: Determination of organ volume by means of ultrasonic B-mode scanning. *J Clin Ultrasound* 2:127–130.

13. Beacock CJM, Roberts EE, Rees RWM, et al: Ultrasound assessment of residual urine. A quantitative method. *Br J Urol* 1985; 57:410–413.

14. Griffiths CJ, Murray A, Ramsden PD: Accuracy and repeatability of bladder volume measurement using ultrasonic imaging. *J Urol* 1986; 136:808–812.

15. Kjeldsen-Kragh J: Measurement of residual urine volume by means of ultrasonic scanning: A comparative study. *Int Med Soc Paraplegia* 1988; 26:192–199.

16. Rifkin MD: Unpublished data, 1988.

Chapter 17

Prostate and Seminal Vesicle Measurements

Matthew D. Rifkin, M.D.

PROSTATE MEASUREMENTS

The prostate, an important organ in the male reproductive system, can undergo benign prostatic hyperplasia in the adult male as well as malignant degeneration. Various pathologic entities may also affect the prostate in the younger individual. Anatomically, the prostate is generally a rounded or ovoid structure situated just superior to the urogenital diaphragm. The margins of the prostate include the levator ani muscles inferolaterally and the obturator internus muscles more superolaterally. The symphysis pubis and pubic bones separated by the anterior prostatic fat and fascia are situated anteriorly and the rectum is positioned posteriorly. The cephalad portion of the prostate is its base, and it abuts the base of the urinary bladder. The inferior portion of the prostate is termed the apex, and its inferior margin is the adjacent urogenital diaphragm.

The seminal vesicles are two paired structures that are situated in the superior-posterior aspect of the prostate between the urinary bladder and the rectum. The two vasa deferentia join the medial aspect of the seminal vesicle to form the ejaculatory ducts.

The posterior (also known as the prostatic) urethra is situated in the midportion of the prostate. The ejaculatory ducts empty into the urethra at the verumontanum.

An accurate estimation of the size and the weight of the prostate is an important determination so that proper medical or surgical intervention can be planned for patients with benign prostatic hyperplasia. The treatment for benign prostatic hyperplasia can vary depending upon the size of the gland, the areas of enlargement, and the patient's clinical symptomatology.

Benign prostatic hyperplasia develops from the periurethral tissues, including the transition zone and the periurethral glandular area. This small area (in the normal prostate) is situated proximal to the verumontanum and inferior to the base of the urinary bladder (Fig 17–1). However, when it enlarges, the gland can assume an appearance of diffuse, often immense, enlargement. The residual normal tissues are compressed by the hyperplastic areas.

In the normal postpubescent male, the prostate weighs approximately 20 g and

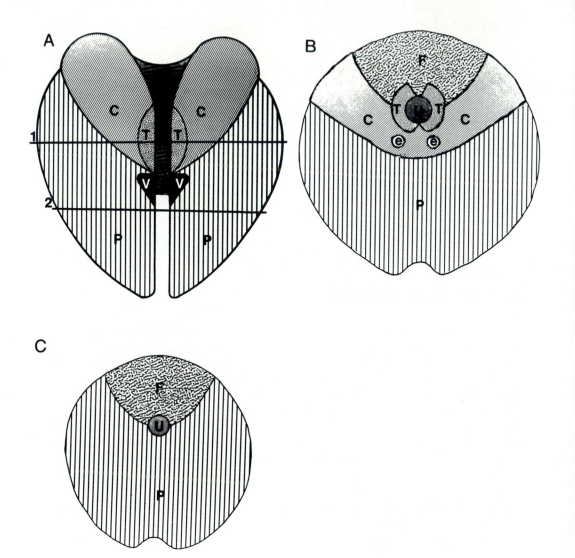

FIG 17–1.
A curved coronal line diagram of the prostate (**A**) with axial diagrams through *line 1* (**B**) and *line 2* (**C**) demonstrates the different zones of the prostate. Note that in the axial scan, the central (*C*) and peripheral (*P*) zones extend quite anteriorly. The absolute anterior portion of the prostate is the anterior prostatic fat and fascia (*F*). The central (*C*) zone surrounds the ejaculatory ducts (*e*). *U* = urethra; *T* = transition zone; *V* = verumontanum.

is about 3.5×4.0 cm in diameter.[1] As the normal male ages, prostatic enlargement may occur, but normal prostates generally do not exceed 30 g in weight.

Symptomatology from hyperplastic changes is not necessarily related to absolute volume. A small hyperplastic nodule impinging upon the prostatic urethra may cause difficulty in urinating, whereas massive hyperplasia (up to and greater than 100 mg) may not necessarily cause significant clinical symptoms.

When patients require surgical intervention for benign prostatic hyperplasia, the surgeon may vary the approach, that is, perform a transurethral, retropubic, or suprapubic prostatectomy, depending upon the size of the gland. The larger glands

TABLE 17–1.

Grades of Prostatic Enlargement
According to Transverse Diameter
and Weight*

Grade	Diameter (cm)	Weight (g)
I	3.0–3.8	<30
II	3.8–4.5	30–50
III	4.5–5.5	50–85
IV	>5.5	>85

*Data from Romero-Aquirre CR, Tallada MB, Mayayo TD, et al: *J Urol* 1980; 86:675–769.

may preclude safe, complete resection by the transurethral approach. Thus, accurate preoperative assessment of the size of the gland is useful to plan surgery.

There are a number of techniques for the determination of prostatic size using ultrasound. These have been developed because clinically the digital rectal examination, intravenous pyelogram, and other clinical methods are inaccurate.[2] This is particularly so when the prostate is asymmetrically enlarged.

Transabdominal ultrasound has been proved to be a useful and accurate technique for estimating volume and weight of the prostate. Charts have been devised to estimate prostate size by degree of enlargement (Table 17–1) or weight (Table 17–2) by measuring a single diameter of the gland[3] obtained on the transverse image (Fig 17–2). Since the specific gravity of prostatic tissue is between 1.0 and 1.05, the size of the prostate in cubic centimeters is equivalent to the weight in grams.

For other formulas, all three measurements of the prostate—the cephalocaudad (also known as the height), the anteroposterior (AP) dimension (also known as the depth), and the transverse dimension (also known as the width)—must be obtained for accurate estimation. This requires, in addition to the transverse image, a longitudinal (sagittal) view (Fig 17–3).

The simplest volumetric calculation for assessing prostatic weight is by using the

TABLE 17–2.

Prostate Weight Estimated by
Ultrasound Measurement of Diameter

Transverse Diameter (cm)	Weight (g)
3.0–3.5	14–22
3.5–4.0	22–33
4.0–4.5	33–47
4.5–5.0	47–65
5.0–5.5	65–87
5.5–6.0	87–113
6.0–6.5	113–143
6.5–7.0	143–179
7.0–7.5	179–220
7.5–8.0	220–276

*Data from Romero-Aquirre CR, Tallada MB, Mayayo, TD, et al: *J Urol* 1980; 86:675–769.

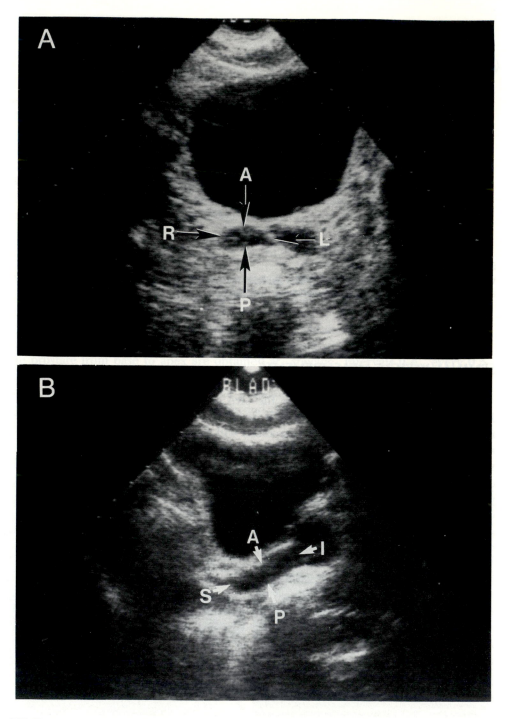

FIG 17–7.
Transabdominal seminal vesicle measurements. The transverse image (**A**) will demonstrate the anterior(*A*)-posterior(*P*) and the right(*R*)-left(*L*) margins. It is important to compare the right and the left seminal vesicles in this measurement. The longitudinal (sagittal) image (**B**) will confirm the AP measurements and allow measurements of the superior(*S*)-inferior (*I*) dimensions. It is also important to compare the right and left side in these cases.

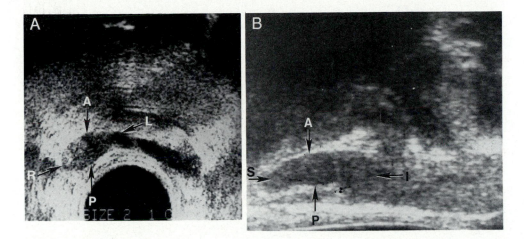

FIG 17–8.
Endorectal measurement of seminal vesicle size. The transverse (**A**) and longitudinal (**B**) images of the prostate using the endorectal technique will allow measurements at the anterior (*A*), posterior (*P*), right (*R*), left (*L*), superior (*S*), and inferior (*I*) margins of the seminal vesicles. It is important to calculate both the right and left measurements. In this patient, the right side (the measured one) is obviously bulkier and larger than the left side.

REFERENCES

1. Leissner KH, Tisell LE: The weight of the human prostate. *Scand J Urol Nephrol* 1979; 13:137–142.
2. Spigelman SS, McNeal JE, Freiha FS, et al: Rectal examination in volume determination of carcinoma of the prostate: Clinical and anatomical correlations. *J Urol* 1986; 136:1228–1230.
3. Romero-Aguirre CR, Tallada MB, Mayayo TD, et al: Evaluation comparative du volume prostatique par l'échographie transabdominale, le profil urètral et la radiologie. *J Urol* 1980; 86:675–769.
4. Vilmann P, Hancke S, Strange-Vognsen HH, et al: The reliability of transabdominal ultrasound scanning in the determination of prostatic volume. *Scand J Urol Nephrol* 1987; 21:5–7.
5. Henneberry M, Carter MF, Neiman HL: Estimation of prostatic size by suprapubic ultrasonography. *J Urol* 1979; 121:615–616.
6. Walz PH, Wenderoth U, Jacobi GH: Suprapubic transvesical sonography of the prostate: Determination of prostate size. *Eur Urol* 1983; 9:148–152.
7. Roehrborn CG, Chinn HKW, Fulgham PF, et al: The role of transabdominal ultrasound in the preoperative evaluation of patients with benign prostatic hypertrophy. *J Urol* 1986; 135:1190–1193.
8. Abu-Yousef MM, Narayana AS: Transabdominal ultrasound in the evaluation of prostate size. *J Clin Ultrasound* 1982; 10:275–278.
9. Hastak SM, Gammelgaard J, Holm HH: Transrectal ultrasonic volume determination of the prostate—A preoperative and postoperative study. *J Urol* 1982; 127:1115–1118.
10. Miyazaki Y, Yamaguchi A, Hara S: The value of transrectal ultrasonography in preoperative assessment for transurethral prostatectomy. *J Urol* 1983; 129:48–50.
11. Rifkin MD: *Ultrasound of the Prostate.* Raven Press, New York, 1988.
12. Rönnberg L, Ylöstalo P, Jouppila P: Estimation of the site of the seminal vesicles by means of ultrasonic B–scanning: A preliminary report. *Fertil Steril* 1978; 30:474–475.

Chapter 18

Measurements of Scrotal Contents

Matthew D. Rifkin, M.D.

The scrotum includes a number of structures, the two largest being the testes and the epididymis. Smaller contents include the skin and fascial layers, and the spermatic cord and its contents (Fig 18–1).

The testis is an ovoid structure that may, on occasion, especially during later life, assume a more rounded appearance. The tunica albuginea is a tightly adherent fibrous membrane surrounding the testis. The testicle is smoothly rounded except for a small testicular appendix, a remnant of the müllerian duct. This appendage, situated superiorly, is present in up to 93% of all males (Fig 18–2). The testicle's internal structures consist of multiple lobules containing coiled seminiferous tubules. The lobules are separated by fibrous septa containing the tubules that drain toward the fibrous mediastinum testis, which supports the integrity of the testicle. The seminiferous tubules straighten and anastomose at the mediastinum testis. There they form the rete testis connecting the testicle to the head of the epididymis by efferent ductules (vasa efferentia). The testicle's major function is to produce sperm.

The epididymis, the connecting structure between the testis and the vas deferens, is derived embryologically from the mesonephric duct. The epididymis serves as a transport organ for sperm and is instrumental in sperm maturation. The mesonephric tubules develop into the efferent ductules connecting the rete testis to the head of the epididymis. The epididymis is divided into three contiguous segments. The largest portion is the head (caput epididymis), also known as the globus major. It is situated superiorly and connected by the efferent ductules in the testis. It may be rounded or triangular in shape. It measures from 6 to 15 mm in diameter (Figs 18–2 and 18–3). The normal diameter of the longest segment, the body or corpus epididymis, is between 2 and 4 mm in thickness (Fig 18–4). It connects the head to the epididymal tail (cauda epididymis), also called the globus minor. The tail connects the epididymis to the vas deferens which inserts into the seminal vesicle and prostate. The epididymis courses along the posterior aspect of the testicle from the superior to inferior aspects. It forms an acute angle at the distal margin and becomes the vas deferens which is not visualized well by ultrasound. A small protuberance, the appendix of the epididymis, present in one third of men, is situated posteriorly on the epididymal head and is also not visualized by ultrasound. This variable structure is a remnant of the cranial end of the mesonephric duct. There are three other

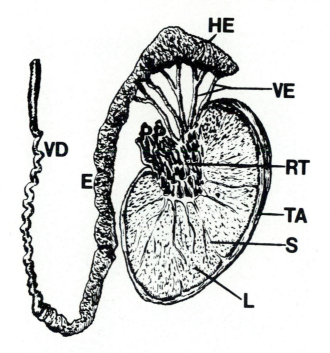

FIG 18–1.
Normal scrotal structures. A diagram of the testis and epididymis demonstrates the various portions of the normal contents of the scrotal sac: *RT* = rete testis; *TA* = tunica albuginea; *S* = septum; *L* = lobule; *VE* = vasa efferentia; *PP* = pampiniform plexus; *HE* = head of epididymis; *E* = epididymis; *VD* = vas deferens.

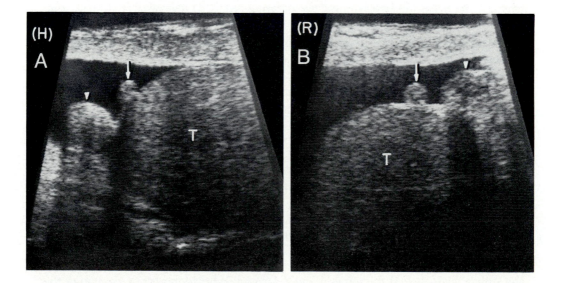

FIG 18–2.
Longitudinal (**A**) and transverse (**B**) images of the normal scrotum demonstrate the testis (*T*), the head of the epididymis (*arrowhead*), and the appendix of the testis (*arrow*). Measurements can be obtained in either view to evaluate size. (*H*) = toward patient's head; (*R*) = patient's right side.

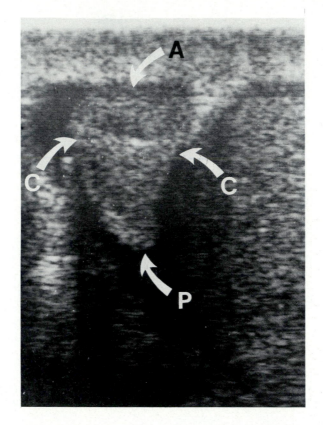

FIG 18–3.
A longitudinal image of the epididymal head (*arrows*) demonstrates the triangular shape of this normal structure. The anterior(*A*)-posterior(*P*) and the cephalocaudad (*C–C*) dimensions can be measured.

testicular appendages: (1) the paradidymis, also known as the organ of Giraldés, and (2) the superior and (3) the inferior vas aberrans of Haller. These appendages are infrequently present and are rarely seen by ultrasound.

Functionally, the epididymis transports, concentrates, stores, and aids in the maturation of sperm. Sperm flow has been calculated to take approximately 10 to 15 days in all male mammals. Sperm motility increases during this period as they travel from the epididymal head to the tail. The flow of spermatozoa is secondary to both a hydrostatic pressure which is within the epididymal tubules and to peristaltic-like contractions of the tubules. The epididymis is surrounded by connective tissue. The tubules are tightly coiled in the in vivo state (measuring about 5 cm in length) and, when stretched, measure up to 4 to 5 m in length.

The testicle is surrounded by a thick, tightly adherent fibrous membrane, the tunica albuginea. Both the testicle and epididymis are loosely enveloped by a double membrane, the tunica vaginalis. This is attached to the upper lateral aspect of the testis and the epididymis together at the sinus epididymis. There are two layers of the tunica vaginalis: (1) the visceral layer, formed from the posterior portion of the peritoneal lining of the testis, and (2) the parietal layer, which is derived embryologically from the anterior layer of the peritoneum. The visceral layer is a serous membrane producing secretions. The parietal layer has lymphatic channels which absorb some of this fluid.

The outer covering of the testis and epididymis is the scrotum. This is a continuous pouch with an internal division known as the median raphe. The median raphe is most prominent on both the ventral and inferior surfaces. It extends along the midline to the peritoneum. The scrotum consists of many layers. The outer covering of the skin contains sebaceous follicles, sweat glands, and hair. The next layer is the tunica dartos, a thin layer of vascular tissue which is fibrous, elastic, and has smooth muscle fibers. The external spermatic fascia is a continuation of the external oblique fascia of the abdominal wall. It is bordered by the dartos fascia externally and the cremasteric fascia internally. The latter membrane is a double layer of elastic muscular tissue and is the continuation of the abdominal internal oblique fascia and muscle. The next layer is loose connective tissue, the internal spermatic fascia, a continuation of the transversalis fascia. The innermost layer is the tunica vaginalis.

The spermatic cord is the life line connecting the scrotum to the pelvis and abdomen. Its contents include the arterial supply, venous drainage, lymphatics, nerves, and the vas deferens, and is tightly bound by a fibrous sheath. The two internal spermatic arteries (one on each side) originate from the abdominal aorta

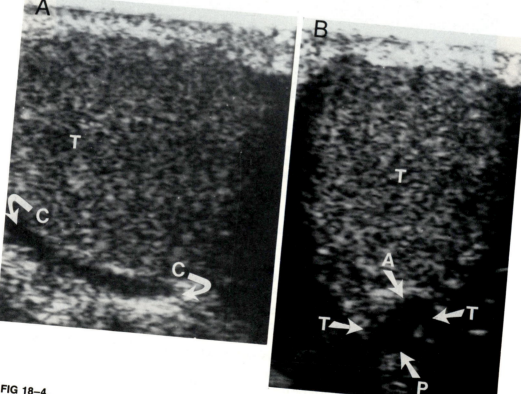

FIG 18–4.
The normal testis (*T*) and normal epididymal body (*arrows*) identified on the longitudinal (**A**) and transverse (**B**) scans. The cephalocaudad (*C–C*) dimension of the epididymis can be measured by the longitudinal view. The anteroposterior image of both the testis and the epididymis (*A–P*) can be measured on either view and the transverse dimension (*T–T*) size of the testis and epididymis is measured on the transverse image.

Chapter 19 _____

Female Pelvic Organ Measurements

Oksana H. Baltarowich, M.D.

Measurements of female reproductive organs vary depending on the physiologic state. Since the organs, mainly the ovaries and uterus, are so dynamic in their function, changes are encountered during the menstrual cycle as well as during the life span of the individual. Therefore it is practical to separate discussion of their measurement into the following categories: prepubertal (premenstrual), premenopausal (adult, childbearing), and postmenopausal.

IMAGING TECHNIQUES

Various imaging techniques have been utilized in the past in order to evaluate pelvic organ sizes. Some techniques have been abandoned, others have not been fully investigated.

Measurements of female organs have been described from pelvic pneumography, which currently is predominantly of historic interest. Pelvic pneumography is a radiographic study of the pelvis obtained after induction of a pneumoperitoneum. This procedure was described over 65 years ago,[1] had attempts at revitalization in the mid-1960s,[2] and subsequently was abandoned in the early 1970s. After introduction of intraperitoneal gas (preferably nitrous oxide or carbon dioxide) plain film radiographs were obtained in the prone Trendelenberg position with several different angulations of the beam to the film. Pneumography was limited to definition of tissue outlines. It did not provide information about homogeneity or composition of tissues. In young patients it could even have required general anesthesia. This technique had inherent problems which preclude establishment of useful absolute measurements for normal female organs.[3] Magnification factors varied for each projection, as well as for the different organs, that is, ovaries and uterus, in the same patient. Organ relationships were altered and distorted by the gravity effect of the prone Trendelenberg position. Summation shadows also caused interpretation problems. Since organ measurements taken on these unusual projections were not absolute values due to the inherent magnification factor, they could not be compared with those of other techniques. This examination was mainly useful in providing a relative approximation of organ sizes in the individual patient.

Hysterosalpingography as a radiographic procedure does not offer useful measurements of ovarian and uterine size. After contrast spills into the peritoneal cavity from the fallopian tubes, it may outline the ovaries and the uterus so that measurements can be attempted. Internal, contrast-lined portions of organs may be measured such as the endocervical canal. Since measurements are mostly a by-product of the examination, they are not clinically useful. They suffer from drawbacks similar to those of pneumography.

Computed tomography (CT) of the pelvis yields no useful measurements for normal ovaries or uterus. Pathology, such as ovarian tumors, is more readily seen. CT is limited in its ability to take measurements since it is a transaxial cross-sectional imaging technique while the organs in the pelvis have variable orientation.

Magnetic resonance imaging (MRI) of the female pelvis offers some advantages over CT.[4] It is nonionizing and produces direct multiplanar images. MRI does not require contrast administration to highlight differences between organ components (such as endometrium and myometrium, uterine corpus and cervix). It is free from artifacts of surgical clips, air interface, or bone. It is, however, costly and complex. The limits of this technique have not been fully realized, and studies of organ measurement have not been reported.

Sonography is the best method of investigating the female pelvis. Ultrasound machines are almost ubiquitous and scans are readily performed. This technique is noninvasive, cost-effective, and acceptable to the patient. Because there is no ionizing radiation, it is a safer technique for imaging the genetically delicate reproductive organs. The real-time equipment is very maneuverable so that an organ may be scanned from various angulations. Sectional images which are suitable for the organ, despite its location, may be obtained, and correct measurements subsequently taken. It has been established numerous times that sonographic measurements are very accurate and have excellent correlation with direct measurement,[5-8] especially when they are performed by experienced personnel using properly calibrated machines.

ULTRASOUND TECHNIQUE

Real-time sector scanning is the optimal ultrasonic technique for pelvic organ visualization. Linear array scanners are not as desirable, mainly because they cannot negotiate the curvature over the pubis. The following technique is considered optimal in evaluation of the uterus and ovaries.

The patient is examined in the supine position with a full bladder that is not overly distended. The pelvis is quickly surveyed in the transverse plane sweeping cephalad and caudad. The uterus is identified approximately in midline and its displacement off the sagittal plane is assessed. The axis of a normal uterus may be altered by changes in posture, intraabdominal pressure, bladder distention, presence of a pelvic mass, presence of adhesions, or rectal fullness. The transducer is then oriented in the longitudinal plane of the uterus, taking into account any inclination from the midline sagittal plane. Demonstration of the entire length of the endometrial and endocervical cavity echoes assures that the proper plane of section for a midline scan of the uterus has been obtained. On longitudinal scans, this is seen as a central linear echo surrounded by a hypoechoic rim. On transverse scans it has the appearance of a rounded "bull's-eye" configuration with a central hyperechoic portion and surrounding hypoechoic halo. The total uterine length (from the top of the fundus to

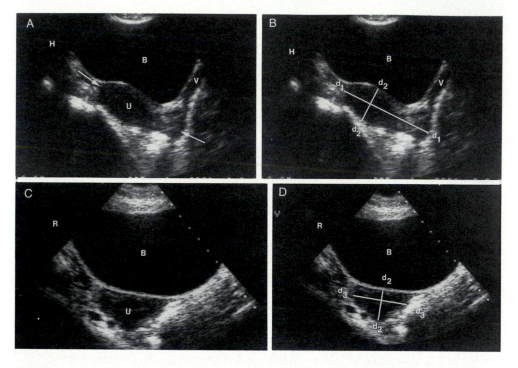

FIG 19–1.
Measurement of the uterus. **A**, midline sagittal scan of the uterus (*U*) showing its maximal length taken from the top of the fundus to the bottom of the cervix, the external cervical os (*arrows*). **B**, same image as **A**, showing the maximal length (d_1) and the maximal AP diameter (d_2) taken perpendicular to d_1 (*solid lines*). **C**, transverse scan taken by rotating the probe 90 degrees from the longitudinal plane of **A** about the d_2 axis. **D**, same image as **C**. The maximal transverse width, d_3, is measured perpendicular to the maximal AP diameter, d_2 (*solid lines*). d_2 is only measured from the long-axis image. *B*, urinary bladder; *V* = vagina; *H* = toward patient's head; *R* = patient's right side.

the external cervical os) is recorded. The maximal anteroposterior (AP) diameter is measured perpendicular to the maximal length (Fig 19–1). The transducer is then rotated 90 degrees at the level of the maximal AP diameter where the maximal transverse width is measured (see Fig 19–1).

The ovaries are found as ovoid structures between the uterus and muscular pelvic side wall. Despite biologic variation, the ovary, when considered as a geometric shape, is best represented by an ellipsoid. By definition, this is a three-dimensional surface in the orthogonal *x, y, z* Cartesian coordinate system, such that when its axes are along the *x-, y-, z*-axes, each cross section in the planes xy, xz, and yz describes an ellipse. Orientation of these ellipsoids (ovaries) in the pelvis varies greatly from one body to the next, as well as in the same individual. One should begin by establishing *its longest diameter*, no matter how the ovary is positioned. Usually this is obtained as follows: After the uterus is located in the longitudinal plane, the transducer is moved away from midline parasagittally and the beam is directed to the contralateral side of the pelvis, therefore maximizing the bladder sonic window. The beam is then inclined and/or rotated, in order to display the longest diameter of the ovary (d_1) (Fig 19–2). Such rotation and inclination are necessary because rarely does the longest axis of the ovary correspond with the body's longitudinal axis. In some situations, the ovaries may lie completely laterally so that the longest diameter would be found on a standard transverse section of the pelvis. Most ovaries, however, are angled in various directions, not corresponding to standard planes of body sections.

When an image of the longest diameter (d_1) of the ovary is found, the *maximal* AP diameter or height (d_2) is measured perpendicular to d_1. The transducer is then rotated 90 degrees to the longitudinal axis of the ovary and the maximal transverse (d_3) diameter can be measured. The AP (d_2) measurement should be reconfirmed on this projection and then d_3 is measured perpendicular to d_2 (see Fig 19–2). It is important that these three measurements be taken 90 degrees to each other. In such a fashion, the beam is directed to find the diameters on the principal axes of this ellipsoid. These diameters are subsequently used for ovarian volume and other calculations.

Sonographically, ovarian volume is the best and most reproducible method of evaluating ovarian size. An ovary compressed by a full bladder has different linear dimensions than when in a noncompressed state. The volume, however, remains constant. Calculation of ovarian volume depends on precise measurements of all three maximal diameters. The formula for the volume (V) of an ellipsoid is used:

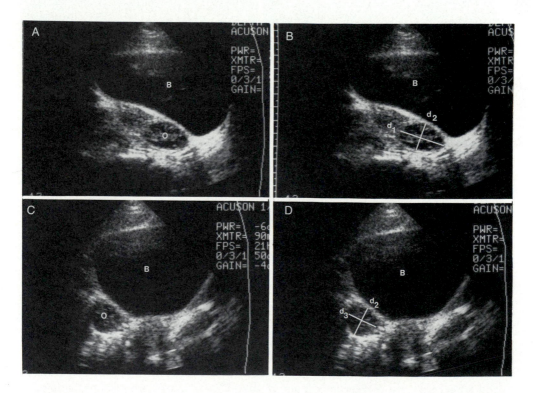

FIG 19–2.
Measurement of the ovary. **A**, the longest diameter of the ovary (*O*) is identified. **B**, same image as **A** shows the longest diameter of the ovary as its reference plane and maximal longitudinal diameter, d_1 (*solid line*). The maximal AP diameter, d_2, is taken perpendicular to d_1 (*solid lines*). **C**, the transverse scan of the ovary is found by rotating the probe 90 degrees from the longitudinal plane of **A** about the d_2 axis. **D**, same image as **C**. The maximal transverse width of the ovary, d_3, is then taken perpendicular to d_2 (*solid lines*). d_2 is only measured from the long-axis image. *B* = urinary bladder.

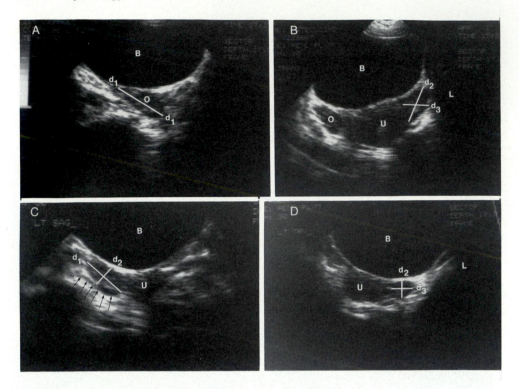

FIG 19–3.
Incorrect and correct ovarian measurements resulting in a large calculated volume difference. **A,** the longest diameter, d_1, of the left ovary (*O*) is slightly overestimated at 5.2 cm (*solid line*). **B,** the AP (d_2) and transverse (d_3) diameters of the same ovary are incorrectly taken, 3.7 and 2.5 cm, respectively. The three measurements were not taken perpendicular to each other. The resultant calculated volume, 25.2 cc, is thus too high. **C,** the longest diameter, d_1, of the same ovary is correctly taken with the AP diameter, d_2, taken perpendicularly (*solid lines*). *Small arrows* delineate internal iliac vessel. **D,** the maximal transverse diameter, d_3, of the same ovary is taken perpendicular to d_2 (*solid lines*). The respective measurements, 4.3, 1.9, and 2.4 cm, yield a volume of 10.3 cc. This is only 41% of the volume calculated from incorrect measurements. *B* = urinary bladder; *U* = uterus; *L* = patient's left side.

$$V = 4/3 \ \pi \times d_1/2 \times d_2/2 \times d_3/2$$

or more simply,

$$V = d_1 \times d_2 \times d_3 \times 0.523$$

where d_1, d_2, and d_3 are the maximal perpendicular diameters.

Measurements on standard projections oriented with respect to the body (sagittal and transverse) are correct only if any of the ellipsoid's axes are oriented along any of the body's standard axes. This occurs if the ovary points directly laterally, directly posteriorly, or directly superiorly. If the ovaries are inclined with respect to the body's major planes, it is incorrect to use the standard planes of section. If this is done anyway, then the diameters obtained are oblique. Computation of volumes from these diameters yield erroneous results, which may be falsely high or low. Improper technique will generate improper measurements (Fig 19–3), unless they are corrected for all angles of inclination from the principal axes of the ellipsoid. Such correction becomes mathematically complicated and impractical.

Using this technique and after gaining some experience, finding the correct longitudinal axis of the ovary should not be very difficult. Hackelöer and Nitschke-Dabelstein have described an ovarian reference plane which is the ovary's longitudinal axis.[9] Because position of the ovarian vessels within the infundibulopelvic ligament is stable in relation to the ovary, they claim that these vessels should be used as the reference plane for the ovary. In our experience, observation of these small ovarian vessels is difficult and time-consuming. Doppler may be necessary for confirmation.

Several anatomic markers for the ovary are more useful than the ovarian vessels. The internal iliac vessels are usually located posteriorly. This relationship, however, is not constant since the anatomic association may be altered by adhesions, pathologic masses, or after bearing children. The distal ureter may be seen posterior to these vessels. Pelvic muscles are less helpful as markers and in addition should not be mistaken for ovaries. Muscles are best identified by looking for symmetry and continuity in cephalad and caudad directions. Confirmation is performed by scanning in parasagittal directions.

When transabdominal scanning is unsuccessful due to obesity, bowel gas, scarring, or adhesions, intravaginal pelvic sonography can be performed.[10] Information about pelvic structures can be obtained with better resolution because the organs are closer to the transducer whose frequency is higher (5.0–7.5 MHz) than that of transabdominal probes. The intravaginally placed transducer is not as maneuverable, however. This limits proper ovarian measurements if one attempts to seek their major axes. The planes obtained are actually oblique and modified coronal, transverse, and sagittal planes. Uterine length determination is also compromised since the uterus assumes a more anatomic anteverted position and is not flattened out by bladder compression as on transabdominal scans. Actual measurements by this technique, other than follicle sizes,[11] have not been reported as of this writing.

THE OVARY

The Prepubertal Ovary

Before discussing prepubertal ovarian measurements, certain definitions are needed. The neonatal period is considered to last from birth to 6 weeks. Infancy then commences and lasts until 2 years of age. Childhood encompasses the ages from 2 to menarche, with early childhood generally designated from 2 to 8 years of age. Late childhood is usually between 8 to 12 years when the first evidence of hormonally influenced changes becomes clinically noted. Since the average age of onset of menarche in the United States is 13 years old, statistically, childhood is considered to end at this age. Menses normally occurs any time between 9 and 17 years of age.

Until recently there has been a paucity of anatomic and physiologic information concerning the development of the female genital tract from the neonatal period to the onset of menarche. Manual physical examinations are difficult and not routinely performed on the young girl. Autopsy material is also not abundant. Ultrasound has made significant contributions to knowledge in the area of pediatric gynecology. Real-time sector scanners enable the routine imaging of neonatal and pediatric ovaries and the morphologic study of the growing human ovary.

TABLE 19–6.
Normal Uterine Dimensions and Volumes in Pediatric Age Groups*

Age (yr)	Length (cm) (Mean ± SD)	AP Corpus (cm) (Mean ± SD)	AP Cervix (cm) (Mean ± SD)	Transverse Corpus (cm) (Mean)†	Volume (cc) (Mean ± SD)
≤6 wk	2.5 ± 5.0	0.25		1.0	
2–7	3.3 ± 0.4	0.7 ± 0.2	0.8 ± 0.2	1.7	2.0 ± 1.2
8	3.6 ± 0.7	0.9 ± 0.3	0.8 ± 0.2	1.8	3.1 ± 1.5
9	3.7 ± 0.4	1.0 ± 0.3	0.9 ± 0.2	1.9	3.7 ± 1.6
10	4.0 ± 0.6	1.3 ± 0.5	1.1 ± 0.3	2.4	6.5 ± 3.8
11	4.2 ± 0.5	1.3 ± 0.3	1.1 ± 0.3	2.3	6.7 ± 2.9
12	5.4 ± 0.8	1.7 ± 0.5	1.4 ± 0.5	3.4	16.2 ± 9.2
13	5.4 ± 1.1	1.6 ± 0.4	1.5 ± 0.2	2.9	13.2 ± 5.6

*From Orsini LF, Salardi S, Pilo G, et al: *Radiology* 1984; 153:113–116. Used by permission.
†Transverse width is calculated backward from the volume by using length and AP corpus dimensions, that is volume is divided by length × AP corpus × 0.523.

(n = 2)[12] (Table 19–6). The range in length probably results from measurements taken on subjects at different times in the newborn period, some before and others after the postnatal involution. The length varies, but not the other two dimensions, because most of the growth at this age occurs longitudinally.

In general, most studies find that during childhood there is no significant growth of the uterus until age 7 or 8 years, after which time a measurable, although small, age-related increase in size is observed.[12,18,19,92] Growth of the uterus increases markedly after approximately age 10 or 11 in most series. Most sources report only length and AP diameter. Unfortunately, the transverse dimension is rarely reported. This third dimension is important in ultrasonic evaluation of uterine measurements since the uterus is subject to compression by the bladder. A compressed uterus may have a decreased AP dimension but its transverse dimension may increase compensatorily.

The measurements of Sample et al.[16] were widely used as a standard until more recent data were known. For ages 1 to 12 they reported a mean uterine length of 2.8 cm (range 2.0–3.8 cm) and a mean uterine AP diameter of 0.8 cm (range 0.5–1.0 cm). Their series is small (only 20 patients) and the age groups are lumped into one category, leaving very few subjects per childhood year (1–12 years old). Therefore, the age-related uterine growth is not appreciated.

The measurements of Orsini et al.[18] of the total uterine length are recommended for use between ages 2 and 13. Since there is no significant change in the total uterine length between ages 2 and 7, one may lump these age groups into one group using 3.3 ±0.4 cm for the average of the means and standard deviations. Thereafter the uterus increases in length from 3.6 ±0.7 cm at age 8 to 5.4 ±1.1 cm at age 13. Orsini et al. also report AP diameters of both the uterine body and cervix for each corresponding age group. As in uterine length, there is no significant difference between the ages of 2 and 7 in the thickness of the uterine body; therefore the average of the means and standard deviations is included (see Table 19–6). No significant change occurs in the thickness of the cervix between ages 2 and 9; however, an average of the diameters for ages 2 to 7 is included in Table 19–6 since uterine length and body thickness are so reported. Unfortunately, the transverse dimensions of the uteri in the different age groups were not reported. They were calculated backward from the measurements of the uterine volumes by using the other two listed dimensions (see Table 19–6). A standard deviation is not given.

Uterine volumes in the pediatric age group have been reported assuming that the uterus is an ellipsoid. Volumes have been calculated using the three maximal diameters of the uterus in three perpendicular planes by the formula $V = d_1 \times d_2 \times d_3 \times 0.523$. Although accurate for volume determination of other organs, for example, kidneys and ovaries,[93, 94] the volume measurements of the premenarchal uterus may not be accurate, since the uterus is not truly an ellipsoid. Up to five-sixths of the uterine length is a narrow cylindrical cervix in premenarchal girls. Orsini et al.[18] have reported uterine volumes for ages 2 through 13. These are included in Table 19–6 for reference, although the calculations may not be precise based on the mathematical considerations of uterine geometry. It is interesting, however, that the calculated uterine volumes are similar to the reported uterine weights, which are related to each other by density. The specific gravity of the human uterine tissue is known to be 1.052[12]; therefore, 1 cc of volume equals approximately 1g of uterine tissue.

More precise methods for measuring volumes of premenarchal uteri may be used. The parallel planimetric area method, also called serial area-volume determination, is more accurate for volume determination than the prolate ellipsoid method.[94–98] This type of volume determination for the nonpregnant uterus has not been performed. In order to calculate volume by this method, parallel transverse scans should be performed at 0.5- to 1.0-cm intervals from the top of the fundus to the cervical tip. The volume is subsequently calculated:

$$V = D (A_1 + A_2 + A_3 + \ldots A_n)$$

where V = volume, D = distance between the scans, A = section area in square centimeters of each respective transverse section. Each sectional area is calculated by:

$$A = \pi/4 \times d_2 \times d_3$$

where d_2 and d_3 are the AP thickness and transverse width, respectively, for each sectional ellipse. Better results from more fixed and rigid intervals are achieved by static scanners, but these are practically obsolete. Overall, the method is very cumbersome.

Another theoretical way of measuring the volume of the nonpregnant uterus would be to presume that the uterus is actually composed of two geometric shapes, one being an ellipsoid and a second being an elliptic cylinder. The total volume (V_T) would be the sum of the respective volumes of the two geometric shapes, $V_1 + V_2$. The volume of the ellipsoid (V_1) is well known:

$$V_1 = d_1 \times d_2 \times d_3 \times 0.523$$

where d_1, d_2, and d_3 are the perpendicular diameters of the ellipsoid. The volume of the elliptical cylinder (V_2) is

$$V_2 = \pi/4 \times d_4 \times d_5 \times d_6$$

238   *Gynecology*

REFERENCES

1. Goetze O: Die Roentgendiagnostik bei gasgefüllter Bauchhöhle: Eine neue Methode. *MMW* 1918; 65:1275–1280.
2. Stevens GM, Weigen JF, Lee RS: Pelvic pneumography. *Med Radiogr Photogr* 1966; 42:82–91.
3. Zemlyn S: Comparison of pelvic ultrasonography and pneumography for ovarian size. *J Clin Ultrasound* 1974; 2:331–339.
4. Hricak H, Lacey C, Schriock E, et al: Gynecologic masses: value of magnetic resonance imaging. *Am J Obstet Gynecol* 1985; 153:31–37.
5. DeLand M, Fried A, van Nagell JR, et al: Ultrasonography in the diagnosis of tumors of the ovary. *Surg Gynecol Obstet* 1979; 148:346–348.
6. Campbell S, Goessen L, Goswamy R, et al: Real-time ultrasonography for determination of ovarian morphology and volume: A possible screening test for ovarian cancer? *Lancet* 1982; 1:425–426.
7. Flickinger L, D'Ablaing G III, Mishell DR Jr: Size and weight determinations of nongravid enlarged uteri. *Obstet Gynecol* 1986; 68:855–858.
8. Platt JF, Bree R, Schwab R, et al: Ultrasound of the normal nongravid uterus: Correlation with gross and histopathology, in Proceedings of the American Roentgen Ray Society 86th Annual Meeting, Miami, March 1987.
9. Hackelöer, B-J, Nitschke-Dabelstein S: Ovarian imaging by ultrasound: an attempt to define a reference plane. *J Clin Ultrasound* 1980; 8:497–500.
10. Schwimer SR, Lebovic J: Transvaginal pelvic ultrasonography. *J Ultrasound Med* 1984; 3:381–383.
11. Schwimer SR, Lebovic J: Transvaginal pelvic ultrasonography: Accuracy in follicle and cyst size determination. *J Ultrasound Med* 1985; 4:61–63.
12. International Commission on Radiological Protection. Task Group on Reference Man: *Report of the Task Group on Reference Man.* Prepared by the Task Group Committee no. 2, International Commission on Radiological Protection, Snyder WS (chairman). New York, Pergamon Press, 1975.
13. Haller JO, Friedman AP, Schaffer R, et al: The normal and abnormal ovary in childhood and adolescence. *Semin Ultrasound* 1983; 4:206–225.
14. Krantz KE, Atkinson JP: Gross anatomy. *Ann NY Acad Sci* 1967; 142:551–575.
15. Simkins CS: Development of the human ovary from birth to sexual maturity. *Am J Anat* 1932; 51:465–505.
16. Sample WF, Lippe BM, Gyepes MT: Gray-scale ultrasonography of the normal female pelvis. *Radiology* 1977; 125:477–483.
17. Stanhope R, Adams J, Jacobs HS, et al: Ovarian ultrasound assessment in normal children, idiopathic precocious puberty, and during low dose pulsatile gonadotrophin releasing hormone treatment of hypogonadotrophic hypogonadism. *Arch Dis Child* 1985; 60:116–119.
18. Orsini LF, Salardi S, Pilu G, et al: Pelvic organs in premenarchal girls: real-time ultrasonography. *Radiology* 1984; 153:113–116.
19. Ivarsson S-A, Nilsson KO, Persson P-H: Ultrasonography of the pelvic organs in prepubertal and postpubertal girls. *Arch Dis Child* 1983; 58:352–354.
20. Gamberini MR, DeSanctis V, Vullo C, et al: Pelvic ultrasound in perimenarchal period. *Riv Ital Pediatr* 1986; 12:698–703.
21. Spivak M: Polycystic ovaries in the newborn and early infancy and their relation to the structure of the endometrium. *Am J Obstet Gynecol* 1934; 27:157–173.
22. Polhemus DW: Ovarian maturation and cyst formation in children. *Pediatr J* 1953; 11:588–594.
23. Merrill JA: The morphology of the prepubertal ovary: Relationship to the polycystic syndrome. *South Med J* 1963; 56:225–231.
24. Peters H, Himelstein-Braw R, Faber M: The normal development of the ovary in childhood. *Acta Endocrinol* 1976; 82:617–630.
25. Peters H, Byskov AG, Grinsted J: The development of the ovary during childhood in health and disease, in Coutts JRT (ed): *Functional Morphology of the Human Ovary,* Lancaster, England, Lancaster MTP Press, 1981, pp 26–34.
26. Clemente CD (ed): *Gray's Anatomy of the Human Body,* ed 28. Philadelphia, Lea & Febiger, 1985.
27. Saphir O: Weights and measurements of organs, in Saphir O (ed): *Autopsy Diagnosis and Technic,* ed 4. New York, Paul B Hoeber, Inc, 1958, pp 511–515.
28. Kistner RW: *Gynecology: Principles and Practice,* ed 4. Chicago, Year Book Medical Publishers, 1986, p 289.
29. Green B: Pelvic ultrasonography, in Sarti DA, Sample WF (eds): *Diagnostic Ultrasound: Text and Cases,* Boston, GK Hall & Co, 1980, p 503.

30. Granberg S, Wikland M: A comparison between ultrasound and gynecologic examination for detection of enlarged ovaries in a group of women at risk for ovarian carcinoma. *J Ultrasound Med* 1988; 7:59–64.
31. Gershon-Cohen J, Hermel MB: Pelvic pneumoperitoneum. The x-ray appearance of the normal female pelvic organs. *Am J Obstet Gynecol* 1952; 64:184–187.
32. Strauss HA, Cohen MR: Gynecography simplified. *Am J Obstet Gynecol* 1955; 70:572–581.
33. Parisi L, Tramonti M, Derchi LE, et al: Polycystic ovarian disease: Ultrasonic evaluation and correlations with clinical and hormonal data. *J Clin Ultrasound* 1984; 12:21–26.
34. Yeh HC, Futterweit W, Thornton JC: Polycystic ovarian disease: US features in 104 patients. *Radiology* 1987; 163:111–116.
35. Andolf E, Jorgensen C, Svalenius E, et al: Ultrasound measurement of the ovarian volume. *Acta Obstet Gynecol Scand* 1987; 66:387–389.
36. Nicolini U, Ferrazzi E, Bellotti M, et al: The contributions of sonographic evaluation of ovarian size in patients with polycystic ovarian disease. *J Ultrasound Med* 1985; 4:347–351.
37. Venturoli S, Paradisi R, Saviotti E, et al: Ultrasound study of ovarian and uterine morphology in women with polycystic ovary syndrome before, during and after treatment with cyproterone acetate and ethinyloestradiol. *Arch Gynecol* 1985; 237:1–10.
38. Munn CS, Kiser LC, Wetzner SM, et al: Ovary volume in young and premenopausal adults: US determination. Work in progress. *Radiology* 1986; 159:731–732.
39. Munn CS: Normal ovary volume in adults of ovulatory age: US determination. *J Ultrasound Med* (in press).
40. Goswamy RK, Campbell S, Royston JP, et al: Ovarian size in postmenopausal women. *Br J Obstet Gynaecol* 1988; 95:795–801.
41. Rodriguez MH, Platt LD, Medearis AL, et al: The use of transvaginal sonography for evaluation of postmenopausal ovarian size and morphology. *Am J Obstet Gynecol* 1988; 159:810–814.
42. Hall DA, Hann LE, Ferrucici JT Jr, et al: Sonographic morphology of the normal menstrual cycle. *Radiology* 1979; 133:185–188.
43. Anderson CF, Jasso L, Giles HR, et al: Cyclic variations in ultrasonographic evaluation of the female pelvis, in White D, Lyons EA (eds): *Ultrasound in Medicine*, vol 4. Proceedings of the 22nd Annual Meeting of the American Institute of Ultrasound in Medicine, Dallas, Texas. New York, Plenum Press, 1978, pp 235–236.
44. Pupols AZ, Wilson SR: Ultrasonographic interpretation of physiological changes in the female pelvis. *J Assoc Canad Radiol* 1984; 35:34–39.
45. Fleischer AC, Kalemeris GC, Machin JE, et al: Sonographic depiction of normal and abnormal endometrium with histopathologic correlation. *J Ultrasound Med* 1986; 5:445–452.
46. Bryce RL, Shuter B, Sinosich MJ, et al: The value of ultrasound, ganodotropin, and estradiol measurements for precise ovulation predication. *Fertil Steril* 1982; 37:42–45.
47. Geisthovel F, Skubsch W, Zabel G, et al: Ultrasonographic and hormonal studies in physiologic and insufficient menstrual cycles. *Fertil Steril* 1983; 39:277–283.
48. Hackelöer BJ, Robinson HP: Ultrasound examination of the growing ovarian follicle. *Geburtshilfe Frauenheilkunde* 1978; 38:163–168.
49. Hackelöer BJ, Fleming R, Robinson HP, et al: Correlation of ultrasonic and endocrinologic assessment of human follicular development. *Am J Obstet Gynecol* 1979; 135:122–128.
50. Hackelöer BJ: The role of ultrasound in female infertility management. *Ultrasound Med Biol* 1984; 10:35–50.
51. Kerin JF, Edmonds DK, Warnes GM, et al: Morphological and functional relations of graafian follicle growth to ovulation in women using ultrasonic, laparoscopic, and biochemical measurements. *Br J Obstet Gynaecol* 1981; 88:81–90.
52. Lenz S: Ultrasonic study of follicular maturation, ovulation and development of corpus luteum during normal menstrual cycles. *Acta Obstet Gynecol Scand* 1985; 64:15–19.
53. Nitschke-Dabelstein S, Hackelöer BJ, Sturm G: Ovulation and corpus luteum formation observed by ultrasonography. *Ultrasound Med Biol* 1981; 7:33–39.
54. Polan ML, Totora M, Caldwell BV, et al: Abnormal ovarian cycles as diagnosed by ultrasound and serum estradiol levels. *Fertil Steril* 1982; 37:342–347.
55. Renaud RL, Macler J, Dervain I, et al: Echographic study of follicular maturation and ovulation during the normal menstrual cycle. *Fertil Steril* 1980; 33:272–276.
56. Robertson RD, Picker RHL, Wilson PC, et al: Assessment of ovulation by ultrasound and plasma estradiol determination. *Obstet Gynecol* 1979; 54:686–691.

57. Smith DH, Picker RH, Sinosich M, et al: Assessment of ovulation by ultrasound and estradiol levels during spontaneous and induced cycles. *Fertil Steril* 1980; 33:387–390.

58. Ylostalo P, Ronnberg L, Jouppila P: Measurement of the ovarian follicle by ultrasound in ovulation induction. *Fertil Steril* 1979; 31:651–655.

59. Nilsson L, Wikland M, Hamberger BJ: Recruitment of an ovulatory follicle in the human following follicle-ectomy and luteectomy. *Fertil Steril* 1982; 137:30–34.

60. Renaud R, Macler J, Dervain I: Echographic study of follicular maturation and ovulation during the normal menstrual cycle. *Fertil Steril* 1980; 33:272–276.

61. Hackelöer BJ: Follicular size assessment by ultrasound, in Sanders RC, James AE Jr (eds): *Ultrasound in Obstetrics and Gynecology*, ed 3. Norwalk, Conn, Appleton-Century-Crofts, 1985, pp 517–529.

62. Orsini LF, Rizzo N, Calderoni P, et al: Ultrasound monitoring of ovarian follicle development: A comparison of real-time and static scanning techniques. *J Clin Ultrasound* 1983; 11:207–213.

63. Fleischer AC, Daniell JF, Rodier J, et al: Sonographic monitoring by ovarian follicular development. *J Clin Ultrasound* 1981; 9:275–280.

64. Hata T, Yoshino K, Nagahara Y, et al: Precise day of ovulation determined by real-time ultrasound evidence of graafian follicular development. *Int J Gynaecol Obstet* 1983; 21:435–438.

65. O'Herlihy C, DeCrespigny LJ, Robinson HP: Monitoring ovarian follicular development with real-time ultrasound. *Br J Obstet Gynaecol* 1980; 87:613–618.

66. O'Herlihy C, DeCrespigny LJ, Lopata A, et al: Preovulatory follicular size: A comparison of ultrasound and laparoscopic measurements. *Fertil Steril* 1980; 34:24–26.

67. Queenan JT, O'Brien GD, Bains LM, et al: Ultrasound scanning of ovaries to detect ovulation in women. *Fertil Steril* 1980; 34:99–105.

68. Zegers-Hochochild F, Lira CG, Parada M, et al: A comparative study of the follicular growth profile in conception and nonception cycles. *Fertil Steril* 1984; 41:244–247.

69. Mendelson EB, Friedman H, Neiman HL, et al: The role of imaging in infertility management. *AJR* 1985; 144:415–420.

70. McArdle C, Seibel M, Weinstein F, et al: Induction of ovulation monitored by ultrasound. *Radiology* 1983; 148:809–812.

71. Dornbluth NC, Potter JL, Shepard MK, et al: Assessment of follicular development by ultrasound and total serum estrogen in human menopausal gonadotropin-stimulated cycles. *J Ultrasound Med* 1983; 2:407–412.

72. Sallam HN, Marinho AO, Collins WP, et al: Monitoring gonadotropin therapy by real-time ultrasonic scanning by ovarian follicles. *Br J Obstet Gynaecol* 1982; 89:155–159.

73. Mantzavinos T, Garcia JE, Jones HW: Ultrasound measurement of ovarian follicles stimulated by human gonadotropins for oocyte recovery and in vitro fertilization. *Fertil Steril* 1983; 40:461–465.

74. O'Herlihy C, Pepperell RJ, Robinson HP: Ultrasound timing of human chorionic gonadotropin administration in clomiphene stimulated cycles. *Obstet Gynecol* 1982; 59:40–45.

75. O'Herlihy C, Evans JH, Bronn JB, et al: Use of ultrasound in monitoring ovulation induction with human pituitary gonadotropins. *Obstet Gynecol* 1982; 60:577–582.

76. Ylostalo P, Lindgren PG, Nillius SJ: Ultrasonic measurement of ovarian follicles, ovarian and uterine size during induction of ovulation with human gonadotropins. *Acta Endocrinol* 1981; 98:592–598.

77. Garcia JE, Jones GS, Acosta AA, et al: Human menopausal gonadotropinol human chorionic gonadotropin follicular maturation for oocyte aspiration, phase I, 1981. *Fertil Steril* 1983; 39:167–173.

78. Cabau A, Bessis R: Monitoring of ovulation induction with human menopausal gonadotropin and human chorionic gonadotropin by ultrasound. *Fertil Steril* 1981; 36:178–182.

79. Haning RV, Zweibel WJ: Ultrasound assistance in clinical management of infertility. *Semin Ultrasound* 1983; 4:226–233.

80. Vargyas JM, Marrs RP, Kletzky DA, et al: Correlation of ultrasonic measurement of ovarian follicle size and serum estradiol levels in ovulatory patients following clomiphene citrate for in vitro fertilization. *Obstet Gynecol* 1982; 144:569–573.

81. Rankin RN, Hutton LC: Ultrasound in the ovarian hyperstimulation syndrome. *J Clin Ultrasound* 1981; 9:473–476.

82. McArdle C, Seibel M, Hann LE, et al: The diagnosis of ovarian hyperstimulation: The impact of ultrasound. *Fertil Steril* 1983; 39:464–467.

83. Marrs RP, Vargyas JM, Saito H, et al: Clinical applications of techniques used in human in vitro fertilization research. *Am J Obstet Gynecol* 1983; 146:477–481.

84. Barber HRK, Graber EA: The PMPO syndrome (postmenopausal palpable ovary syndrome). *Obstet Gynecol* 1971; 38:921–923.

85. Hall DA, McCarthy KA, Kopans DB: Sonographic visualization of the normal postmenopausal ovary. *J Ultrasound Med* 1985; 5:9–11.

86. Moyle JW, Rochester D, Sider L, et al: Sonography of ovarian tumors: Predictability of tumor type. *AJR* 1983; 141:985–991.

87. Goswamy RK, Campbell S, Whitehead MI: Establishment of normal ranges for ovarian volumes and identification of enlarged ovaries by real-time mechanical sector sonar in postmenopausal women, in Lerski RA, Marley P (eds): *Ultrasound 82* Proceedings of the Third Meeting of the World Federation of Ultrasound in Medicine and Biology. Oxford, Pergamon Press, 1983, pp 615–619.

88. Goswamy RK, Campbell S, Whitehead MI: Screening for ovarian cancer. *Clin Obstet Gynaecol* 1983; 10:621–643.

89. Scammon RE: The prenatal growth and natal involution of the human uterus. *Proc Soc Exp Biol Med* 1926; 23:687–690.

90. Krantz KE, Phillips WP: Anatomy of the human uterine cervix. *Ann NY Acad Sci* 1962; 97:551–563.

91. Kangarloo H, Sarti DA, Sample WF: Ultrasound of the pediatric pelvis. *Semin Ultrasound* 1980; 1:51–60.

92. Colle M, Calabet A, Sanciaume C, et al: Contribution of pelvic ultrasonography (P.U.S.) to endocrine investigations in girls. *Pediatr Res* 1984; 18:113.

93. Hricak H, Lieto RP: Sonographic determination of renal volume. *Radiology* 1983; 148:311–312.

94. Jones TB, Price RR, Gibbs SJ: Volumetric determination of placental and uterine growth relationships with B-mode ultrasound by serial area-volume determination. *Invest Radiol* 1981; 16:101–106.

95. Geirsson RT, Christie AD, Patel N: Ultrasound volume measurements comparing a prolate ellipsoid method with a parallel planimetric area method against a known volume. *J Clin Ultrasound* 1982; 10:329–332.

96. Jones TB, Riddick LR, Harpen MD, et al: Ultrasonographic determination of renal mass and renal volume. *J Ultrasound Med* 1983; 2:151–154.

97. Kurtz AB, Shaw WM, Kurtz RJ, et al: The inaccuracy of total uterine volume measurements: Sources of error and a proposed solution. *J Ultrasound Med* 1984; 3:289–297.

98. Kurtz AB, Kurtz RJ, Rifkin MD, et al: Total uterine volume: A new graph and its clinical applications. *J Ultrasound Med* 1984; 3:299–308.

99. Langlois PL: The size of the normal uterus. *J Reprod Med* 1970; 4:221–226.

100. Jouppila P: Ultrasound in the diagnosis of early pregnancy and its complications. *Acta Obstet Gynecol Scand [Suppl]* 1971; 50:15.

101. Zemlyn S: The length of the uterine cervix and its significance. *J Clin Ultrasound* 1981; 9:267–269.

102. Piiroinen O: The use of ultrasound in diagnosis. *Acta Obstet Gynecol Scand* 1975; 46:1–60.

103. Hertig A, Gore H: Female genitalia, in Anderson WAD (ed): *Pathology*, ed 6. St Louis, CV Mosby, 1971, p 1489.

104. Woodburne RT: *Essentials of Human Anatomy*. New York, Oxford University Press, 1970.

105. Moorehead RP: *Human Pathology*. New York, McGraw-Hill Book Co, 1975.

106. Blaustein A (ed): *Pathology of the Female Genital Tract*, ed 2. New York, Springer-Verlag, 1977.

107. Platt JF, Bree RL, Davidson D: Ultrasound of the normal non-gravid uterus: correlation with gross and histopathology. *J Clin Ultrasound* 1990; 18:15–19.

108. Piiroinen O, Kaihola HL: Uterine size measured by ultrasound during the menstrual cycle. *Acta Obstet Gynecol Scand* 1975; 54:247–250.

109. Lavery J, Shaw L: Sonography of the puerperal pelvis. *Ultrasound Med* 1989; 8:481–486.

110. Siegler AM: *Hysterosalpingography*, ed 2. New York, Medcom Press, 1974.

111. Callen PW, DeMartini WJ, Filly RA: The central uterine cavity echo: A useful anatomic sign in the ultrasonographic evaluation of the female pelvis. *Radiology* 1979; 131:187–190.

112. Farrer-Brown G, Beilby J: The blood supply of the uterus. 2. Venous pattern. *J Obstet Gynecol Br Commw*, 1970; 77:682.

113. Fleischer AC, Mendelson EB, Bohn-Velex M, et al: Transvaginal and transabdominal sonography of the endometrium. *Semin Ultrasound CT MRI* 1988; 9:81–101.

114. Sakamoto C, Nakano H: The echogenic endometrium and alterations during menstrual cycle. *Int J Gynaecol Obstet* 1982; 20:255–259.

115. Fleischer AC, Pittaway DE, Beard LA, et al: Sonographic depiction of endometrial changes occurring with ovulation induction. *J Ultrasound Med* 1984; 3:341–346.

116. Duffield SE, Picker RH: Ultrasonic evaluation of the uterus in the normal mentrual cycle. *Med Ultrasound* 1981; 5:70–74.

117. Fleischer AC, Kalemeris GC, Entman SS: Sonographic depiction of the endometrium during normal cycles. *Ultrasound Med Biol* 1986; 12:271–277.

118. Sakamoto C: Sonographic criteria of phasic changes in human endometrial tissue. *Int J Gynaecol Obstet* 1985; 23:7–12.

119. Johnson MA, Graham MF, Cooperberg PL: Abnormal endometrial echoes: Sonographic spectrum of endometrial pathology. *J Ultrasound Med* 1982; 1:161–166.

120. Fleischer AC: Personal communication, 1987.

121. Glissant A, de Mouzon J, Frydman R: Ultrasound study of the endometrium during in vitro fertilization cycles. *Fertil Steril* 1985; 44:786–790.

122. Rabinowitz R, Laufer N, Lewin A, et al: The value of ultrasonographic endometrial measurement in the prediction of pregnancy following *in vitro* fertilization. *Fertil Steril* 1986; 45:824.

123. Imoedemhe DAG, Shaw RW, Kirkland A, et al: Ultrasound measurement of endometrial thickness on different ovarian stimulation regimens during in-vitro fertilization. *Hum Reprod* 1987; 2:545–547.

124. Hackelöer BJ: Ultrasound screening of the ovarian cycle. *In Vitro Fertil Embryo Transfer* 1984; 1:217–220.

125. Thickman D, Arger P, Tureck R, et al: Sonographic assessment of the endometrium in patients undergoing in vitro fertilization. *J Ultrasound Med* 1986; 5:197–201.

126. Miller EI, Thomas RH, Lines P: The atrophic postmenopausal uterus. *J Clin Ultrasound* 1977; 5:261–263.

127. Van Dongen L: Ultrasonography of the cervix. *S Afr Med J* 1984; 65:82–85.

128. Asplund J: The uterine cervix and isthmus under normal and pathological condition; a clinical and roentgenological study. *Acta Radiol* 1952; 38(suppl 91).

129. Sweeney WJ III: The interstitial portion of the uterine tube: Its gross anatomy course and length. *Obstet Gynecol* 1962; 19:3.

130. Kurtz AB, Rifkin MD: Normal anatomy of the female pelvis, in Sanders RC, James AE, (eds): *The Principles and Practice of Ultrasonography and Gynecology*, ed 3. Norwalk, Conn, Appleton-Century-Crofts, 1985; p 118.

131. Sample WF: Gray scale ultrasonography of the normal female pelvis, in Sanders RC, James AE (eds): *The Principles and Practice of Ultrasonography in Obstetrics and Gynecology*, ed 2. Norwalk, Conn, Appleton-Century-Crofts, 1980, pp 75–89.

132. Hricak H, Chang YCCF, Thurnher S: Vagina: Evaluation with MR imaging. Part I. Normal anatomy and congenital anomalies. *Radiology* 1988; 169:169–174.

PART VI

First Trimester Obstetrical Measurements

Chapter 20

Uterine Length
Alfred B. Kurtz, M.D.
Barry B. Goldberg, M.D.

Articles have been published describing the increase in size of the overall uterine length and the greatest anteroposterior (AP) diameter of the uterine fundus from 6 to 20 gestational weeks.[1-4] The measurements were performed on bistable equipment. Although the exact measurement points were not discussed, in general the uterine length increased from 8.5 cm at 6 weeks to 11 cm at 10 weeks to 13 cm at 12 weeks, while the AP diameter increased from 5 cm at 6 weeks to 6 cm at 10 weeks to 7 cm at 12 weeks.

The articles proposed that these measurements provided an accurate evaluation of the early gestational period with a variation of plus or minus slightly more than 1 week.[4] Two other first trimester measurements, the gestational sac and crown-rump length, however, have been more extensively evaluated and have been shown to have the same or greater accuracy. Uterine size measurements are therefore not necessary. In addition, measurements of the uterus are only an indirect evaluation of the growing fetus and could be very inaccurate if uterine masses are present.

REFERENCES

1. Hellman LF, Kobayashi M, Fillisti L, et al: Growth and development of the human fetus prior to the twentieth week of gestation. *Am J Obstet Gynecol* 1969; 103:784–800.
2. Hoffbauer H: The importance of ultrasonic diagnosis in early pregnancy. *Electromedia* 1970; 3:227–230.
3. Piiroinen O: Studies in diagnostic ultrasound. *Acta Obstet Gynecol Scand [Suppl]* 1975; 55:1–60.
4. Jouppila PC: Length and depth of the uterus and the diameter of the gestation sac in normal gravidas during early pregnancy. *Acta Obstet Gynecol Scand* 1971; 50(suppl 15):29–31.

Chapter 21

Gestational Sac

Alfred B. Kurtz, M.D.

Barry B. Goldberg, M.D.

The gestational sac from 5 to 13 gestational weeks has been evaluated in six articles.[1-6] Five articles used linear measurements, two with actual numbers[2,4] and three in graph form.[1,3,5] The sixth article[6] gave gestational sac volumes in numeric form with the volume obtained by taking parallel scans at 0.5- to 1.0-cm intervals. A planimeter was used to calculate the area of each scan, with the areas then added together to obtain a volume. No article adequately stated the landmarks used in measuring the gestational sac. In addition, the linear measurement articles failed to state whether an average diameter or the longest diameter of the gestational sac was used. This is important since the linear measurement articles do not take into account the potential effect that a distended urinary bladder would have on the shape of the sac, usually changing its shape from round to ovoid or less commonly to the shape of a teardrop (Figs 21–1 to 21–4). Only an average linear or a volume measurement would compensate for this distortion.

The overall accuracy of this method has been studied by one group and found to be approximately ±1 week.[4] While not substantiated, if correct it would be slightly better than uterine size but inferior to crown-rump length measurements. The measurement is still valuable, however, particularly in the early part of the first trimester. By transabdominal approach, the gestational sac can be routinely imaged by 5 weeks while the crown-rump length is frequently not seen until the seventh week. Although not completely studied, it seems that endovaginal imaging will permit routine identification of the gestational sac and crown-rump length at least 1 week earlier (Fig 21–5).

An average linear measurement seems to be as accurate as a volume measurement and is therefore preferable since it is less cumbersome to obtain. It is recommended that this measurement be performed from inner edge to inner edge. If the sac is round, only one measurement is needed (see Fig 21–1). If ovoid or teardrop-shaped, three measurements are obtained and averaged (see Fig 21–2 to 21–4). Two of these measurements are taken from the long axis of the uterus, the length and the AP dimension perpendicular to the length. By turning into a transaxial projection at the point of the AP dimension, the width measurement is obtained. It is recommended that the measurements obtained from the endovaginal approach, while oriented differently, be similarly performed (Figs 21–5, 21–6).

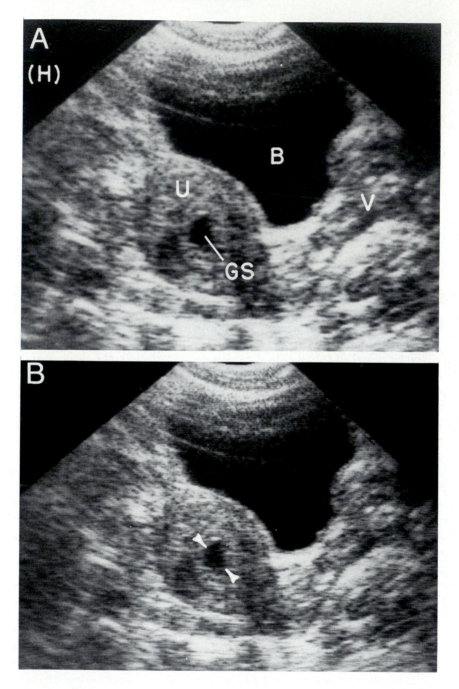

FIG 21–1.
A, long-axis ultrasound image of a round gestational sac (*GS*) within the uterus (*U*) at 5 weeks. Since the sac is round, only one measurement is needed. **B,** same image as **A**. *Arrowheads* denote inner edges of rounded sac to be measured. *V* = vagina; *B* = maternal bladder; (*H*) = toward patient's head.

TABLE 22–1.
Crown-Rump L[...]

Mean Predicte Crown-Rump Length (mm)
6.7
7.4
8.0
8.7
9.5
10.2
11.0
11.8
12.6
13.5
14.4
15.3
16.3
17.3
18.3
19.3
20.4
21.5
22.6
23.8
25.0
26.2
27.4
28.7
30.0
31.3
32.7

*From Robins[...]
measuremen[...]
†Values deriv[...]

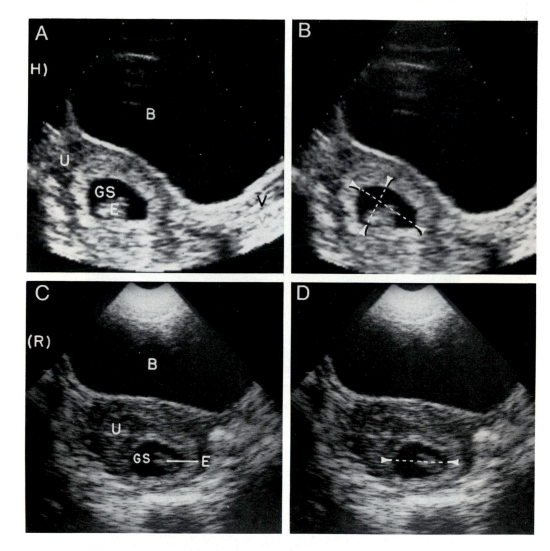

FIG 21–2.
Ultrasound images of an 8-week pregnancy within an ovoid gestational sac (*GS*). **A**, long-axis scan showing the uterus (*U*) with a living embryo (*E*) within the gestational sac. **B**, same image as **A** showing the length measurement (*arrowheads* and *dotted line* along the long axis of the uterus) and the AP measurement (*arrowheads* and *dotted line*) perpendicular to the length. **C**, transaxial scan taken perpendicular to the point where the AP measurement was obtained. Within the uterus (*U*) is the gestational sac (*GS*) containing the living embryo (*E*). **D**, same image as **C** showing the width measurement (*arrowheads* and *dotted line*). *B* = maternal bladder; *V* = vagina; (*H*) = toward patient's head; (*R*) = toward patient's right.

and occasionally ear[...]
heart motion (Fig 22-[...]
however, by 9 to 10[...]
imaging seems to pe[...]
22–3). All measure[...]
top of the head (cro[...]

The accuracy of[...]
Robinson and Flem[...]
with a 95% probabi[...]

Chapter 22

Crown-

Al

Ba

Initial work in 197:
evaluate fetal age i
gestational weeks
with known menstr
was found with an
and Fleming[2] and
five of the six articl
obtained their me
fetus was accepted
was initially felt t
with measuremer
age.[2]

All of the earli
small fetal size an
that a high degre
static scanning. 1
study[9] proposed
obtained withoul
fetal measureme
week in 75% of

More recent
curacy, easier to
used. Static ima
ularly when an
time facilitates
measurements.
from real-time (
They felt that th
sion analysis sh
of fetal dating
regression anal
proach, the cr(

254

REFERENCES

1. Robinson HP: Sonar measurement of fetal crown-rump length as means of assessing maturity of first trimester of pregnancy. *Br Med J* 1973; 4:28–31.
2. Robinson HP, Fleming JEE: A critical evaluation of sonar "crown-rump length" measurements. *Br J Obstet Gynaecol* 1975; 82:702–710.
3. Drumm JE, Clinch J, MacKenzie G: The ultrasonic measurement of fetal crown-rump length as a method of assessing gestational age. *Br. J Obstet Gynecol* 1976; 83:417–421.
4. Kurjak A, Cecuk S, Breyer B: Prediction of maturity in first trimester of pregnancy by ultrasonic measurement of fetal crown-rump length. *J Clin Ultrasound* 1976; 4:83–84.
5. Hoffbauer H, Pachaly J, Arabin B, et al: Control of fetal development with multiple ultrasonic body measures. *Contrib Gynecol Obstet* 1979; 6:147–156.
6. Pedersen JF: Fetal crown-rump length measurement by ultrasound in normal pregnancy. *Br J Obstet Gynaecol* 1982; 89:926–930.
7. Parker AJ: Assessment of gestational age of the Asian fetus by the sonar measurement of crown-rump length and biparietal diameter. *Br J Obstet Gynaecol* 1982; 89:836–838.
8. Drumm JE: The prediction of delivery date by ultrasonic measurement of fetal crown-rump length. *Br J Obstet Gynaecol* 1977; 84:1–5.
9. Higginbottom J, Slater J, Porter G: Assessment of gestational age in the first trimester of pregnancy by maximum fetal diameter. *Ultrasound Med Biol* 1977; 3:47–51.
10. Parker AJ, Docker MF, Davies P, et al: The reproducibility of fetal crown rump length measurements obtained with real time ultrasound systems compared with those of a conventional B-scanner. *Br J Obstet Gynaecol* 1981; 88:734–738.
11. Sande HA, Reiertsen O: Crown rump length: A comparison of real time scanning and conventional compound scanning. The interindividual measuring variation between two operators. *Ultrasound Med Biol* 1979; 5:279–281.
12. Adam AH, Robinson HP, Dunlop C: A comparison of crown-rump length measurements using a real-time scanner in an antenatal clinic and a conventional B-scanner. *Br J Obstet Gynaecol* 1979; 86:521–524.
13. Deter RL, Harrist RB, Hadlock FP, et al: Longitudinal studies of fetal growth with the use of dynamic image ultrasonography. *Am J Obstet Gynecol* 1982; 143:545.
14. Deter RL, Harrist RB, Hadlock FP, et al: The use of ultrasound in the assessment of normal fetal growth: A review. *J Clin Ultrasound* 1981; 9:481–493.
15. Nelson LH: Comparison of methods for determining crown-rump measurement by real-time ultrasound. *J Clin Ultrasound* 1981; 9:67–70.
16. Chervenak FA, Brightman RC, Thornton J, et al: Crown-rump length and serum human chorionic gonadotropin as predictors of gestational age. *Obstet Gynecol* 1986; 67:210–213.
17. Smazal SF, Weisman LE, Hoppler KD, et al: Comparative analysis of ultrasonographic methods of gestational age assessment. *J Ultrasound Med* 1983; 2:147–150.
18. Kopta MM, May RR, Crane JP: A comparison of the reliability of the estimated data of confinement predicted by crown-rump length and biparietal diameter. *Am J Obstet Gynecol* 1983; 145:562–565.
19. Selbing A, Fjallbrant B: Accuracy of conceptual age estimation from fetal crown-rump length. *J Clin Ultrasound* 1984; 12:343–346.
20. van de Velde EHE, Broeders GHB, Horbach JGM, Esser-Rath VWCJ: Estimation of pregnancy duration by means of ultrasonic measurements of the fetal crown-rump length. *Europ J Obstet Gynecol Reprod Biol* 1980; 10:225–230.
21. Bovicelli L, Orsini LF, Rizzo N, et al: Estimation of gestational age during the first trimester by real-time measurement of fetal crown-rump length and biparietal diameter. *J Clin Ultrasound* 1981; 9:71–75.
22. Selbing A: Ultrasound in first trimester shows no difference in fetal size between the sexes. *Br Med J* 1985; 290:750.
23. Dubowitz LMS, Goldberg C: Assessment of gestation by ultrasound in various stages of pregnancy in infants differing in size and ethnic origin. *Br J Obstet Gynaecol* 1981; 88:255–259.
24. Pedersen JF: Ultrasound evidence of sexual difference in fetal size in first trimester. *Br Med J* 1980; 281:1253.
25. Pedersen LM, Tygstrup I, Pedersen J: Congenital malformations in newborn infants of diabetic women. *Lancet* 1964; 1:1124–1126.

26. Tchobroutsky C, Breart GL, Rambaud DC, et al: Correlation between fetal defects and early growth delay observed by ultrasound. *Lancet* 1985; 1:706–707.

27. Berger GS, Edelman DA, Kerenyi TD: Fetal crown-rump length and biparietal diameter in the second trimester of pregnancy. *Am J Obstet Gynecol* 1975; 122:9–12.

28. Campbell S, Warsof SL, Little D, et al: Routine ultrasound screening for the prediction of gestational age. *Obstet Gynecol* 1985; 65:613–620.

Chapter 23

Trunk Circumference
Alfred B. Kurtz, M.D.
Barry B. Goldberg, M.D.

Recently Reece et al.[1] measured the circumference of the fetal trunk from 7 to 12 weeks in both number and graph form using real-time ultrasound. The trunk circumference was obtained from the transaxial image at a point just caudad to the cardiac pulsation by taking the average abdominal diameter times π. Comparison was then made to crown-rump lengths obtained in the same study. Both were similar in their prediction of gestational age. When combined, the accuracy did not increase. Therefore while this is a new and interesting first trimester measurement, the much more thoroughly studied crown-rump length is still recommended.

REFERENCE

1. Reece EA, Scioscia AL, Green J, et al: Embryonic trunk circumference: A new biometric parameter for estimation of gestational age. *Am J Obstet Gynecol* 1987; 156:713–715.

PART VII

Second and Third Trimester Obstetrical Measurements

Chapter 24

Fetal Head Measurements

Alfred B. Kurtz, M.D.

Barry B. Goldberg

BIPARIETAL DIAMETER

The biparietal diameter (BPD) is one of the most discussed and documented obstetrical ultrasound measurements. Starting as far back as 1964, in utero BPDs were compared to caliper measurements of the newborn head. Similar results were obtained.[1-7] These studies were performed using A-mode alone,[1-4] a combination of A-mode and bistable B-mode,[5, 6] and gray-scale B-mode alone.[7] While there were slight discrepancies, all modalities showed an equal accuracy with no method superior. In general, more than 90% of the cases were only ±2 mm apart, with some variations approaching 4 to 5 mm. Ultrasound and caliper measurements of the heads of aborted fetuses were also compared and found to be less than 3 mm different.[8] There were inherent errors, however, in scanning aborted fetuses, including the collapse of the fetal skull.

Despite the close correlation of fetal to newborn head measurements, inaccuracies exist among in utero ultrasound studies. These inaccuracies can be subdivided into those created by inability of observers to measure consistently, errors caused by failure to image the head in the correct anatomic plane, and errors in instrumentation. A number of articles have discussed observers' inability to measure consistently.[5, 9-14] These studies were performed using A-mode, a combination of A-mode and bistable B-mode, and gray-scale B-mode, including real-time. The smallest measurement error found in any series was by Campbell[5] where a standard deviation of ±0.25 mm was obtained between scans. This is surprisingly low. Cooperberg et al.[13] showed a standard deviation of ±0.69 to 0.91 mm. The remainder of the standard deviations were higher with errors approaching 2% per reading,[12] ultrasound "experts" having a smaller error than trainees.[14] The two best-controlled studies[9, 10] found that paired readings (two readings 15 minutes apart) had an average error of 1.53 mm. When three BPD readings were taken during any one examination, a standard deviation of ±1.21 mm was obtained. If the measurements were taken either 24 hours or 4 weeks apart, the standard deviation increased to ±2.54 mm. Real-time ultrasound equipment was determined to be easier to use and as accurate as static scanners.[11, 13] When a single observer performed all the measurements, accuracy seemed better than when measurements were performed by different ob-

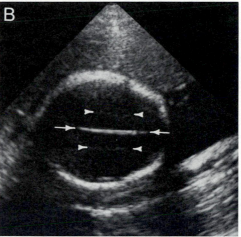

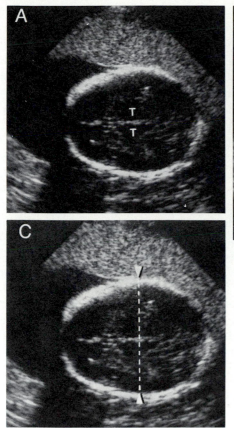

FIG 24–1.
Transaxial (BPD) ultrasound images of a late second trimester fetus. **A,** scan taken at the level of the thalami (*T*). The thalami are imaged in the midline, equidistant from the lateral walls (parietal tables) of the calvarium. **B,** scan taken more cephalad at the level of the falx midline echo (*arrows*) and bodies of the lateral ventricles (*arrowheads*). **C,** same image as **A** showing the outer edge to inner edge (leading edge to leading edge) measurement, denoted by *arrowheads* and *dotted line.*

servers.[10, 11] From these articles it can be appreciated that an error is introduced every time a measurement is taken. While this error is minimized if the observer is skilled and also if the same observer performs all the measurements, an error of as little as 1 mm and as much as 2 mm occurs with each examination. When interval measurements are taken, the error could double and approach 4 mm.

Technical factors involved in measuring the fetal head in the correct anatomic plane were also evaluated with static and real-time equipment. Using both A-mode and B-mode on aborted fetuses, Watmough et al.[15] showed that the imaging of a midline echo alone was not sufficient to obtain an accurate BPD measurement. Instead they showed that scanning at various angles, even if a midline echo were still imaged, caused the BPD to vary by as much as 19 mm. Therefore, Johnson et al.,[16] using gray-scale equipment, recommended that transaxial scans (BPDs) be performed at the thalamus at the level of the thalamobasal ganglia (Fig 24–1,A). If scans were taken at a slightly more cephalad level, at the bodies of the lateral ventricles, the BPDs were found to be smaller on an average of 3 mm with a range of 0 to 9 mm (Fig 24–1,B). Shepard and Filly[17] further refined the anatomic positions at the thalamus and brain stem to take the optimum BPD measurements. They found that an image taken at either the level of the third ventricle with the quadrigeminal cisterns or at the top third ventricle (with visualization of the cavum septi pellucidi) were highly consistent, with correlation coefficients to the maternal age of greater than .99 (Fig 24–2). Similarly, Hadlock et al.[18] found that the maximum measurements of BPD, fronto-occipital diameter (FOD), and head circumference should all be obtained at the same level, at the level of the thalamus and the cavum septi pellucidi. More cephalad images decreased the BPD measurement from 0 to 9 mm while more caudad images gave a decreased measurement of 0 to 10 mm.

Errors in instrumentation include the machine calibration for velocity of sound, the amplification settings (power or gain), and the type of B-mode ultrasound imager, that is, bistable or gray-scale, static or real-time. The calibrated velocity of sound to which the machine is set varies in different countries. It can be corrected by a simple ratio of that velocity divided by the standard (1540 m/sec) used in most countries, including the United States and Canada. The machine amplification settings are also important.[19] As the amplification is increased, the calvarial echoes artifactually widen, increasing from 1 to 2 mm at low settings to 3 to 5 mm at medium settings to 6 to 10 mm at high settings. This is of particular importance if outer to outer BPD measurements are used since the widening of both calvarial echoes will increase the measurement. Most tables, however, use outer to inner measurements (leading edge to leading edge), which avoids this error (see Fig 24–1,A and C). Nevertheless, medium amplification settings are still recommended since it is difficult to find the exact points to measure when high amplification is used, and the medium amplification settings correlated best with the true BPD measurements of neonates.[19] Lastly, the evaluation of different types of ultrasound imagers, B-mode, bistable or gray-scale, static or real-time, has been studied.[11, 13, 19] All have been found to be equally accurate. It is recommended, however, that real-time gray-scale B-mode equipment be used because of the ability of even inexperienced observers to obtain accurate reproducible results, comparable to the expert examiner.[11]

The accuracy of BPD measurements in predicting gestational age continues to be of major importance. While it had been stated that a crown-rump length measurement obtained from 7 to 13 weeks was the most accurate for establishing fetal age,[20] recent articles have shown that the BPD measurement between 20 and 24 weeks has comparable accuracy.[21–23] Therefore, the first and second trimester measurements taken from an early crown-rump length at 7 weeks to a biparietal diameter at 24 weeks are of equal accuracy, equivalent to ±5 to 7 days with close correlation to maternal dating when accurate menstrual history is known.[22, 23] Campbell[24] and Sabbagha et al.[25] even felt that this accuracy could be extended to 30 gestational weeks.

Later on in the pregnancy, in the third trimester, the BPD becomes more inaccurate in predicting gestational age. Some observers have stated that these inaccuracies approach ±3 to $3^{1}/_{2}$ weeks at term.[17, 26, 27] If these stated inaccuracies at term are correct, potential errors would be quite extensive, resulting in an equal probability that a fetus at 37 weeks could be either 34 or 40 weeks. At the present time, this observation of inaccuracy at term is not substantiated by all observers. In an article by Wiener et al.[28] the standard deviation of the BPD was evaluated from 15 weeks to term in six works (five previous articles and their own). In two of these studies, the standard deviation increased toward term. In two others, however, the standard deviation did not significantly increase, and in the last two, the standard

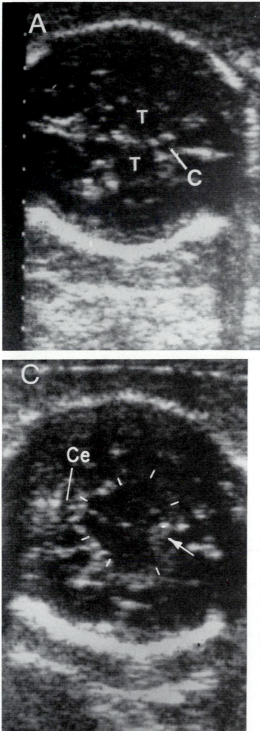

FIG 24–2.
Transaxial (BPD) ultrasound images of a mid–third trimester fetus. These three levels are all acceptable for obtaining a correct measurement, provided that the thalami or midbrain structures are imaged equidistant from the lateral walls (parietal tables) of the calvarium. **A**, at the level of the upper thalami (*T*). **B**, at the level of the mid- to lower thalami (*arrows*). *Arrowheads* denote slitlike third ventricle. **C**, at the level of the midbrain (denoted by *lines*). Note the heart or arrow-shaped appearance, with point aimed posteriorly toward the cerebellum (*Ce*). Arrow denotes anterior surface of midbrain. C = cavum septi pellucidi.

deviation significantly decreased toward term. Similarly, another article showed that while the BPD variation was greater in the third trimester, a variation of only ±2 weeks was observed up to 33 weeks.[22] Although not exactly comparable, this variation of ±2 weeks continued to term when a range of 90% of the average measurements was compared in 17 tables.[29] In addition, despite all these reported inaccuracies in the use of the BPD, two articles analyzing multiple fetal parameters in the second and third trimesters found that the head measurements, and in particular the BPD, were the most reliable indicators of gestational age.[30, 31]

To date, there have been 60 published comparisons of BPD to gestational age. Of these, 31 compared a single BPD measurement in millimeters to a single gestational age in weeks.[12, 26, 32–60] (Two of these presented only graphs in their original articles, namely, Hellman et al.[32] and Garrett and Robinson,[52] with the numbers subsequently published by Kurtz et al.[29]). An additional article by Wladimiroff et al.[38] presented a graph that appeared identical to the graph that accompanied the numbers by Wladimiroff et al.[37] and therefore will not be discussed further.

Of the 30 remaining articles,[12, 26, 32–37,39–60] all showed an increase in the BPD as the gestation progressed toward term (17 of these studies are shown in figure 1 of Kurtz et al.[29]). Twenty-six evaluated the second and third trimesters, with two[33, 34] analyzing only the second trimester and two[42, 43] evaluating only the third. There was an equal distribution of the BPD, evaluated by A-mode, B-mode, or a combination of the two. The calculated velocity of the sound of the ultrasound machine was known in 26 articles and not discussed in the other four.[48–50, 57] The outer to inner diameter was used to measure the fetal head in 25 articles, the outer to outer diameter used in only four,[33, 35, 41, 52] with no discussion of where the measurements were taken in one.[57]

Twenty-four of the 60 articles compared the BPD to gestational age in graph form.[3, 8, 24, 25, 31, 61–79] Seventeen of these 24 studies evaluated the BPD in both the second and third trimesters with the other seven analyzing the third trimester only. While it is difficult to accurately extrapolate curves back to their original numbers and to compare these numbers to the previous 30 articles in table form, 17 of the graphs were within the range of these 30 articles, 5 were consistently high,[3, 24, 31, 64, 65] and two were consistently low.[63, 73]

Four of the above articles in graph form evaluated pregnant diabetic women.[71–74] Two of these,[71, 72] while not specifically stating the severity of the diabetes, found no difference in BPD growth throughout the second and third trimesters. The other two articles,[73, 74] one evaluating class A to C diabetics and the other class A to D diabetics, found no difference in BPD growth from 13 to 38 weeks. After that time, the BPD was observed to increase more than the normal nondiabetic group.

At least part of the variation in BPD measurements is due to biologic growth that occurs normally in any single population group.[80] Studies on different ethnic and racial groups and between the sexes are limited, but in general do not show marked differences. Two studies suggested that female fetuses were only slightly smaller than male fetuses, with the difference increasing toward term both in BPD[77, 81] and in head circumference.[77] While most of the information was in graph form, numbers given at 36 weeks for males and females revealed a minimal difference with overlap in BPD measurements of 90.6 ±3.1 mm versus 88.2 ±4.0 mm respectively.[77] Ethnic and racial studies have shown varied results. Four studies found no significant difference in head size either of black versus white fetuses[58] or of mixed groups,[82–84] although Dubowitz and Goldberg[83] and Okupe et al.[85] did show a slight shift of blacks toward the upper end of the normal curve after 34 and 38 weeks, respectively. Munoz et al.[86] showed the reverse—a decrease in BPD of blacks (Zulus) after 34 weeks when compared to whites. This study is suspect, however, since the authors failed to take into account fetal head shape even though the newborn head circumference and birth weight of both groups were similar. Others have found small differences. Walton[78] compared Polynesian to white fetuses in New Zealand and found a slight but consistent difference. On average, the Polynesian BPDs measured 1.89 mm greater throughout the second and third trimester. Osefo and Chukudebelu[56] compared BPD measurements of Nigerian fetuses to measurements from previous articles and found them to have, on average, 4-mm smaller BPDs from 20 weeks to term. While more work is clearly needed in this area, it is surprising how close the BPD measurements are in different racial and ethnic groups.

A newer approach to correlating BPD with gestational age has been proposed. Because of the variations outlined above, it would be unlikely that a specific BPD could ever be anticipated to equal a specific gestational age. Rather, a BPD number would be expected to encompass a range of gestational ages. Although the midpoint would be slightly more probable, the fetus would be equally likely to be anywhere within that range. This has been termed a range table where a BPD represents a range in days or weeks. This type of study was performed in the remaining five of the 60 articles.[17, 23, 28, 29, 87] Of these Kurtz et al.[29] is a compilation of 17 previous articles comprising more than 10,000 patients and 27,000 measurements. This table evaluated the average numbers from other tables and included 90% of their variation. The other four range tables used much smaller numbers and were compiled in their home institutions. One of these, Kopta et al.,[23] did not state their confidence limits, while the other three used limits of 95% in two,[17, 28] and 66% in one series.[87]

In comparing these range tables, the range would be expected to be narrowest in the table with the largest number of measurements. The Kurtz et al. table[29] should therefore have the narrowest range. This was found to be true with all except the comparison to the Kopta et al. article[23] between 40 and 80 mm in diameters. Since the confidence limits were not shown on this last table, it is difficult to make an adequate evaluation. In addition, the ranges of two of the other three tables did not entirely overlap. While Shepard and Filly's[17] upper limits were always outside those of the Kurtz et al. (as would be expected since fewer measurements were used), their lower limits were slightly above those of Kurtz et al., from a BPD of 46 to 88 mm. Similarly, while the Sabbagha range table[87] had a larger range, the range was uniformly lower from 85 mm to term. Despite these discrepancies, it is felt that the Kurtz et al. range table should be used when comparing BPD to gestational age (Table 24–1). In addition to the range, the average number of weeks was calculated from the equation and is also included for each BPD measurement.

The most frequent use of the BPD measurement is in gestational age estimation. The BPD can also be used to evaluate whether the head is too large or too small. If another fetal measurement (independent of the BPD) or the last menstrual period is known, the head can be established as normal, large, or small for gestational age. When fetal head enlargement is present, it is almost always secondary to hydrocephalus. This is a relatively straightforward diagnosis since dilated lateral ventricles can be easily imaged in utero. A small fetal head, termed microcephaly, however, is a much more complicated topic and will be discussed under ratios of the head and body.

TABLE 24–1.
Composite Biparietal Diameter Table*

Biparietal Diameter (mm)	Gestational Age (wk)		Biparietal Diameter (mm)	Gestational Age (wk)	
	Mean[†]	Range (90% Variation)[‡]		Mean[†]	Range (90% Variation)[‡]
20	12.0	12.0			
21	12.0	12.0	61	24.2	22.6–25.8
22	12.7	12.2–13.2	62	24.6	23.1–26.1
23	13.0	12.4–13.6	63	24.9	23.4–26.4
24	13.2	12.6–13.8	64	25.3	23.8–26.8
25	13.5	12.9–14.1	65	25.6	24.1–27.1
26	13.7	13.1–14.3	66	26.0	24.5–27.5
27	14.0	13.4–14.6	67	26.4	25.0–27.8
28	14.3	13.6–15.0	68	26.7	25.3–28.1
29	14.5	13.9–15.2	69	27.1	25.8–28.4
30	14.8	14.1–15.5	70	27.5	26.3–28.7
31	15.1	14.3–15.9	71	27.9	26.7–29.1
32	15.3	14.5–16.1	72	28.3	27.2–29.4
33	15.6	14.7–16.5	73	28.7	27.6–29.8
34	15.9	15.0–16.8	74	29.1	28.1–30.1
35	16.2	15.2–17.2	75	29.5	28.5–30.5
36	16.4	15.4–17.4	76	30.0	29.0–31.0
37	16.7	15.6–17.8	77	30.3	29.2–31.4
38	17.0	15.9–18.1	78	30.8	29.6–32.0
39	17.3	16.1–18.5	79	31.1	29.9–32.5
40	17.6	16.4–18.8	80	31.6	30.2–33.0
41	17.9	16.5–19.3	81	32.1	30.7–33.5
42	18.1	16.6–19.8	82	32.6	31.2–34.0
43	18.4	16.8–20.2	83	33.0	31.5–34.5
44	18.8	16.9–20.7	84	33.4	31.9–35.1
45	19.1	17.0–21.2	85	34.0	32.3–35.7
46	19.4	17.4–21.4	86	34.3	32.8–36.2
47	19.7	17.8–21.6	87	35.0	33.4–36.6
48	20.0	18.2–21.8	88	35.4	33.9–37.1
49	20.3	18.6–22.0	89	36.1	34.6–37.6
50	20.6	19.0–22.2	90	36.6	35.1–38.1
51	20.9	19.3–22.5	91	37.2	35.9–38.5
52	21.2	19.5–22.9	92	37.8	36.7–38.9
53	21.5	19.8–23.2	93	38.8	37.3–39.3
54	21.9	20.1–23.7	94	39.0	37.9–40.1
55	22.2	20.4–24.0	95	39.7	38.5–40.9
56	22.5	20.7–24.3	96	40.6	39.1–41.5
57	22.8	21.1–24.5	97	41.0	39.9–42.1
58	23.2	21.5–24.9	98	41.8	40.5–43.1
59	23.5	21.9–25.1			
60	23.8	22.3–25.5			

*From Kurtz AB, Wapner RJ, Kurtz RJ, et al: *J Clin Ultrasound* 1980; 8:319–326. Used by permission.

[†]From weighted least mean square fit equation: $Y = -3.45701 + 0.50157x - 0.00441x^2$.

[‡]For each biparietal diameter, 90% of gestational age data points fell within this range.

UNUSUAL HEAD SHAPE: DETECTION AND CORRECTION FACTORS

The following are measurements used to evaluate and correct unusual head shapes: fronto-occipital diameter, cephalic index, "corrected" biparietal diameter.

The distance from the frontal to the occipital bone, termed the fronto-occipital diameter (FOD), is another measurement of the fetal head. It is measured in the transaxial view, on the same image that is used to obtain the biparietal diameter (BPD).[88] Nine articles have been published comparing the FOD to the BPD,[35, 44, 51, 52, 54, 55, 60, 89, 90] with one additional article comparing the FOD to menstrual age.[91] Since this last article did not compare the FOD to the BPD, it will not be discussed further. Of the remaining nine articles, five were performed on static scanners, three giving actual numbers,[35, 44, 90] with the other two in graph form.[89, 52] The other four were obtained with real-time images, all giving numbers.[51, 54, 55, 60] While one article evaluated the FOD only in the second trimester,[52] the others evaluated it in both the second and third trimesters. There are two shortcomings in these articles: (1) Although the aritcles described whether the BPD was obtained by an outer-to-outer or outer-to-inner measurement, only three articles stated where to measure the FOD, one using outer to outer measurements,[90] one outer to inner,[60] and the other middle to middle.[55] (2) Only three articles[51, 54, 90] described the internal head landmarks used to define the plane of section necessary to obtain these measurements, with one[90] using a plane of section at the level of the falx echo, slightly higher than the accepted level of the thalamus to obtain the measurements.

Notwithstanding these shortcomings, the main reason for obtaining the fronto-occipital measurement is to determine if the fetal head is correctly shaped. If it is, then a BPD is a valid measurement. If not, then another measurement of the fetal head should be substituted. The correct transaxial head shape can be computed from the BPD and the FOD by using the formula called the cephalic index (CI) (Table 24–2). An equally useful reason for obtaining the FOD is that the BPD and FOD can be used to calculate the "corrected" BPD (discussed in this section) and the head circumference (discussed in the next section).

This CI has been previously employed to evaluate the shape of the newborn head. In transaxial view, the head is usually ovoid. However, on occasion, it may be more rounded (brachycephaly) or more elongated (dolichocephaly or scaphocephaly). *Dorland's Illustrated Medical Dictionary* defines a normal CI as being between 75.9 and 81.[92] When the CI is below 75.9, the head is dolichocephalic. When the CI is greater than 81, the head is brachycephalic. Two studies on neonates using direct caliper measurements, one after cesarean section and the other 2 days after vaginal delivery,

---

TABLE 24–2.
Cephalic Index Formula*†

$$\text{Cephalic Index} = \frac{\text{short axis (biparietal diameter)}}{\text{long axis (fronto-occipital diameter)}} \times 100 = 78.3$$

Normal range
   At 1 SD = 74–83
   At 2 SD = 70–86

*Data from Hadlock FP, Deter RL, Carpenter RJ, et al: *AJR* 1981; 137:83–85.
†Measurements of short and long axis taken from outer to outer margins of head.

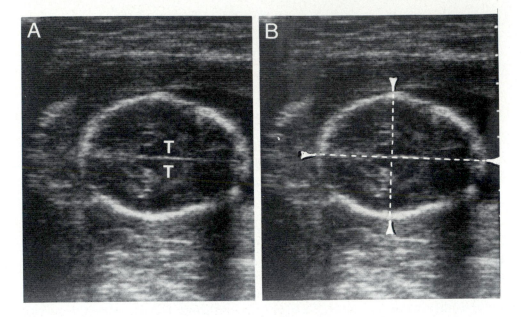

FIG 24–3.
Transaxial ultrasound image of a 32-week fetus. **A,** scan taken at the level of the thalami (*T*), the same level used to measure the BPD. **B,** same image as **A** showing the outer to outer measurements for both the short axis (BPD) and long axis (FOD). Measurements denoted by *arrowheads* and *dashed lines.*

revealed comparable numbers with a normal mean CI of 80 and a range of 75.6 to 85.0 at ±2 SD.[93, 94] The CI from radiographic evaluation of infants less than 4 weeks of age was somewhat higher, however, with a mean of 81.5 and a range of 79.4 to 85.7,[95] a finding attributed by the author to radiographic distortion of the breadth more than the length measurement.

Using real-time ultrasound, in two articles this same CI has been measured on fetuses between 14 and 42 gestational weeks.[96, 97] The measurements were taken in transaxial view from the widest transverse and longitudinal dimensions of the calvarium.[88, 96] In three articles, the optimum place to measure was at the level used to obtain the BPD, at the thalamus or upper part of the brain stem, in the region of the cavum septi pellucidi.[44, 51, 88] While the measurements are supposed to be taken from the outer margins of the calvarium for both the BPD and the FOD[96] (Fig 24–3), it is not certain that all observers adhered to this standard.[97] Instead, they may have used the standard BPD measurement of leading edge to leading edge, which makes the BPD approximately 2 to 3 mm smaller. This minor difference probably has no clinical significance.

The BPD, termed the "short axis," divided by the FOD, termed the "long axis," times 100 was found to be equal to 78.3 (see Table 24–2).[96] The range at 1 SD was 74 to 83 and at 2 SD was 70 to 86.[96] Almost identical results obtained by Shields et al.[97] showed a CI range of 59.3 to 89.5. The median was 78.8 with a 2-SD range of 68.4 to 89.2. These numbers are very similar to the neonatal measurements.[93, 94] It should be stressed that an abnormal CI does not, by itself, imply the head is abnormal. An "abnormal" shape only means that a correction measurement of the fetal head is needed and that careful evaluation of the internal fetal head anatomy should be performed (Fig 24–4). It has been found that fetal heads in normal breech presentation and following premature rupture of membranes with oligohydramnios are more likely to be dolichocephalic.[98, 99]

When the CIs were computed from the BPDs and FODs in the nine articles on FOD,[35, 44, 51, 52, 54, 55, 60, 89, 90] the numbers varied considerably. Levi and Erbsman[90] obtained a mean CI of 72 at 18 gestational weeks, gradually increasing to 77.8 by 38 weeks. Fescina et al.[51] and Jeanty et al.[54] detected a CI of 100 at 10 to 30 weeks, gradually decreasing to 79 to 80 by term. Hoffbauer et al.,[35] Hannsman,[44] Chevernak et al.,[55] and Persson and Weldner[60] obtained intermediate CIs varying from 79 to 88 throughout gestation while the mean CIs from the graphs[52, 89] ranged from 75 to 82.5.

The Hadlock et al.[96] CI numbers are recommended, because of their close correlation to the newborn CI. The numbers of Shields et al.[97] would have also been acceptable. The only question that remains is whether to use 1 SD between 74 and 83 or enlarge the range to encompass 2 SD between 70 and 86 (see Table 24–2). Hadlock et al.[96] gave both but recommended using only 1 SD, so that only two thirds of normal fetal heads would be encompassed within the normal range. While many

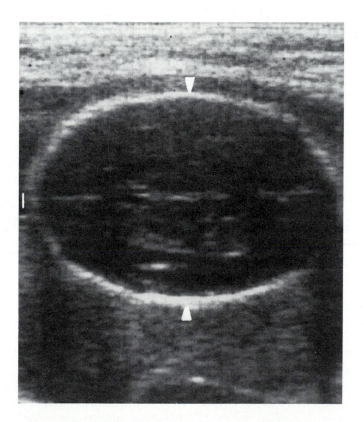

FIG 24–4.
Transaxial ultrasound image of an unusually ovoid fetal head at 30 gestational weeks. When the outer to outer dimension of the short axis (denoted by *arrowheads*) was compared to the same dimension of the long axis (denoted by *lines*), the CI was low at 68. The internal head anatomy was normal.

TABLE 24–3.
Corrected Biparietal Diameter (BPD)*

Area-corrected BPD (BPDa)

$$BPDa = \sqrt{(BPD \times FOD)/1.265}$$

*Data from Doubilet PM, Greenes RA: *AJR* 1984;
142:797–800.

normal cases (34%) fell outside the normal head shape range, it ensured that few, if any, abnormal head shapes would be missed. To make the ratio more clinically useful, however, it is recommended that 2 SD, encompassing 95% of normal cases, be used instead.

A possible new approach to the problem of unusual head shape has been recently proposed. When the FOD and BPD do not have the correct ratio, rather than employing a different head measurement such as circumference,[96] the head shape can be "corrected" so that each BPD is ideal for a CI of 78.3.[100] The formula proposed is termed the "area-corrected BPD" (Table 24–3). While this approach has theoretical appeal, further work will be necessary to prove its practical usefulness.

HEAD CIRCUMFERENCE

In the prediction of third trimester fetal age, the in utero measurement of head circumference has been found to be accurate to ±2 to 3 weeks.[96] Head circumference measurements have also been found to correlate closely with the true gestational age (±1 week) based on the menstrual history and postnatal evaluation.[101–103] In particular, the head circumference of premature infants has been found to correlate with, but be consistently higher by 1 cm than, the third trimester ultrasound examinations.[101–103] This overestimation is probably caused by the incorporation of the newborn soft tissues surrounding the calvarium into the circumference measurements. Ultrasound disregards these soft tissues and measures only the outer edge of the bone.

While a digitizer or map reader can be employed as the standard way of tracing the outer part of the calvarium to obtain a circumference (Fig 24–5), work had been performed using equations.[104–107] Initially, it was felt that multiplying the BPD by a factor of 3.5 would give a fairly accurate head circumference measurements.[104] Later, two well-controlled studies compared the head circumferences obtained by tracing the margins of the head with an electronic digitizer to those computed by the equation for a circumference (the average of the BPD and FOD, taken from the outer rims, multiplied by 1.57) (Table 24–4). One study found an insignificant mean error of, at most, 6% between these two methods at 2 SD.[105] The other found a small but constant overestimation in the head circumference, which was also not significant.[106]

DeVore and Platt[107] and Birnholz[108] pointed out that this formula was really a circumference measurement of a circle. They felt that this equation was not always accurate in obtaining measurements of ovoid fetal heads and compared it to equations which they claimed to be the true equations for an ellipse circumference. While the authors were correct in their statements that an equation of a circumference of a circle may not be precise, the equations that were chosen[107, 108] were not true ellipse circumference equations but only approximations and were not more accurate than

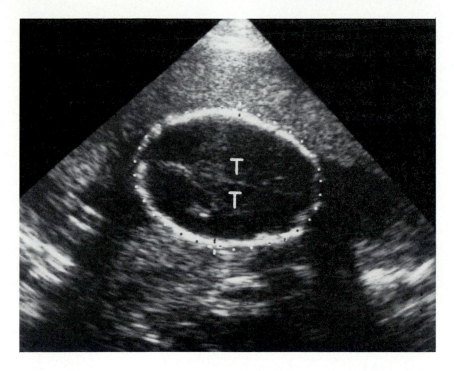

FIG 24–5.
Transaxial ultrasound image of a 28-week fetus. Scan taken at the level of the thalami (*T*), the same level used to measure the BPD. *Dotted line* denotes outer margin of calvarium used to calculate the head circumference with a digitizer or map reader.

the circle circumference equation.[106] In addition, DeVore and Platt[107] correctly recommended that a circle circumference equation be used until the CI fell below 70. Since the CI is unlikely to be below 70, the circle circumference equation will suffice in most instances and has been found to be as accurate as other proposed equations.[97, 106]

There are sixteen articles evaluating head circumference to gestational age.[31, 35, 51, 54, 55, 62, 90, 109–117] Ten give specific numbers,[35, 51, 54, 55, 90, 112–114, 116, 117] two of which were performed with static scanners[35, 90] and the rest with real-time scanners. The other six articles were given in graph form only[62, 109–111, 115] or as an equation only[31] and will not be discussed further. Since reference 112 is preliminary work by Athey and Hadlock with the more definitive work in Hadlock et al.,[113] the former will also not be discussed further. Since van Egmond-Linden et al.[117] gave numbers

---

TABLE 24–4.
Circumference Computations

1. Planimetry
2. Equation for a circle

$$\left(\frac{BPD + FOD}{2}\right) \pi = (BPD + FOD) \times 1.57$$

TABLE 24–5.
Head Circumference Measurement Table*

Head Circumference (mm)	Gestational Age (wk)		Head Circumference (mm)	Gestational Age (wk)	
	Predicted Mean Values†	95% Confidence Limits‡		Predicted Mean Values†	95% Confidence Limits‡
80	13.4	12.1–14.7	230	24.9	22.6–27.2
85	13.7	12.4–15.0	235	25.4	23.1–27.7
90	14.0	12.7–15.3	240	25.9	23.6–28.2
95	14.3	13.0–15.6	245	26.4	24.1–28.7
100	14.6	13.3–15.9	250	26.9	24.6–29.2
105	15.0	13.7–16.3	255	27.5	25.2–29.8
110	15.3	14.0–16.6	260	28.0	25.7–30.3
115	15.6	14.3–16.9	265	28.1	25.8–30.4
120	15.9	14.6–17.2	270	29.2	26.9–31.5
125	16.3	15.0–17.6	275	29.8	27.5–32.1
130	16.6	15.3–17.9	280	30.3	27.6–33.0
135	17.0	15.7–18.3	285	31.0	28.3–33.7
140	17.3	16.0–18.6	290	31.6	28.9–34.3
145	17.7	16.4–19.0	295	32.2	29.5–34.8
150	18.1	16.5–19.7	300	32.8	30.1–35.5
155	18.4	16.8–20.0	305	33.5	30.7–36.2
160	18.8	17.2–20.4	310	34.2	31.5–36.9
165	19.2	17.6–20.8	315	34.9	32.2–37.6
170	19.6	18.0–21.2	320	35.5	32.8–38.2
175	20.0	18.4–21.6	325	36.3	32.9–39.7
180	20.4	18.8–22.0	330	37.0	33.6–40.4
185	20.8	19.2–22.4	335	37.7	34.3–41.1
190	21.2	19.8–22.8	340	38.5	35.1–41.9
195	21.6	20.0–23.2	345	39.2	35.8–42.6
200	22.1	20.5–23.7	350	40.0	36.6–43.4
205	22.5	20.9–24.1	355	40.8	37.4–44.2
210	23.0	21.4–24.6	360	41.6	38.2–45.0
215	23.4	21.8–25.0			
220	23.9	22.3–25.5			
225	24.4	22.1–26.7			

*From Hadlock FP, Deter RL, Harrist RB, et al: *AJR* 1982; 138:649–653. Used by permission.
†Data from Table 3 of Hadlock et al.
‡Data from Table 4 of Hadlock et al.

from 16 to 28 weeks without third trimester measurements, this article too will not be discussed further.

The remaining eight articles[35, 51, 54, 55, 90, 113, 114, 116] presented measurements obtained throughout the second and third trimesters from 10 weeks until term. For proper selection of the measurement plane, the midline echo was used in one,[90] the midline echo and third ventircle in four,[51, 113, 114, 116] with the remaining articles not stating a specific anatomic plane. In comparing six of the most recent articles,[51, 54, 55, 113, 114, 116] all except Ott[116] were fairly closely grouped, with the numbers from Ott, close at 15 weeks, becoming progressively smaller 35 mm less at term. Hoffbauer et al.[35] had numbers smaller before 17 weeks and much larger after 38 weeks and Levi and Erbsman[90] had uniformly larger numbers until 40 weeks by as much as 22 mm. These last two articles[35, 90] will not be discussed further.

These six recent articles[51, 54, 55, 113, 114, 116] appear to have employed good technique, although the technique was stated in only four.[51, 113, 114, 116] The articles not only had a mean head circumference for menstrual age but also 95% or greater confidence limits. The major difference among these studies is that only one[113] gave its data in a clinically useful form, with a variation in weeks for each head circumference. The remaining articles present a range of head circumferences in centimeters for each gestational week, a method which has little practicality. It is recommended that the table by Hadlock et al.[113] (Table 24–5) be used.

The reproducibility of the head circumference measurements has been analyzed. The intraobserver error has been found to be insignificant except if technical factors, particularly the use of different measuring devices, are considered. Measuring devices gave varied results, and, in addition, investigators used these devices differently.[118] The interobserver error was found in one study[113] to be approximately 1% with a mean error by three independent readings in the third trimester of only 1.8 mm (<0.75%). Another study,[118] however, showed the interobserver error to be larger, with a mean of 1.2% and a range of ±4.3% at 1 SD with no systematic differences between prenatal and postnatal measurements.

The overall accuracy of head circumference measurements, in comparison to the BPD measurements, has also been evaluated. Hadlock et al.[113] stated that the head circumference was a good predictor of gestational age but not as good as the BPD. They felt that it still should be used, however, particularly with unusual head shapes. Three other observers[116, 119, 120] stated that the head circumference was more accurate in predicting gestational age, probably secondary to changes in head shape caused by pressure of the uterine wall or external forces on the pliable skull. While an article by Law and MacRae[120] showed strong statistical evidence that the head circumference was more accurate than the BPD, especially in the third trimester, a major flaw in this work was the omission of the CI to determine if the heads were unusually shaped.

HEAD AREA

Eight articles have been published comparing the area of the head to the gestational age,[31, 51, 52, 90, 121–124] with actual numbers given in three.[51, 90, 122] Six articles utilized static scanners from the late second through the third trimesters, two giving numbers,[90, 122] three in graph form,[52, 121, 123] and one as an equation.[31] The last article[51] analyzed the head area with real-time throughout the second and third trimesters. The intraobserver error was found to be larger than that for head circumferences: ±2.6 weeks.[52] In addition, while all articles showed an expected increase in head area as the gestation progressed, the four articles in graph form[52, 121, 123, 124] had much lower numbers for head areas than the three in numeric form.[51, 90, 122] Of interest is the article by Wladimiroff et al.[122] where head areas where calculated by squaring the BPD rather than by using a planimeter tracing. Despite this unusual approach, the numbers were quite close to the numbers of Levi and Ebsman[90] and Fescina et al.[51]

The reasons for the discrepancies between studies cannot be ascertained. Since, however, the accuracy is not better than either the BPD or the head circumference measurements and since the variation may be greater, it is felt that the head area is not a useful or proven method.

HEAD VOLUME

Four articles have been published calculating the volume of the fetal head.[125–128] In one[125] the volume was obtained by considering the head as an ellipsoid volume and calculating it in the transaxial view by multiplying the fronto-occipital diameter (FOD) times biparietal diameter (BPD) times a constant. The volumes increased from 30 cc at 18 weeks to 514 cc at term. In two other articles,[126, 127] the volume was computed from the cube of an average transaxial diameter, the average diameter calculated as a square root of FOD × BPD. The head volume increased from 16 cc at 12 weeks to 1,191 cc at term. Lastly, Dubose[128] calculated the head volume by three parameters: the BPD, FOD, and vertical calvarial diameter. The last-named was measured from the interpetrosal portion of the base of the skull to the vertex in coronal view. It is this measurement that makes the calculated head volumes theoretically more accurate. By using an equation for a sphere, head volumes increased from 10 to 350 cc throughout the second and third trimester.

Despite the theoretical probability that a volume measurement is better for evaluating brain mass and overall head size, this method has not as yet been proved. It should, therefore, at present not be considered in the routine examination of the fetal head. It may have a place in future analysis if it can be shown to be more accurate than the BPD and head circumference measurements. A problem that head volume might have been able to solve became apparent in a recent article on fetuses with premature rupture of the membranes and oligohydramnios.[129] While the BPD was unreliable, the FOD and CI were only able to predict which fetal heads were abnormally shaped in 45% of cases. It is possible that the fetal head had been misshapen by the oligohydramnios primarily in the craniocaudal dimension.

VENTRICULAR SIZE

Ultrasound has been shown to be accurate in the evaluation of lateral ventricular size in both children and adults. In infants, a comparison of computed tomography (CT) to real-time ultrasound revealed close correlation.[130, 131] To date there have been 12 ultrasound articles analyzing the in utero size of the lateral ventricles.[121, 132–142]

Four articles measured the bodies of the lateral ventricles,[132–134, 141] three in numeric[132, 134, 141] and one in graph and equation form.[133] All used real-time equipment, two from 12 weeks to term,[132, 133] one from 15 to 25 weeks,[141] and one from 27 weeks to term.[134] In addition to obtaining linear measurements, a ratio of the lateral ventricle bodies to intracranial hemidiameter was also obtained. The lateral ventricle is measured from the falx midline echo to the widest part of the lateral wall of the body of the lateral ventricle, and the intracranial hemidiameter is measured on the same side, parallel to the first line, from the falx midline echo to the widest part of the inner surface of the calvarium[132] (Fig 24–6).

Recently there has been discussion about what produces the echo at the lateral wall of the body of the lateral ventricle. Hertzberg and co-workers[143] have shown that the echo is created by interfaces with branches of the internal cerebral vein at the outer edge of the lateral ventricle, rather than by the lateral ventricular wall itself. Since these veins fan out into the brain from the edge of the ventricle, images obtained superiorly and perhaps also laterally could show sonographic parallel lines that might be mistaken for the outer edge of the lateral ventricles. Nevertheless, at

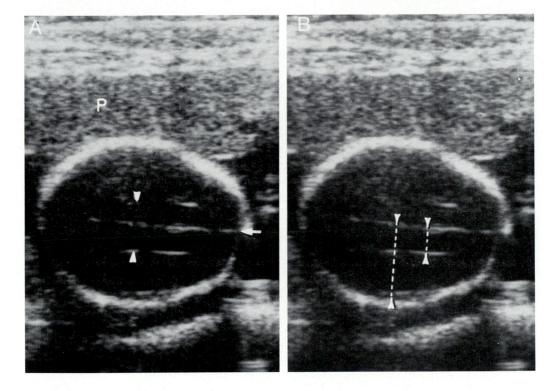

FIG 24–6.
Transaxial scan of the fetal head near term at the region of the bodies of the lateral ventricles. **A,** the two linear lines (*arrowheads*) of the lateral ventricular bodies are parallel to the falx midline echo (*arrow*). **B,** same image as **A** showing the measurements of the bodies of the lateral ventricles (LV) on the right and the intracranial hemidiameter (ICHD) on the left, both denoted by *arrowheads* and *dotted lines.* The LV and the ICHD measurements should be taken at their widest points, parallel to each other. Note that the LV/ICHD ratio is small near term, only 33%. *P* = placenta.

the level of the lateral ventricles, the echo originates at the outer margin of the ventricle and is reproducible. The validity of this ratio has been confirmed in newborn infants, 25 term and 41 preterm.[144] For the term infants, the ratio is 28%, with a range of 24% to 30%, while the ratio in the preterm infants is slightly larger at 31% with a range of 24% to 34%, both comparable to the in utero ratios of Johnson et al.[132] and Jeanty et al.[133]

The work by Hadlock et al.[134] is confined solely to the third trimester and has consistently larger ventricular numbers and wider ratio ranges than do Johnson et al.[132] and Jeanty et al.[133] Hadlock et al. attributed these larger numbers to the way in which their measurements were obtained, measuring the bodies of the lateral ventricles from the outer margin of the falx echo to the outer border of the body of the lateral ventricle, rather than from the middle of the falx echo to the inner border of the body of the lateral ventricle. Since these margins are thin structures, it would not seem that such small measurement changes alone should be responsible for such large differences in the ventricular numbers or in their ratios. Therefore this article will not be considered further.

The articles of Johnson et al.[132] and Jeanty et al.[133] correlate closely in both lateral ventricle measurements and in ratios from the early gestation period until term.

Only the work by Johnson et al. is recommended because its results are in numeric form. The main weakness in their data, however, is in the early second trimester. There were not even enough data points to calculate a ventricular width or a ratio at 19 weeks. Pretorius et al.,[141] from the same institution, reevaluated the second trimester with 122 normal fetuses and directly analyzed their work against that of Johnson et al. Since the two compare closely, a combined table using the original work by Johnson et al.[132] from 26 weeks to term and the later work by Pretorius et al.[141] from 15 to 25 weeks is recommended (Table 24–6).

In the early second trimester, the lateral ventricles are very prominent and take up most of the inner area of the calvarium, as much as 74% of the head at 15 weeks. At this stage of gestation, from approximately 12 to 18 weeks, the hyperechoic choroid plexus almost completely fills the lateral ventricular bodies[145] (Fig 24–7). As the

TABLE 24–6.

Lateral Ventricular Body Measurement Table*†

Menstrual Age (wk)	Measurements (mm)		
	LVW, 2 SD	HW, 2 SD	(LVW/HW), 2 SD
15	8 (6–10)	15 (12–18)	56 (38–74)
16	9 (7–11)	15 (13–17)	57 (46–68)
17	9 (8–10)	15 (14–16)	58 (49–67)
18	9 (8–10)	18 (17–19)	51 (41–61)
19	9 (7–11)	20 (19–21)	49 (41–57)
20	9 (7–11)	19 (17–20)	46 (38–54)
21	9 (7–11)	21 (20–22)	42 (31–53)
22	9 (7–11)	23 (21–25)	40 (29–51)
23	8 (7–9)	24 (22–26)	34 (26–42)
24	9 (8–10)	25 (23–27)	35 (27–43)
25	9 (8–10)	28 (25–31)	33 (29–37)
26	9	30	30 (24–36)
27	9	30	28 (23–34)
28	11	33	31 (18–45)
29	10	34	29 (22–37)
30	10	34	30 (26–34)
31	10	34	29 (23–36)
32	11	36	31 (26–36)
33	11	34	31 (25–37)
34	11	38	28 (23–33)
35	11	38	29 (26–31)
36	11	39	28 (23–34)
37	12	41	29 (24–34)
Term	12	43	28 (22–33)

*Combined table of two articles from the same group: Fifteen to 25 gestational weeks: Pretorius DH, Drose JA, Manco-Johnson ML: *J Ultrasound Med* 1986; 5:121–124. Used by permission. Twenty-six gestational weeks to term: Johnson ML, Dunne MC, Mack LA, et al: *J Clin Ultrasound* 1980; 8:311–318. Used by permission.
†LVW = lateral ventricular body width; HW = hemispheric width.

pregnancy progresses toward term, the cerebral cortex grows, causing the head to enlarge and the choroid plexus and the lateral ventricles to become relatively less prominent. By 21 weeks, the bodies of the lateral ventricles have decreased to a maximum of 53% (Fig 24–8), further decreasing to 33% by term (see Fig 24–6).

The atrium or trigone of the lateral ventricle connects anteriorly to the body, posteriorly to the occipital horn, and inferiorly to the temporal horn. It has been evaluated in five articles,[134–138] all with real-time from early to mid–second trimester to term in three,[135–137] in the third trimester in one,[134] and randomly in the last.[138] A measurement of this region could be more clinically useful than a measurement of the body since early hydrocephalus has been shown to enlarge the atrial regions prior to affecting either the bodies or frontal horns of the lateral ventricles.[135]

Identification of the atrial region is performed in a transaxial plane, somewhat similar to the plane of section used to obtain the thalami.[137] The transducer is rotated posteriorly and inferiorly about 1.5 to 2.0 cm.[134, 136] The atria can be visualized consistently from 12 weeks to term, with identification facilitated by imaging the hyperechoic choroid plexuses within them[134, 136] (Fig 24–9). The width of the atrium,[135–137] the amount of choroid plexus within it,[136, 138] and the distance from the midline to the outer border of the atrium[135, 136] have been measured and three ratios obtained, namely, the width of the atrium to the midline-outer atrial border,[136] the atrial width to intracranial hemidiameter,[135, 136] and the midline-outer atrial border to the intracranial hemidiameter.[134–136]

All of these six parameters have merit. The atrial width seems to be as useful as any. The earliest article, by McGahan and Phillips,[135] showed a progressive increase of 8 mm at 19 weeks to 16 mm at term. The other two, however, showed no significant change in atrial width throughout the second and third trimester,[136, 137] a mean and 2 SD of 6.9 $\pm$ 1.3 mm[136] and 7.6 $\pm$ 1.2 mm.[137] The last two results showing no significant change in atrial width are more likely to be correct since the telencephalon cleaves at about 6 gestational weeks and remains unchanged thereafter.[136] Similarly, the width of the lateral ventricular bodies also shows very little variation, 8 mm at 15 weeks to 12 mm at term[132, 141] (see Table 24–6).

The only difficulty with the work on atrial width has been the cut-off number that can be used to consistently diagnose ventriculomegaly. Cardoza and co-workers[137] felt that an atrial diameter of greater than 10 mm, greater than 4 SD from the mean, was sufficient to suggest ventricular enlargement. However, in graph form, Pilu and co-workers[136] showed that a considerable number of atrial width measurements can be above 10 mm at 4 SD. Nevertheless, the work by Cardoza and co-workers[137] is recommended with the caveat that there may be instances when an atrial width greater than 10 mm can be normal (Table 24–7).

The amount of choroid plexus within the atria of the lateral ventricle has also been evaluated. Pilu and co-workers[136] found that the choroid plexus should always occupy at least 60% of the atrial width and in most cases completely fill the atria. Mahony and co-workers[138] felt that the choroid plexus should not be separated from the atrial wall by a space of more than 2 mm with mild lateral ventriculomegaly diagnosed by a separation of 3 to 8 mm.

The distance of the midline-outer border of atrium, its ratios to the intracranial hemidiameter and the atrial width, and the ratio of atrial width to intracranial hemidiameter[134–136] closely correlate with the BPD and gestational age. These numbers change throughout the second and third trimester. While these numbers may be of future value in identifying the growth of the hippocampus and deep cerebral

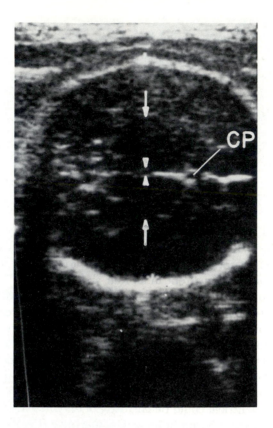

FIG 24–10.
Transaxial scan of the fetal head at 36 weeks. Note the third ventricle (*arrowheads*) between the thalami (*arrows*). The cavum septi pellucidi (*CP*) is located anteriorly.

OCULAR DIMENSIONS

The fetal eye can be routinely imaged.[146–148] Two articles have evaluated the eye[147, 148] throughout the second and third trimester, one in numeric form[147] and one in equation and graph form.[148] In the second and third trimesters, a view of one or both eyes could be obtained in 96% of cases and the eyeball (globe), lens, iris, pupil, and cornea routinely identified.[147] While the hyaloid artery, between the lens and posterior choroid, could be identifed prior to 20 weeks, it is generally absent after 25 weeks.[147]

The globe appears as a rounded structure with less than a 5% variation between the major diameters in two views, sagittal and base.[147] The globe is surrounded by hyperechoic retrobulbar fat so that its measurement can easily be taken from its anechoic borders (Fig 24–11). By examining 157 normal fetuses, it was found that the average diameter increased continually throughout the second and third trimester with periods of accelerated growth between 12 and 20 weeks, 28 and 32 weeks, and at term.[147] In contradistinction, Jeanty et al.[148] showed a more asymptotic growth near term. Numeric measurements were presented in one article, comparing favorably to a previous pathologic series referenced within the article.[147] While these

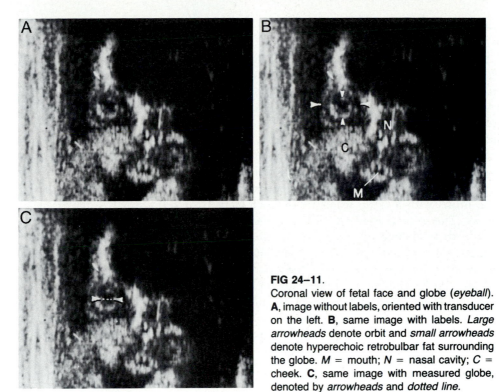

FIG 24–11.
Coronal view of fetal face and globe (*eyeball*).
A, image without labels, oriented with transducer on the left. **B,** same image with labels. *Large arrowheads* denote orbit and *small arrowheads* denote hyperechoic retrobulbar fat surrounding the globe. *M* = mouth; *N* = nasal cavity; *C* = cheek. **C,** same image with measured globe, denoted by *arrowheads* and *dotted line.*

values are slightly lower than those shown by Jeanty et al.,[148] approximately 1 to 2 mm after 20 weeks, the measurements are considered close enough that a table is recommended[147] (Table 24–8). Further work is needeed to confirm these measurements.

TABLE 24–8.
Fetal Globe (Eyeball) Diameter Measurement Table*

Globe Diameter (mm)		Gestational Age (wk)	
Mean Diameter	Range of 16%–84%, 1 SD	Mean Age	Range of 16%–84%, 1 SD
4.7	4.0–5.5	14.5	12.5–16.5
7.4	6.2–8.6	17.9	16.5–19.3
9.9	9.6–10.2	22.4	21.4–23.5
11.2	10.3–12.1	25.7	24.6–26.8
13.4	12.5–14.4	30.4	29.2–31.6
14.9	14.5–15.3	33.6	32.6–34.7
16.0	15.1–16.9	38.2	36.8–39.2

*From Birnholz JC: *Early Hum Dev* 1985; 12:199–209. Used by permission.

ORBITAL DIMENSIONS

Three articles have evaluated orbital diameters.[148-150] Jeanty et al.[148] measured the outer orbital diameter (outer to outer orbital distance) and the inner orbital diameter (inner to inner orbital distance) in both equation and graph form. Jeanty et al.[149] measured the outer orbital diameter, also termed "binocular distance," in numeric and equation form. Mayden et al.[150] measured the outer and inner orbital diameters in numeric and graph form. In the same article, aborted fetuses were evaluated in a water bath and their orbital diameters correlated well with in utero measurements obtained on live fetuses of the same gestational age.

All articles used real-time equipment, with Mayden et al.[150] also evaluating the fetal orbits with a static scanner. All used more than 180 normals from 12 to 42 weeks. The criteria used for all the studies were comparable: the sections had to have both orbits imaged symmetrically with each orbit of largest possible diameter (Fig 24–12). Of the three, two[149, 150] demonstrated the outer margins used to obtain the outer orbital diameter taken at the inner margins of the bone. Only one[150] showed the margins for the inner orbital diameter.

There are technical difficulties in obtaining the precise landmarks to make outer orbital diameter measurements. The globe is surrounded by hyperechoic fat and the hyperechoic orbital rim. These tend to blend together, especially when the fetus is

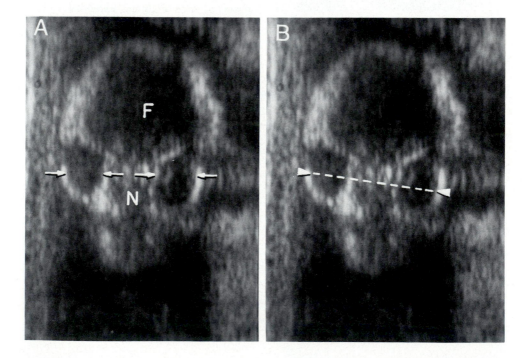

FIG 24–12.
Coronal scan of the face in a 30-week fetus pregnancy. **A,** image oriented with transducer on the left showing the two orbits (*arrows*). N = nasal cavity; F = frontal bone. **B,** same image as **A** showing outer to outer orbital (binocular distance) measurement, denoted by *arrowheads* and *dashed line*. Note that the margins of the orbits are distinct and separable from the hyperechoic bone outside the orbits.

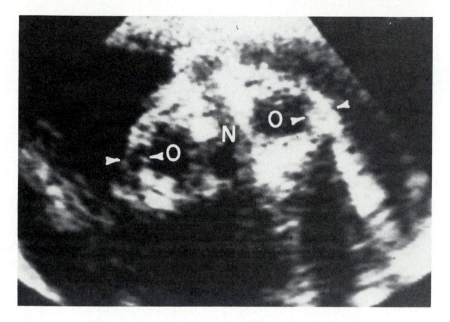

FIG 24–13.
Face-up magnified image of the fetal orbits. While the globes (*O*) can be clearly identified, a combination of hyperechoic retrobulbar fat, bone, and overlying subcutaneous tissue (*arrowheads*) makes the outer borders indistinct. *N* = nasal cavity.

face up or occiput up, causing indistinct margins (Fig 24–13). Nevertheless, when the numbers in these articles were compared, all three demonstrated an outer orbital diameter increase from 13 mm at 12 weeks to 59 mm or greater by term. Their numbers were closely grouped, varying from 0 to 3 mm at each stage of gestation. The outer orbital diameter was shown to closely parallel the increase in biparietal diameter (BPD) as gestation progressed, and therefore to be a useful means of verifying fetal age. In addition, the outer orbital diameter was found to be a good indicator of hypotelorism[150] and perhaps could also be used to diagnose hypertelorism, although no cases were observed. The inner orbital diameter varied very little throughout gestation, 5 mm at 12 weeks to 19 mm at term, did not correlate well with either the BPD or the gestational age,[148, 150] and will not be discussed further.

There are two reasons to obtain an outer orbital (binocular) diameter. First, it is a good method of confirming gestational age and obtaining valid measurements of the face even when the head may be in a difficult position to obtain an accurate BPD. This latter circumstance can be a particular problem near term, especially when the head is in vertex presentation. In this instance, a table comparing the outer orbital diameter to gestational age is needed[149] (Table 24–9). Second, there are circumstances where a facial to calvarial disproportion is suspected. When this is considered, a table comparing the outer orbital diameter to the BPD is needed[150] (Table 24–10). While ideally one table could have all three parameters, that is, the outer orbital diameter, BPD, and gestational age (including range), the articles published have only two of the three and therefore two tables are recommended.

TABLE 24–9.
Outer Orbital Diameter (Binocular Distance) Measurement Table*

| Outer Orbital Diameter (mm) | Gestational Age (wk) | | Outer Orbital Diameter (mm) | Gestational Age (wk) | |
	Predicted Mean Values	Range From 5th to 95th Percentile		Predicted Mean Values	Range From 5th to 95th Percentile
15	10.4	7.1–13.9			
16	11.0	7.7–14.4	41	25.9	22.6–29.1
17	11.6	8.3–15.0	42	26.6	23.1–29.9
18	12.1	8.9–15.6	43	27.1	23.9–30.4
19	12.9	9.6–16.1	44	27.7	24.4–31.0
20	13.4	10.1–16.7	45	28.3	25.0–31.6
21	14.0	10.7–17.3	46	28.9	25.6–32.1
22	14.6	11.3–17.9	47	29.6	26.1–32.9
23	15.1	11.9–18.6	48	30.1	26.9–33.4
24	15.9	12.6–19.1	49	30.7	27.3–34.0
25	16.4	13.1–19.7	50	31.3	27.9–34.6
26	17.0	13.7–20.3	51	31.9	28.6–35.1
27	17.6	14.3–20.9	52	32.6	29.1–35.9
28	18.1	14.9–21.6	53	33.0	29.7–36.4
29	18.9	15.6–22.1	54	33.6	30.3–37.0
30	19.4	16.1–22.7	55	34.1	30.9–37.6
31	20.0	16.6–23.3	56	34.9	31.6–38.1
32	20.6	17.1–23.9	57	35.4	32.1–38.7
33	21.1	17.9–24.6	58	36.0	32.7–39.3
34	21.7	18.4–25.1	59	36.6	33.3–39.9
35	22.3	19.0–25.7	60	37.1	33.9–40.6
36	22.9	19.6–26.3	61	37.9	34.6–41.1
37	23.6	20.1–26.9	62	38.4	35.1–41.7
38	24.1	20.6–27.4	63	39.0	35.7–42.3
39	24.7	21.4–28.0	64	39.6	36.3–42.9
40	25.3	22.0–28.6	65	40.1	36.9–43.5

*From Jeanty P, Cantraine F, Cousaert E, et al: *J Ultrasound Med* 1984; 3:241–243. Used by permission.

TABLE 24–10.
Outer Orbital Diameter (Binocular Distance) Measurement Table*

Predicted Outer Orbital Diameter (mm)	Biparietal Diameter (mm)	Mean Gestational Age (wk)	Predicted Outer Orbital Diameter (mm)	Biparietal Diameter (mm)	Mean Gestational Age (wk)
13	19	11.6	41	57	23.8
14	20	11.6	41	58	24.3
15	21	12.1	42	59	24.3
16	22	12.6	43	60	24.7
17	23	12.6	43	61	25.2
17	24	13.1	44	62	25.2
18	25	13.6	44	63	25.7
19	26	13.6	45	64	26.2
20	27	14.1	45	65	26.2
21	28	14.6	46	66	26.7
21	29	14.6	46	67	27.2
22	30	15.0	47	68	27.6
23	31	15.5	47	69	28.1
24	32	15.5	48	70	28.6
25	33	16.0	48	71	29.1
25	34	16.5	49	73	29.6
26	35	16.5	50	74	30.0
27	36	17.0	50	75	30.6
27	37	17.5	51	76	31.0
28	38	17.9	51	77	31.5
30	40	18.4	52	78	32.0
31	42	18.9	52	79	32.5
32	43	19.4	53	80	33.0
32	44	19.4	54	82	33.5
33	45	19.9	54	83	34.0
34	46	20.4	54	84	34.4
34	47	20.4	55	85	35.0
35	48	20.9	55	86	35.4
36	49	21.3	56	88	35.9
36	50	21.3	56	89	36.4
37	51	21.8	57	90	36.9
38	52	22.3	57	91	37.3
38	53	22.3	58	92	37.8
39	54	22.8	58	93	38.3
40	55	23.3	58	94	38.8
40	56	23.3	59	96	39.3
			59	97	39.8

*From Mayden KL, Tortora M, Berkowitz RL, et al: Orbital diameters: *Am J Obstet Gynecol* 1982; 144:289–297. Used by permission.

CEREBELLAR DIMENSIONS

The cerebellum has been evaluated in three articles,[151–153] two in numeric form throughout the second and third trimester[151, 153] and one as a graph from 14 to 32 weeks.[152] With real-time ultrasound, all used the standard transaxial image of the head, obtaining the cavum septi pellucidi and thalamus as midline structures and then rotating the transducer slightly posterior and inferior to image the posterior fossa (Fig 24–14). All measured the transaxial cerebellar diameter, with Smith et al.[153] also measuring the anteroposterior (AP) diameter. McLeary et al.[151] compared the cerebellum to the biparietal diameter (BPD), Goldstein et al.[152] compared it to the BPD, FOD, head circumference, and gestational age, while Smith et al.[153] compared the cerebellum only to the menstrual age. All showed a continual growth of the cerebellum throughout the second and third trimester with slowing near term. McLeary et al.[151] and Goldstein et al.[152] claimed to have been able to image the cerebellum in at least 95% of cases, with difficulty arising in markedly obese patients, fetuses in occiput-posterior position, or late in the third trimester when the fetus is in vertex presentation and often engaged. Smith et al.[153] found the cerebellum was more difficult to image and less reproducible after 30 weeks, perhaps due to its borders becoming less distinct as the bones of the base of the skull further ossify.

The usefulness of the cerebellar measurements is fourfold: (1) The cerebellar measurement can be used to establish a gestational age. While this is not often necessary, McLeary and co-workers[151] felt that the posterior fossa would not be affected by the external pressures that could distort the head and, therefore, in some cases, would be more reliable than a head measurement. (2) It can be compared to the BPD. Since both the BPD and cerebellum are imaged using the same scanning technique, the cerebellum becomes a potentially useful measurement to confirm the

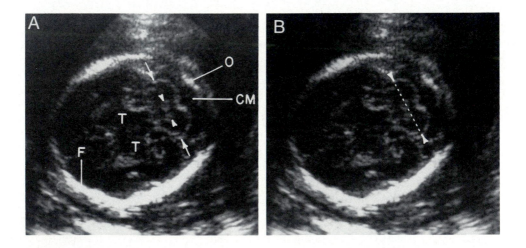

FIG 24–14.
Transaxial image of the fetal head at 30 weeks, rotated slightly posterior and inferior to image the cerebellum (denoted by *arrows*). **A,** the cerebellum is located immediately posterior to the thalami (*T*). The hyperechoic midline cerebellar structure is the vermis (*arrowheads*). **B,** same image as **A** showing the transverse dimension of the cerebellum, denoted by *arrowheads* and *dotted line*. *F* = frontal bone; *O* = occipital bone; *CM* = cisterna magna.

BPD. (3) Imaging and measuring the cerebellum may help to determine if there is abnormality in the posterior fossa. Failure to demonstrate all or part of the cerebellum could be a sign of cerebellar hypoplasia. (4) It has recently been shown that the cerebellum continues to grow normally from 26 weeks to term, even in well-documented cases of intrauterine growth retardation (presumably the asymmetric type).[154] This was found to be true despite significant growth slowing of the BPD, abdominal circumference, and femur length. If this last finding can be confirmed, then the transverse cerebellar measurement would be a very important means of determining the actual age of the fetus, even when the rest of the fetus is small, and thus in diagnosing growth retardation.

A table comparing the transverse dimension of the cerebellum to the BPD is recommended. In all three articles, the numbers are similar (within 3 mm) until 32 weeks.[151–153] After that time, only the two articles with numbers[151, 152] will be compared. Discrepancies continue to increase, although it is not certain why these differences are present. Both articles have good-sized series of patients and both use a predicted statistical mean (rather than a true mean) and a calculated range. In the

TABLE 24–11.

Fetal Cerebellar Transverse Diameter Measurement Table*

Cerebellar Transverse Diameter (mm)	Biparietal Diameter (mm)		Cerebellar Transverse Diameter (mm)	Biparietal Diameter (mm)	
	Predicted Mean Value	Range of 16%–84% (1 SD)		Predicted Mean Value	Range of 16%–84% (1 SD)
15	34.7	31.5–38.0	35	74.4	70.7–78.2
16	37.2	34.0–40.6	36	75.8	72.1–79.5
17	39.8	36.4–43.2	37	77.1	73.4–80.8
18	42.2	38.8–45.7	38	78.3	74.4–82.0
19	44.6	41.1–48.1	39	79.5	75.9–83.1
20	46.9	43.4–50.5	40	80.6	77.0–84.2
21	49.2	45.6–52.8	41	81.7	78.1–85.2
22	51.4	47.8–55.0	42	82.6	79.1–86.2
23	53.5	49.9–57.2	43	83.6	80.1–87.1
24	55.6	51.9–59.3	44	84.4	81.0–87.9
25	57.6	53.9–61.3	45	85.3	81.9–88.6
26	59.5	55.8–63.3	46	86.0	82.7–89.3
27	61.5	57.7–65.2	47	86.7	83.5–89.9
28	63.3	59.5–67.1	48	87.3	84.2–90.5
29	65.1	61.3–68.8	49	87.9	84.8–91.0
30	66.8	63.0–70.6	50	88.4	85.4–91.4
31	68.4	64.7–72.2	51	88.8	85.9–91.8
32	70.0	66.3–73.8	52	89.2	86.4–92.1
33	71.6	67.8–75.3	53	89.6	86.8–92.3
34	73.0	69.3–76.8	54	89.8	87.2–92.5

*From McLeary RD, Kuhns LR, Barr M Jr: *Radiology* 1984; 151:439–442. Used by permission.

article by McLeary and co-workers,[151] the cerebellar diameters increase up to 54 mm, equal to a BPD of 90 mm or a mean gestational age of 36.6 weeks. No further measurements into the last month of pregnancy are available. The article by Goldstein et al.[152] continues to a BPD of 92 mm, a mean gestational age of 37.8 weeks. However, the cerebellar numbers do not increase steadily. In fact, over the 4-week period between 31 and 35 weeks, the mean cerebellar diameters increased by only 2.5 mm.[152] In addition, in the article by Goldstein and co-workers, a mean and range from 10% to 90% are presented for both variables, making their work somewhat cumbersome to use. As a result, the work by McLeary et al. is recommended[151] (Table 24–11). More data are needed to confirm the measurements after 32 weeks, however.

SUBARACHNOID CISTERNS

The fetal subarachnoid cisterns have been studied extensively throughout the second and third trimesters.[155] Visualization of the cisterns is variable. Some are more successfully identified in the second trimester, some in the third trimester, and some throughout both trimesters.[155] Knowledge of these cisterns is important so that their identification as normal fluid-filled spaces avoids the incorrect diagnosis of abnormality. In addition, if these cisterns are prominent and dilated ventricles are present, the diagnosis of communicating hydrocephalus can be suggested.[155]

Of particular importance is the large cistern of the posterior fossa, the cisterna magna. It is located caudad to the cerebellum, between the cerebellum and the base of the occipital bone. Images of this region are obtained in the same manner as that used to visualize the cerebellum. After obtaining the standard BPD image with the cavum septi pellucidi and thalamus as midline structures, the transducer is angled posteriorly and inferiorly (Fig 24–15,A).

Two articles evaluated the normal cisterna magna,[153,156] one in numeric form from 15 weeks to 36 weeks[156] and the other in graph form from 14 to 32 weeks.[153] It was noted that this cistern could be identified in greater than 90% of fetuses from 15 to 28 weeks.[156] After 29 and 33 weeks, respectively, the ability to image this region declined sharply to 58% and 33%.[156] Nevertheless, when imaged, the depth of the cisterna magna from the posterior aspect of the cerebellum to the occipital bone measured 5 mm in average diameter with a range of ±3 mm[156] (Fig 24–15,B) (Table 24–12). No cisterna magna measured more than 10 mm in size.[156] Although the graph of Smith et al.[153] tended to confirm these observations, it shows a 2-SD maximum of 15 mm at 30 weeks! It is not certain whether this was an actual measurement or more probably a calculated theoretical number.

TABLE 24–12.
Cisterna Magna Measurements*
(Range 15–36 wk)

Anteroposterior Depth (mm)		
Mean	Range	Maximum
5	2–8	10

*From Mahony BS, Callen PW, Filly RA, et al: *Radiology* 1984; 153:773–776. Used by permission.

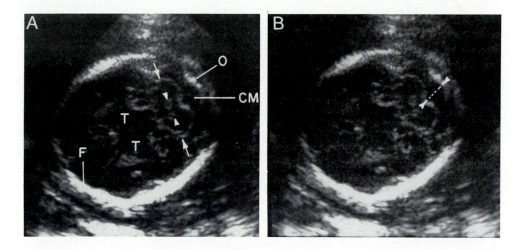

FIG 24–15.
Transaxial image of the fetal head at 30 weeks, rotated slightly posterior and inferior to image the cerebellum (denoted by *arrows*) and the cisterna magna (*CM*). **A,** the cisterna magna is located immediately posterior to the cerebellum, between it and the occipital bone (*O*). *Arrowheads* denote vermis of cerebellum. **B,** same image as **A** showing the depth of the cisterna magna, denoted by *arrowheads* and *dotted line. F* = frontal bone; *T* = thalami.

The value of both imaging and measuring the cisterna magna is important, since it can be used to detect and confirm posterior fossa abnormalities. Cerebellar hypoplasia, communicating hydrocephalus, and Dandy-Walker cysts could enlarge this space.[156, 157] Conversely, if the cisterna magna cannot be imaged or is less than 2 mm in size, especially prior to 28 weeks, this would suggest a spinal abnormality with secondary Arnold-Chiari type II malformation.[156] It must be emphasized, though, that a prominent cisterna magna without any other findings might also be a normal variant.[156]

REFERENCES

1. Durkan JP, Russo GL: Ultrasonic fetal cephalometry: accuracy, limitations, and applications. *Obstet Gynecol* 1966; 27:399–403.
2. Willocks J, Donald I, Duggan TC, et al: Fetal cephalometry by ultrasound. *J Obstet Gynaecol Br Commw* 1964; 71:11–20.
3. Kohorn EI: An evaluation of ultrasonic fetal cephalometry. *Am J Obstet Gynecol* 1967; 97:553–559.
4. Taylor ES, Holmes JH, Thompson HE, et al: Ultrasound diagnostic techniques in obstetrics and gynecology. *Am J Obstet Gynecol* 1964; 90:655–671.
5. Campbell S: Ultrasonic fetal cephalometry during the second trimester of pregnancy. *J Obstet Gynaecol Br Commw* 1970; 77:1057–1063.
6. Sabbagha RE: Assessment of differences in sonar biparietal diameter values regarding fetal age and weight. *J Clin Ultrasound* 1973; 1:68–74.
7. Hohler CW, Inglis J, Collins H, et al: Ultrasound biparietal diameter. Defining relationships in normal pregnancy. *NY State J Med* 1976; 76:373–376.
8. Hern WA: Correlation of fetal age and measurements between 10 and 26 weeks of gestation. *Obstet Gynecol* 1984; 63:26–32.
9. Lunt RM, Chard L: Reproducibility of measurement of fetal biparietal diameter by ultrasonic cephalometry. *J Obstet Gynaecol Br Commw* 1974; 81:682–685.

10. Davison JM, Lint T, Farr V, et al: The limitations of ultrasonic fetal cephalometry. *J Obstet Gynaecol Br Commw* 1981; 80:769–775.
11. Docker MF, Settatree RS: Comparison between linear array real time ultrasonic scanning and conventional compound scanning in the measurement of the fetal biparietal diameter. *Br J Obstet Gynaecol* 1977; 84:924–929.
12. Levi S, Smets P: Intra-uterine fetal growth studied by ultrasonic biparietal measurements: the percentiles of biparietal distribution. *Acta Obstet Gynecol Scand* 1973; 52:193–198.
13. Cooperberg PL, Chow T, Kite V, et al: Biparietal diameter: a comparison of real time and conventional B-scan techniques. *J Clin Ultrasound* 1976; 4:421–423.
14. Fescina RH, Ucieda FJ: Reliability of fetal anthropometry by ultrasound. *J Perinat Med* 1980; 8:93–98.
15. Watmough D, Crippin D, Mallard JR: A critical assessment of ultrasonic fetal cephalometry. *Br J Radiol* 1974; 47:24–33.
16. Johnson ML, Dunne MG, Mack LA, et al: Evaluation of fetal intracranial anatomy by static and real-time ultrasound. *J Clin Ultrasound* 1980; 8:311–318.
17. Shepard M, Filly RA: A standardized plane for biparietal diameter measurement. *J Ultrasound Med* 1982; 1:145–150.
18. Hadlock FP, Deter RL, Harrist RB, et al: Fetal biparietal diameter: rational choice of plane of section for sonographic measurement. *AJR* 1982; 138:871–874.
19. Hughey M, Sabbagha RE: Cephalometry by real-time imaging: a critical evaluation. *Am J Obstet Gynecol* 1978; 131:825–830.
20. Drumm JE: The prediction of delivery date by ultrasonic measurement of fetal crown-rump length. *Br J Obstet Gynaecol* 1977; 84:1–5.
21. Campbell S, Warsof SL, Little D, et al: Routine ultrasound screening for the prediction of gestational age. *Obstet Gynecol* 1985; 65:613–620.
22. Smazal SF, Weisman LE, Hoppler KD, et al: Comparative analysis of ultrasonographic methods of gestational age assessment. *J Ultrasound Med* 1983; 2:147–150.
23. Kopta MM, May RR, Crane JP: A comparison of the reliability of the estimated date of confinement predicted by crown-rump length and biparietal diameter *Am J Obstet Gynecol* 1983; 145:562–565.
24. Campbell S: The prediction of fetal maturity by ultrasonic measurement of the biparietal diameter. *J Obstet Gynecol Br Commw* 1969; 76:603–609.
25. Sabbagha RE, Turner H, Rockett H, et al: Sonar BPD and fetal age: Definition of the relationship. *Obstet Gynecol* 1974; 43:7–14.
26. Campbell S, Newman GB: Growth of the fetal biparietal diameter during normal pregnancy. *J Obstet Gynaecol Br Commw* 1971; 78:518–519.
27. Sabbagha RE, Hughey M: Standardization of sonar cephalometry and gestational age. *Obstet Gynecol* 1978; 52:402–406.
28. Wiener SN, Flynn MJ, Kennedy AW, et al: A composite curve of ultrasonic biparietal diameters for estimating gestational age. *Radiology* 1977; 122:781–786.
29. Kurtz AB, Wapner RJ, Kurtz RJ, et al: Analysis of biparietal diameter as an accurate indicator of gestational age. *J Clin Ultrasound* 1980; 8:319–326.
30. Levi S, Erbsman F: Antenatal fetal growth from the nineteenth week: Ultrasonic study of 12 head and chest dimensions. *Am J Obstet Gynecol* 1975; 121:262–268.
31. Weinraub Z, Schneider D, Langer R, et al: Ultrasonographic measurement of fetal growth parameters for estimation of gestational age and fetal weight. *Isr J Med Sci* 1979; 15:829–832.
32. Hellman LF, Kobayashi M, Fillisti L, et al: Growth and development of the human fetus prior to the twentieth week of gestation. *Am J Obstet Gynecol* 1969; 103:784–800.
33. Hoffbauer H: The importance of ultrasonic diagnosis in early pregnancy. *Electromedia* 1970; 3:227–230.
34. Piiroinen O: Studies in diagnostic ultrasound. *Acta Obstet Gynecol Scand [Suppl]* 1975; 55:1–60.
35. Hoffbauer H, Pachaly J, Arabin B, et al: Control of fetal development with multiple ultrasonic body measures. *Contrib Gynecol Obstet* 1979; 6:147–156.
36. Hadlock FP, Deter RL, Harrist RB, et al: Fetal biparietal diameter: a critical re-evaluation of the relation to menstrual age by means of real-time ultrasound. *J Ultrasound Med* 1982; 1:97–104.
37. Wladimiroff JW, Bloemsma CA, Wallenburg HCS: Ultrasonic assessment of fetal head and body sizes in relation to normal and retarded fetal growth. *Am J Obstet Gynecol* 1978; 131:857–860.
38. Wladimiroff JW, Bloemsma CA, Wallenburg HCS: Ultrasonic diagnosis of the large-for-dates infant. *Obstet Gynecol* 1978; 52:285–288.

39. Varma TR: Prediction of delivery date by ultrasound cephalometry. *J Obstet Gynaecol Br Commw* 1973; 80:316–319.
40. Brown RE: *Ultrasonography: Basic Principles and Clinical Applications.* St Louis, Warren H Green Inc, 1967, p 116.
41. Winsberg F: Personal communications; Hobbins J, Winsberg F: *Ultrasonography in Obstetrics and Gynecology.* Baltimore, Williams & Wilkins Co, 1977, p 165.
42. Lee BO, Major FJ, Weingold AB: Ultrasonic determination of fetal maturity at repeat cesarean section. *Obstet Gynecol* 1971; 38:294–297.
43. Hibbard LT, Anderson GV: Clinical applications of ultrasonic fetal cephalometry. *Obstet Gynecol* 1967; 29:842–847.
44. Hansmann M: A critical evaluation of the performance of ultrasonic diagnosis in present-day obstetrics. *Gynakologe* 1974; 7:26–35.
45. Aantaa K. Forss M: Determination of biparietal diameter by the ultrasonic B-scan technique. *Acta Obstet Gynecol Scand* 1974; 53:121–124.
46. Hassani SN: *Ultrasound in Gynecology and Obstetrics.* New York, Springer-Verlag, 1979, pp 91–92.
47. Hobbins JC: *Yale Nomogram.* Iselin, NJ, Siemens Corp, Electro Medical Division, 1979.
48. Flamme P: Ultrasonic fetal cephalometry: percentiles curve. *Br Med J* 1972; 3:384–385.
49. Yiu-Chiu V, Chiu L: Ultrasonographic evaluation of normal fetal anatomy and congenital malformations. *CT* 1981; 5:367–381, 508–509.
50. Persson PH, Grennert L, Gennser G, et al: Normal range curves for the intrauterine growth of the biparietal diameter. *Acta Obstet Gynecol Scand* 1978; 78:15–20.
51. Fescina RH, Ucieda FJ, Cordano MC, et al: Ultrasonic patterns of intrauterine fetal growth in a Latin American country. *Early Hum Dev* 1982; 6:239–248.
52. Garrett W, Robinson D: Assessment of fetal size and growth rate by ultrasonic echoscopy. *Obstet Gynecol* 1979; 38:525–534.
53. Eriksen PS, Secher NJ, Weis-Bentzon M: Normal growth of the fetal biparietal diameter and the abdominal diameter in a longitudinal study. *Acta Obstet Gynecol Scand* 1985; 64:65–70.
54. Jeanty P, Cousaert E, Hobbins JC, et al: A longitudinal study of fetal head biometry. *Am J Perinatol* 1984; 1:118–128.
55. Chervenak FA, Jeanty P, Cantraine F, et al: The diagnosis of fetal microcephaly. *Am J Obstet Gynecol* 1984; 149:512.
56. Osefo NJ, Chukudebelu WO: Sonar cephalometry and fetal age relationship in the Nigerian woman. *East Afr Med J* 1983; 60:98–102.
57. Oman SD, Wax Y: Estimating fetal age by ultrasound measurement: an example of multivariate calibration. *Biometrics* 1984; 40:947–960.
58. Sanders M: Personal communications; 1979: Sabaggha RE, Barton FA, Barton BA: Sonar biparietal diameter: I. Analysis of percentile growth differences in two normal populations using same methodology. *Am J Obstet Gynecol* 1976; 126:479–484.
59. Yagel S, Adoni A, Oman S, et al: A statistical examination of the accuracy of combining femoral length and biparietal diameter as an index of fetal gestational age. *Br J Obstet Gynaecol* 1986; 93:109–115.
60. Persson PH, Weldner BM: Normal range growth curves for fetal biparietal diameter, occipitofrontal diameter, mean abdominal diameters and femur length. *Acta Obstet Gynecol Scand* 1986; 65:759–761.
61. Kossoff G, Garrett WJ, Radovanovich G: Grey scale echography in obstetrics and gynaecology. *Australas Radiol* 1974; 18:63–111.
62. Deter RL, Harrist RB, Hadlock FP, et al: Longitudinal studies of fetal growth with the use of dynamic image ultrasonography. *Am J Obstet Gynecol* 1982; 143:545–554.
63. Thompson HE, Holmes JH, Gottesfeld KR, et al: Fetal development as determined by ultrasonic pulse echo techniques. *Am J Obstet Gynecol* 1965; 92:44–52.
64. Campbell S, Dewhurts CJ: Diagnosis of the small-for-dates fetus by serial ultrasonic cephalometry. *Lancet* 1971; 2:1002–1006.
65. Willocks J, Dunsmore IR: Assessment of gestational age and prediction of dysmaturity by ultrasonic fetal cephalometry. *J Obstet Gynaecol Br Commw* 1971; 78:804–808.
66. Bartolucci L: Biparietal diameter of the skull and fetal weight in the second trimester: an allometric relationship. *Am J Obstet Gynecol* 1975; 122:439–445.
67. Willocks J: The study of fetal growth by serial cephalometry and estriol measurements. *J Reprod Med* 1971; 6:84–88.

68. Queenan JT, Kubarych SF, Cook LN, et al: Diagnostic ultrasound for detection of intrauterine growth retardation. *Am J Obstet Gynecol* 1976; 124:865–873.

69. Chapman MG, Sheat JH, Furness ET, et al: Routine ultrasound screening in early pregnancy. *Med J Aust* 1979; 2:62–63.

70. Issel EP, Prenzlau P, Bayer H, et al: The measurement of fetal growth during pregnancy by ultrasound (B-scan). *J Perinatol Med* 1975; 3:269–275.

71. Aantaa K, Forss M: Growth of the fetal biparietal diameter in different types of pregnancies. *Radiology* 1980; 137:167–169.

72. Ogata ES, Sabbagha R, Metzger BE, et al: Serial ultrasonography to assess evolving fetal macrosomia: studies in 23 pregnancy diabetic women. *JAMA* 1980; 243:2405–2408.

73. Ojala A, Ylostalo P, Jouppila P, et al: Fetal cephalometry by ultrasound in normal and complicated pregnancy. *Ann Chir Gynaecol Fenn* 1970; 59:71–75.

74. Murata Y, Martin CB: Growth of the biparietal diameter of the fetal head in diabetic pregnancy. *Am J Obstet Gynecol* 1973; 115:252–256.

75. Pap G, Pap L: Ultrasonic estimation of gestational age and fetal weight. *Paediatr Acad Sci Hung* 1979; 20:119–135.

76. Pap G, Szoke J, Pap L: Intrauaterine growth retardation: ultrasonic diagnosis. *Acta Paediatr Hung* 1983; 24:7–15.

77. Parker AJ, Davies P, Mayho AM, et al: The ultrasound estimation of sex-related variations of intrauterine growth. *Am J Obstet Gynecol* 1984; 149:665–669.

78. Walton SM: Ethnic considerations in ultrasonic scanning of fetal biparietal diameters. *Aust NZ J Obstet Gynaecol* 1981; 21:82–83.

79. Wittman BK, Robinson HP, Aitchison T, et al: The value of diagnostic ultrasound as a screening test for intrauterine growth retardation: comparison of nine parameters. *Am J Obstet Gynecol* 1979; 134:30–35.

80. Jordan HVF: Biological variation in the biparietal diameter and its bearing on clinical ultrasonography. *Am J Obstet Gynecol* 1978; 131:53–58.

81. Pedersen JF: Ultrasound evidence of sexual difference in fetal size in first trimester. *Br Med J* 1980; 281:1253.

82. Parker AJ: Assessment of gestational age of the Asian fetus by the sonar measurement of crown-rump length and biparietal diameter. *Br J Obstet Gynaecol* 1982; 89:836–838.

83. Dubowitz LMS, Goldberg C: Assessment of gestation by ultrasound in various stages of pregnancy in infants differing in size and ethnic origin. *Br J Obstet Gynaecol* 1981; 88:255–259.

84. Meire HB, Farrant P: Ultrasound demonstration of an unusual fetal growth pattern in Indians. *Br J Obstet Gynaecol* 1981; 88:260–263.

85. Okupe RF, Coker OO, Gbajumo SA: Assessment of fetal biparietal diameter during normal pregnancy by ultrasound in Nigerian women. *Br J Obstet Gynaecol* 1984; 91:629–632.

86. Munoz WP, Moore PJ, MacKinnon A, et al: Biparietal diameter and menstrual age in the black population attending Edendale Hospital. *J Clin Ultrasound* 1986; 14:681–688.

87. Sabbagha RE: *Ultrasound in High-Risk Obstetrics.* Philadelphia, Lea & Febiger, 1979, p 38.

88. Hadlock FP, Deter RL, Harrist RB, et al: Fetal biparietal diameter: rational choice of plane of section for sonographic measurement. *AJR* 1982; 138:871–874.

89. Kossoff G, Garrett WJ, Radovanovich G: Grey scale echography in obstetrics and gynaecology. *Australas Radiol* 1974; 18:63–111.

90. Levi S. Erbsman F: Antenatal fetal growth from the nineteenth week: ultrasonic study of 12 head and chest dimension. *Am J Obstet Gynecol* 1975; 121:262–268.

91. Deter RL, Harrist RB, Hadlock FP, et al: The use of ultrasound in the assessment of normal fetal growth: A review. *J Clin Ultrasound* 1981; 9:481–493.

92. *Dorland's Illustrated Medical Dictionary,* ed 24. Philadelphia, WB Saunders Co, 1957, pp 217, 444.

93. Hastings Ince JG: On the value of cephalometry in the estimation of foetal weight: Based on measurements of 1010 infants. *J Obstet Gynaecol Br Emp* 1939; 46:1003–1009.

94. Jordaan HVF: The differential enlargement of the neuro-cranium in the full-term fetus. *S Afr Med J* 1976; 50:1978–1981.

95. Haas LL: Roentgenological skull measurements and their diagnostic applications. *AJR* 1952; 67:197–209.

96. Hadlock FP, Deter RL, Carpenter RJ, et al: Estimating fetal age: Effect of head shape on BPD. *AJR* 1981; 137:83–85.

97. Shields JR, Medearis AL, Bear MB: Fetal head and abdominal circumferences: Effect of profile shape on the accuracy of ellipse equations. *J Clin Ultrasound* 1987; 15:241–244.

98. Kasby CB, Poll V: The breech head and its ultrasound significance. *Br J Obstet Gynaecol* 1982; 89:106–110.

99. Wolfson RN, Zador IE, Halvorsen P, et al: Biparietal diameter in premature rupture of membrane: Errors in estimating gestational age. *J Clin Ultrasound* 1983; 11:371–374.

100. Doubilet PM, Greenes RA: Improved prediction of gestational age from fetal head measurements. *AJR* 1984; 142:797–800.

101. Usher R, McLean F: Intrauterine growth of live-born Caucasian infants at sea level: Standards obtained from measurements in 7 dimensions of infants born between 25 and 44 weeks of gestation. *Pediatrics* 1969; 74:901–910.

102. Lubchenco LO, Hansmann C, Boyd E: Intrauterine growth in length and head circumference as estimated from live births at gestational ages from 26 to 42 week. *Pediatrics* 1966; 37:403–408.

103. Babson SG, Benda GI: Growth graphs for the clinical assessment of infants of varying gestational age. *Pediatrics* 1976; 89:814–820.

104. Gairdner D: Ultrasonic fetal cephalometry. *Br Med J* 1972; 3:585.

105. Hadlock FP, Kent WR, Loyd JL, et al: An evaluation of two methods for measuring fetal heads and body circumferences. *J Ultrasound Med* 1982; 1:359–360.

106. Shields JR, Medearis AL, Bear MB: Fetal head and abdominal circumferences: Ellipse calculations versus planimetry. *J Clin Ultrasound* 1987; 15:237–239.

107. DeVore GR, Platt LD: Choosing the correct equation for computing the head circumference from two diameters: the effect of head shape. *Am J Obstet Gynecol* 1984; 148:221.

108. Birnholz JC: On calculating the perimeter of an ellipse. *J Clin Ultrasound* 1984; 12:55–56.

109. Deter RL, Harrist RB, Hadlock FP, et al: The use of ultrasound in the assessment of normal fetal growth: A review. *J Clin Ultrasound* 1981; 9:481–493.

110. Parker AJ, Davies P, Mayho AM, et al: The ultrasound estimation of sex-related variations of intrauterine growth. *Am J Obstet Gynecol* 1984; 149:665–669.

111. Campbell S, Thoms A: Personal communications; Fetal head circumference against gestational age, in Metrewelli: *Practical Clinical Ultrasound*. Chicago, 1978, p 114.

112. Athey PA, Hadlock FP, Appendix, in Harshberger SE (ed): *Ultrasound in Obstetrics and Gynecology*. St Louis, CV Mosby Co, 1981, p 269.

113. Hadlock FP, Deter RL, Harrist RB, et al: Fetal head circumference: relation to menstrual age. *AJR* 1982; 138:649–653,

114. Deter RL, Harrist RB, Hadlock RP, et al: Fetal head and abdominal circumferences: II. A critical reevaluation of the relationship to menstrual age. *J Clin Ultrasound* 1982; 10:365–372.

115. Fescina RH, Martell M: Intrauterine and extrauterine growth of cranial perimeter in term and preterm infants. *Am J Obstet Gynecol* 1983; 147:928–932.

116. Ott WJ: The use of ultrasonic fetal head circumference for predicting expected date of confinement. *J Clin Ultrasound* 1984; 12:411–415.

117. van Egmond-Linden A, Wladimiroff JW, Niermeijer MF, et al: Fetal hydrocephaly: Diagnosis, prognosis and management. *Ultrasound Med Biol* 1986; 12:939–944.

118. Deter RL, Harrist RB, Hadlock FP, et al: Fetal head and abdominal circumferences: I. Evaluation of measurement errors. *J Clin Ultrasound* 1982; 10:357–363.

119. Crane JP, Kopta MM: Prediction of intrauterine growth retardation via ultrasonically measured head/abdominal circumference ratios. *Obstet Gynecol* 1979; 54:597–601.

120. Law RG, MacRae KD: Head circumference as an index of fetal age. *J Ultrasound Med* 1982; 1:281–288.

121. Kossoff G, Garrett WJ, Radovanovich G: Grey scale echography in obstetrics and gynaecology. *Australas Radiol* 1974; 18:63–111.

122. Wladimiroff JW, Bloemsma CA, Wallenburg HCS: Ultrasonic assessment of fetal growth. *Acta Obstet Gynecol Scand* 1977; 56:37–42.

123. Varma TR, Taylor H, Bridges C: Ultrasound assessment of fetal growth. *Br J Obstet Gynaecol* 1979; 86:623–632.

124. Rossavik IK, Deter RL, Hadlock FP: Mathematical modeling of fetal growth: III. Evaluation of head growth using the head profile area. *J Clin Ultrasound* 1987; 15:23–30.

125. Marinez DA, Bartown JL: Estimation of fetal body and fetal head volumes: description of technique and nomograms for 18 to 41 weeks of gestation. *Am J Obstet Gynecol* 1980; 137:78–84.

126. Rossavik IK, Deter RL: Mathematical modeling of fetal growth: I. Basic principles. *J Clin Ultrasound* 1984; 12:529–533.

127. Rossavik IK, Deter RL: Mathematical modeling of fetal growth: II. Head cube (A), abdominal cube (B) and their ratio (A/B). *J Clin Ultrasound* 1984; 12:535–545.

128. DuBose TJ: Fetal biometry. Vertical calvarial diameter and calvarial volume. *J Diagn Med Sonogr* 1985; 1:205–217.

129. O'Keeffe DF, Garite TJ, Elliott JP, et al: The accuracy of estimated gestational age based on ultrasound measurement of biparietal diameter in preterm premature rupture of membranes. *Am J Obstet Gynecol* 1985; 151:309–312.

130. Hanson J, Levander B, Liliequist B: Size of the intracerebral ventricles as measured with computer tomography, encephalography and echoventriculography. *Acta Radiol [Suppl] (Stockh)* 1975; 346:98–106.

131. Skolnick ML, Rosenbaum AE, Matzuk T, et al: Detection of dilated cerebral ventricles in infants: a correlative study between ultrasound and computed tomography. *Radiology* 1979; 131:447–451.

132. Johnson ML, Dunne MG, Mack LA, et al: Evaluation of fetal intracranial anatomy by static and real-time ultrasound. *J Clin Ultrasound* 1980; 8:311–318.

133. Jeanty P, Dramaix-Wilmet M, Delbeke D, et al: Ultrasonic evaluation of fetal ventricular growth. *Neuroradiology* 1981; 21:127–131.

134. Hadlock FP, Deter RL, Park SK: Real-time sonography: ventricular and vascular anatomy of the fetal brain in utero. *Am J Neuroradiol* 1980; 1:507–511.

135. McGahan JP, Phillips HE: Ultrasonic evaluation of the size of the trigone and the fetal ventricle. *J Ultrasound Med* 1983; 2:315–319.

136. Pilu G, Reece EA, Goldstein I, et al: Sonographic evaluation of the normal developmental anatomy of the fetal cerebral ventricles: II. the atria. *Obstet Gynecol* 1989; 73:250–256.

137. Cardoza JD, Goldstein RB, Filly RA: Exclusion of fetal ventriculomegaly with a single measurement: the width of the lateral ventricular atrium. *Radiology* 1988; 169:711–714.

138. Mahony BS, Nyberg DA, Hirsch JH, et al: Mild idiopathic lateral cerebral ventricular dilatation in utero: sonographic evaluation. *Radiology* 1988; 169:715–721.

139. Denkhaus H, Winsberg F: Ultrasonic measurement of the fetal ventricular system. *Radiology* 1979; 131:781–787.

140. Jorgensen C, Ingemarsson I, Svalenius E, et al: Ultrasound measurement of the fetal cerebral ventricles: A prospective, consecutive study. *J Clin Ultrasound* 1986; 14:185–190.

141. Pretorius DH, Drose JA, Manco-Johnson ML: Fetal lateral ventricular ratio determination during the second trimester. *J Ultrasound Med* 1986; 5:121–124.

142. Goldstein I, Reece EA, Pilu GL, et al: Sonographic evaluation of the normal developmental anatomy of fetal cerebral ventricles: I. The frontal horn. *Obstet Gynecol* 1988; 72:588–592.

143. Hertzberg BS, Bowie JD, Burger PC, et al: The three lines: origin of sonographic landmarks in the fetal head. *AJR* 1987; 149:1009–1012.

144. Johnson ML, Mack LA, Rumack CM, et al: B-mode echoencephalography in the normal and high risk infant. *AJR* 1979; 133:375–381.

145. Chinn DH, Callen PW, Filly RA: The lateral cerebral ventricle in early second trimester. *Radiology* 1983; 148:529–531.

146. Benacerraf BR, Frigoletto Jr. FD, Bieber FR: The fetal face: Ultrasound examination. *Radiology* 1984; 153:495–497.

147. Birnholz JC: Ultrasonic fetal ophthalmology. *Early Hum Dev* 1985; 12:199–209.

148. Jeanty P, Dramaix-Wilmet M, Van Gansbeke N, et al: Fetal ocular biometry by ultrasound. *Radiology* 1982; 143:513–516.

149. Jeanty P, Cantraine F, Cousaert E, et al: The binocular distance: A new way to estimate fetal age. *J Ultrasound Med* 1984; 3:241–243.

150. Mayden KL, Tortora M, Berkowitz RL, et al: Orbital diameters: a new parameter for prenatal diagnosis and dating. *Am J Obstet Gynecol* 1982; 144:289–297.

151. McLeary RD, Kuhns LR, Barr M Jr: Ultrasonography of the fetal cerebellum. *Radiology* 1984; 151:439–442.

152. Goldstein I, Reece EA, Pilu G, et al: Cerebellar measurements with ultrasonography in the evaluation of fetal growth and development. *Am J Obstet Gynecol* 1987; 156:1065–1069.

153. Smith PA, Johansson D, Tzannatos C, et al: Prenatal measurement of the fetal cerebellum and cisterna cerebellomedullaris by ultrasound. *Prenat Diagn* 1986; 6:133–141.

154. Reece EA, Goldstein I, Pilu G, et al: Fetal cerebellar growth unaffected by intrauterine growth retardation: a new parameter for prenatal diagnosis. *Am J Obstet Gynecol* 1987; 157:632–638.

155. Pilu G, DePalma L, Romero R, et al: The fetal subarachnoid cisterns: An ultrasound study with report of a case of congenital communicating hydrocephalus. *J Ultrasound Med* 1986; 5:365–372.

156. Mahony BS, Callen PW, Filly RA, et al: The fetal cisterna magna. *Radiology* 1984; 153:773–776.
157. Comstock CH, Boal DB: Enlarged fetal cisterna magna: Appearance and significance. *Obstet Gynecol* 1985; 66(Suppl):25S–28S.

Chapter 25 _____

Fetal Body Measurements

Alfred B. Kurtz, M.D.

Barry B. Goldberg, M.D.

THORACIC DIAMETER

Seven articles have measured the thoracic diameter, comparing it to gestational age,[1-7] three throughout the second and third trimesters[1, 4, 5] and the others from 21 weeks or beyond to term. Measurements have been obtained from static scanners in five,[1-4, 7] three giving actual numbers,[1, 2, 7] with one in graph[4] and one in equation[3] form. The other two[5, 6] used real-time scanners, both in graph form. All showed an increase in thoracic diameter with increasing gestational age.

Six of the articles obtained thoracic measurements in the transaxial projection at the region of cardiac motion or just above the diaphragm,[2-7] three with standard deviations.[2, 4, 5] In the last article,[1] the thoracic diameter was obtained from a long-axis view of the fetus. Since the exact internal anatomic landmarks and the points of measurement were not mentioned, this article will not be considered further. The anteroposterior (AP) dimension was measured in four,[2-4, 7] with four measuring the transaxial diameter.[2, 5-7] Only three specifically stated that the thoracic measurements were taken from outer edge to outer edge.[2, 5, 6]

The results of these measurements are diverse. The AP dimensions varied among the articles by 6 mm at 24 weeks to 12 mm at term, while the transaxial diameters varied by as much as 20 mm throughout gestation. Because of these discrepancies, it is felt that the thoracic diameter measurements are not accurate enough to be used routinely. The abdominal measurements, on the other hand, have been much more extensively evaluated, have at least the same or smaller standard deviations, and are therefore recommended instead.

THORACIC CIRCUMFERENCE

Seven articles have compared thoracic circumference to gestation age,[1-3, 7-10] three from 16 or less to 40 weeks,[1, 9, 10] three from 20 weeks to postterm,[2, 7, 9] and one from 32 weeks to term.[3] Five[1, 2, 7, 9, 10] presented their data in numeric form, with the other two using equations[3] or graphs[8] instead. Four[2, 8-10] also gave standard deviations. The earlier four[1, 2, 3, 7] were evaluated with static scanners, and the more recent three[8–10] with real-time alone, all giving numbers that increased with increasing gestational age. Six of the seven[2, 3, 7–10] measured the circumference in transaxial projection at the region of cardiac motion from the outer limits of the thoracic cage. The last article[1] measured the fetus in long axis. The authors failed to state at what level the measurements were obtained and whether the outer margins were used.

When the numbers were compared, it was found that Weinreb et al.,[3] Hansmann,[7] Nimrod et al.,[8] Fong et al.,[9] and Chitkara et al.[10] had numbers uniformly below the other two by 5 to 7 cm at every gestational age. The Levi and Erbsman[2] and Hoffbauer et al.[1] articles were fairly close from 22 to 32 weeks but after that time diverged until at term the Hoffbauer et al.[1] measurements were 2.5 cm larger.

When all of these articles were then compared to the newborn measurements of Usher and McLean[11] there were discrepancies either in the second trimester[1, 2] or near term.[3, 7–10] It is therefore felt that the thoracic circumference does not have enough data or close enough grouping to be used in clinical practice. The abdominal measurements have been more widely evaluated, appear to have at least the same, if not smaller, standard deviations, and are recommended instead.

An interesting approach has been proposed by Fong and co-workers.[9] They compared the thoracic circumference to other measurable fetal parameters, the biparietal diameter, head and abdominal circumference, and the femur length in 100 normal pregnancies, and found the closest correlation was with femur length. A table using numbers was constructed comparing the femur length in millimeters to the predicted mean and 2 SD of the thoracic circumference in centimeters. This approach has merit since the thoracic circumference is not needed to establish gestational age. By comparing number to number, symmetry between fetal parts can be predicted instead. Unfortunately, there are few numbers at most femur length points, 16 points from 10 to 81 mm not even being measured. Further work and corroboration is therefore needed.

THORACIC LENGTH

Chitkara et al.[10] measured the length of the thorax in 576 women from 16 to 40 weeks, comparing it to gestational age. The measurement was obtained in a midline view from the cephalic end of the sternum to the diaphragm and showed a mean increase from 20 mm at 16 weeks to 65 mm at 40 weeks. The authors' purpose in obtaining this measurement was the statement that some dysplasias are associated with thoracic shortening in addition to thoracic narrowing.

While not discussed in the article, this measurement appears to be technically difficult to obtain. It would seem that only when the fetus is in a face-up, chin-up presentation could this measurement be consistently obtained. In addition, thoracic length would have limited use since dysplasias with thoracic shortening would also have thoracic narrowing, and a cross-sectional thoracic measurement or a ratio of the thoracic to abdominal circumferences would have equal or greater value.

THORACIC AREA

Six articles have measured the thoracic area comparing it to gestational age.[2,3, 12–15] One was in numeric form,[2] one as an equation,[3] two in numeric and graph form,[13, 14] and the other two in graph form alone.[12, 15] An additional article by Wladimiroff et al.[16] published a graph of the thoracic area which appears to be identical to a graph in another of their articles[20] and will not be discussed further.

All obtained their data on static scanners. The measurements started from either the mid–second trimester[2, 13] or the early third trimester[3, 12, 14, 15] and continued until term, all showing increase in thoracic area with increasing gestational age. Five of these articles stated the exact anatomic position used to obtain the measurements,[2, 3, 13–15] two at the level of the heart[2, 3, 15] and two below the cardiac pulsations.[13, 14] This latter position, below the cardiac pulsations, while termed thoracic, is more likely to be in the upper abdomen. These two articles[13, 14] will therefore be analyzed in both the thoracic area and abdominal area sections. All used a planimeter or map reader to obtain area measurements. While only one stated that the outer margins of the thoracic cage were measured,[2] even that article failed to state exactly where the measurements were obtained and actually referred to the thoracic area as a "trunk" measurement.

The thoracic area numbers were quite discrepant and no definite pattern could be established. Surprisingly, even the numbers from the two articles by Wladimiroff et al.[13, 14] were divergent. Because no definite trend could be established, it is felt that the thoracic area measurement should not be routinely used.

ABDOMINAL DIAMETER

Eight articles have measured the diameter of the fetal abdomen,[1, 3, 17–22] five in numeric form,[1, 17, 19, 20, 22] one as a graph,[21] and one in equation form.[3] All showed an increase in the abdominal diameter with increasing gestational age.

Hoffbauer et al.[1] evaluated the transverse abdominal diameter throughout the second and third trimesters in both the "small and large" dimensions (presumably AP and transverse). Neither the part of the abdomen nor the abdominal boundaries used to take these measurements were described. Weinreb et al.[3] measured the AP diameter of the abdomen but failed to mention the exact anatomic position used and whether the measurements were taken outer to outer diameter. Garrett and Robinson[18] evaluated the fetal abdominal diameter from 23 to 36 weeks, measuring the transaxial abdominal diameter at the area above the kidney and below the heart which is in the region of the liver, presumably outer to outer diameter. Because of these inconsistencies, these three articles will not be considered further.

Of the remaining five articles,[17, 19–22] Fescina et al.[17] evaluated the AP and transverse diameters, Grandjean et al.[21] the transverse diameter, and Eriksen et al.,[19] Persson and Weldner,[20] and Tamura et al.[22] averaged the two diameters perpendicular to each other, all at the level of the umbilical vein, from early second trimester to term. While the umbilical vein is a reproducible landmark, it is only valid if imaged within the liver, not extending to the anterior abdominal wall and equidistant from the right and left sides of the abdomen (Fig 25–1,A). In that position it is termed the umbilical portion of the left portal vein. All measurements should then be taken outer to outer margins since there is not a reproducible inner margin. If the body is round, only one measurement needs to be taken (Fig 25–1,B). If the body is ovoid, however, two measurements perpendicular to one another (preferably transverse and AP) are averaged (Fig 25–2).

Four of these five articles were precise in their anatomic position and in their

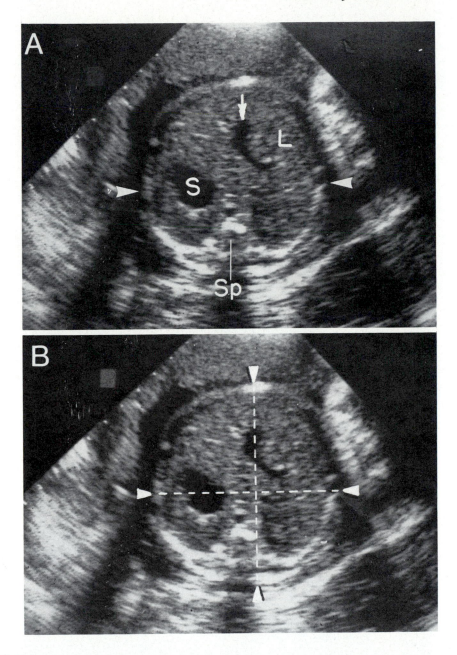

FIG 25–1.
Transaxial scan of the upper fetal abdomen in a 30-week fetus. **A**, round abdomen with the umbilical portion of the left portal vein (*arrow*) positioned within the liver (*L*), not extending to the anterior abdominal wall and equidistant from the lateral abdominal walls (*arrowheads*). *S* = stomach; *Sp* = spine. **B**, same image as **A** showing the outer diameter measurements, denoted by *arrowheads* and *dashed lines*. The two lines are perpendicular to each other, one AP and the other transverse. Since the body is round, only one of the two is needed for an adequate abdominal diameter measurement.

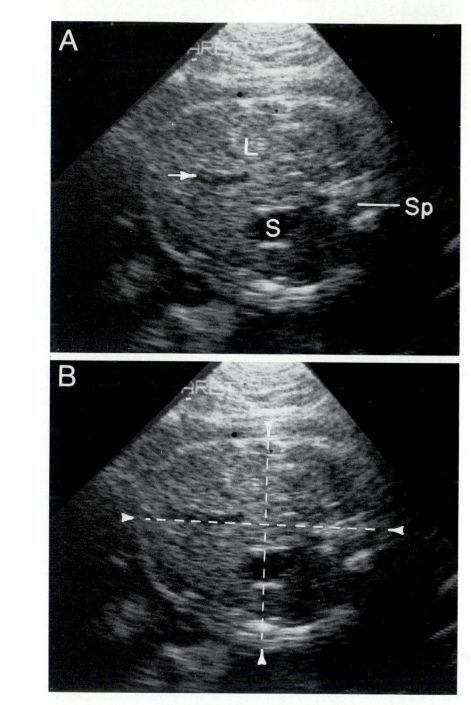

FIG 25–2.
Transaxial scan of the upper abdomen in a 32-week fetus with oligohydramnios. **A,** ovoid abdomen with the umbilical portion of the left portal vein (*arrow*) positioned within the liver (*L*) equidistant from the lateral abdominal walls. *S* = stomach; *Sp* = spine. **B,** same image as **A** showing the outer diameter measurements perpendicular to one another, denoted by *arrowheads* and *dashed lines.* Since the body is ovoid, both measurements should be taken and averaged to obtain the abdominal diameter.

outer to outer measurements[19–22] while the fifth was vague in its description of the umbilical vein position and the margins used.[17] When their numbers were compared, the numbers of Grandjean et al.[21] tapered off after 35 weeks and Fescina et al.[17] did not give a standard deviation with the mean. These latter two articles will therefore also not be considered further.

The remaining three articles, by Eriksen et al.,[19] Persson and Weldner,[20] and Tamura et al.,[22] had closely grouped mean numbers and all gave a standard deviation range. They all compared their measurements to the gestational age; two were longitudinal studies, one examining their patients every 2 to 4 weeks[19] or triweekly.[20] The third study was a cross-sectional analysis.[22] In addition, all showed a close one-to-one relationship (in millimeters) to the biparietal diameter until approximately 30 weeks, the biparietal measurements taken from either their own article[19] or compared to the table of Kurtz et al.[23] In the last trimester, all revealed an increase in body size to 15 mm or more greater than the biparietal diameter by term.

The major differences among these three articles[19, 20, 22] was that Tamura et al.[22] compared their measurements only to gestational age whereas Eriksen et al.[19] and Persson and Weldner[20] compared the mean abdominal measurements to both biparietal diameter and gestational age. This latter approach has more clinical usefulness. Therefore Eriksen et al. and Persson and Weldner are the two preferable studies and either would suffice for appropriate mean abdominal diameter measurements. The only difference in the two articles is that the Erikson et al. article was performed using approximately twice the number of measurements. Because of their larger numbers, the standard deviation of this article would be expected to be smaller. It is not. While this finding is puzzling, the table by Eriksen et al.[19] is nevertheless recommended (Table 25–1).

ABDOMINAL CIRCUMFERENCE

Abdominal circumference measurements, initially used in the evaluation of the newborn,[11] have now been used extensively in utero. In two articles comparing the accuracies of pre- and postnatal ultrasound abdominal circumferences,[24, 25] the measurements were found to correlate closely with errors of no greater than 6%. This percentage is misleading, however, since in one article,[24] the prenatal measurements were always 6% greater, while in the other[25] the fetal measurements were both higher and lower. These inaccuracies contrast sharply with the higher correlation of pre- and postnatal head circumference measurements. At least part of this inaccuracy is technical since (a) the neonatal abdominal circumference measurement is taken only during expiration whereas the respiration phase of the fetus could not be determined,[25] (b) in obtaining the neonatal measurements, there can be slight tightening or relaxing of the measurement tape resulting in neonatal measurement discrepancies of 5 to 10 mm,[25] and (c) the newborn measurements are taken in the midabdomen at the level of the umbilicus,[24] while fetal abdominal measurements are obtained higher, at the level of the fetal liver.[24, 26]

Despite these discrepancies, there have been 15 in utero analyses of abdominal circumference in 16 articles.[1, 3, 17, 25–37] Of these, while Campbell and Wilkin[35] initially presented their data in graph form, their numbers were published by Bree and Mariona.[36] Only the Campbell and Wilkin analysis will be considered further since it could not be determined if the numbers published by Bree and Mariona were

TABLE 25–1.
Abdominal Diameter Measurements*

Gestational Age (wk)	Predicted Mean Biparietal Diameter (mm)	Average Abdominal Diameter (mm)	
		Predicted Mean	Range From 5th to 95th Percentile
13	25.6	22.7	18.2–27.2
14	28.5	26.4	21.7–31.1
15	31.5	30.1	25.3–34.9
16	34.6	33.7	28.6–38.8
17	37.7	37.3	32.0–42.7
18	40.9	40.9	35.4–46.5
19	44.1	44.5	38.7–50.3
20	47.4	48.0	41.9–54.0
21	50.6	51.4	45.2–57.7
22	53.9	54.9	48.3–61.5
23	57.1	58.3	51.4–65.2
24	60.4	61.7	54.5–68.9
25	63.5	65.0	57.5–72.6
26	66.6	68.4	60.5–76.2
27	70.0	71.7	63.4–79.9
28	72.6	74.9	66.3–83.6
29	75.4	78.2	69.1–87.2
30	78.1	81.4	71.9–90.9
31	80.7	84.6	74.6–94.5
32	83.1	87.7	77.2–98.2
33	85.4	90.8	79.8–101.8
34	87.5	93.9	82.4–105.5
35	89.4	97.0	84.8–109.2
36	91.1	100.1	87.3–112.9
37	92.6	103.1	89.5–116.5
38	93.8	106.1	91.9–120.3
39	94.8	109.0	94.1–124.0
40	95.5	112.0	96.2–127.8

*From Eriksen PS, Sechor NJ, Weis-Bentzon M: *Acta Obstet Gynecol Scand* 1985; 64:65–70. Used by permission.

obtained from the original authors or extrapolated from their graph. In addition, Athey and Hadlock[30] will not be considered further since their data were the preliminary results later finalized by Hadlock et al.[26] Lastly, Ogata et al.[27] will be discussed at the end of this section when diabetic effects on abdominal circumference will be evaluated.

The remaining 13 articles[1, 3, 17, 25, 26, 28, 29, 31–35, 37] analyzed abdominal circumference in both the second and third trimester and found it to increase as the gestational age increased. Seven were given in numbers,[1, 17, 25, 26, 31, 34, 35] five in graph

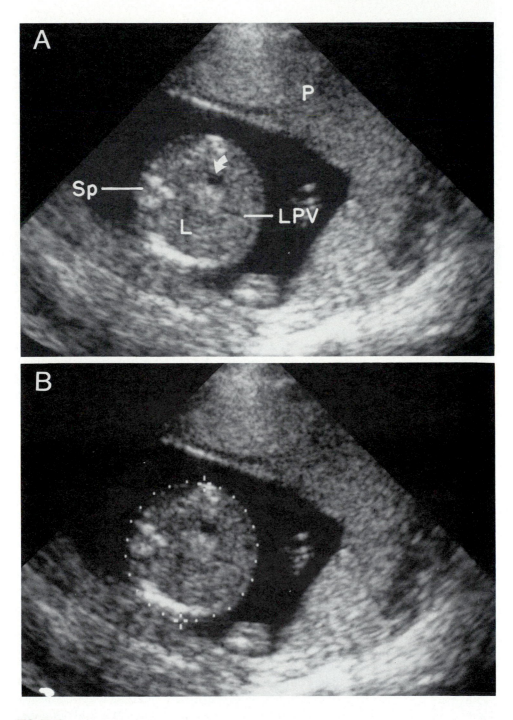

FIG 25–3.
Transaxial image of the upper fetal abdomen in a 22-week fetus. **A,** rounded body with the umbilical portion of the left portal vein (*LPV*) well positioned and midline within the liver (*L*). *Sp* = spine; *P* = placenta; *curved arrow* = stomach. **B,** same image as **A** showing dotted line created by a digitizer around the outer margins of the abdomen to obtain a circumference measurement.

form,[28, 29, 32, 33, 37] and one as an equation.[3] Five used static scans,[1, 3, 25, 35, 37] seven used real-time,[17, 26, 28, 31–34] and one[29] did not state the type of scanner. All the articles except those of Hoffbauer et al.[11] and Meire and Farrant[29] stated that the measurements were obtained at the area of the liver, in particular at either the umbilical portion of the left portal vein or fetal stomach, and that the outer margins of the abdomen were measured with a digitizer (Fig 25–3).

The accuracy in obtaining each measurement has been analyzed. The intraobserver error is not significant, an error of only 0.7% (range 0%–1.7%) when one photograph is used, with the measurement error increasing to 1.9% (range 0.4%–5.9%) from two photographs.[24, 26] The interobserver error is similarly small, 2.4% with a range of 0.8% to 4% at 1 SD, felt to be caused primarily by the use of different measuring devices.[24]

Two questions need to be answered about the abdominal circumference measurements: (1) Are static and real-time scanners equally accurate in obtaining an abdominal circumference? (2) Can the circumference be as accurately measured using an equation as it can with a map reader or digitizer? For the question of real-time versus static scan accuracy, two articles compared the two methods and found no statistical difference.[38, 39] For the question of equation versus digitizer, the answer is not as straightforward. The equation for abdominal circumference is the formula for a circumference of a circle[40] (Table 25–2). This equation should be accurate since in transaxial view the abdomen is either circular or mildly ellipsoidal. In a study of 122 fetal abdomens between 15 and 42 weeks, the abdomens (as expected) were found to be round or mildly ovoid.[41] When the smaller abdominal diameter was divided by the larger abdominal diameter, the range varied from 70.4 to 100 with a median of 89.1 and a 2-SD range of 82.1 to 96.1.[41]

TABLE 25–2.
Circumference Computations

1. Planimetry
2. Equation for a circle

$$\left(\frac{d_1 + d_2}{2}\right) \pi = (d_1 + d_2) \times 1.57$$

Three articles performing both computations found a small error of no greater than 6%.[34, 40, 42] One article presented all the numbers from 18 weeks to term, showing that the digitized numbers were always larger, 1.6% larger at 18 weeks increasing to 6% at term.[34] They calculated this discrepancy to be highly significant at a $P<.0001$. Another article did not show numbers or state in which direction the error occurred, but found the error of 6% not of great significance at a $P<.05$.[40] The third determined that equations slightly and consistently underestimated the abdominal circumference, a finding of no statistical significance.[42] Since all the articles had a small error of no greater than 6%, it is statistically puzzling why one article deemed these discrepancies significant and the other two did not. It would not seem, however, that a maximum error of 6% near term should cause large measurement inconsistencies. In addition, while the numbers are different for digitized versus equation-produced abdominal circumference measurements, they still overlapped in the one article that felt that they were significant at less than 1 SD, 25% to 75%.[34] Near term, the increased error might be due to a more crowded and therefore more ellipsoid body. Perhaps a correction factor in the circle circumference equation is needed to compensate for this small error.

When these 13 articles were compared, Hadlock et al.,[26] Deter et al.,[31] Fescina et al.,[17] and the equation-produced numbers of Tamura et al.[34] were found to be very close in their mean numbers. Tamura and Sabbagha,[25] Deter et al.,[32, 33] Meire and Farrant,[29] and the digitized values of Tamura et al.[34] had uniformly larger numbers by approximately 3% to 4%, approaching 6% near term. Hoffbauer et al.[1] Hobbins et al.,[37] Weinreb et al.,[3] and Parker et al.[28] had uniformly smaller numbers by approximately 5% to 8%. Campbell and Wilkin[35] were fairly close from 26 weeks until 32 weeks and then showed a marked decrease with a variation of -2.9% at term.

It is felt that the Hadlock et al.,[26] Deter et al.,[31] Tamura et al.,[34] and Fescina et al.[17] are the most accurate, since they are in the middle of the mean numbers of all other articles. All four gave a range of standard deviations, Tamura et al.[34] from the 10th to 90th percentile and the other three at least at 2 SD.[17, 26, 31] Of these four articles, Hadlock et al.[26] showed mean abdominal circumferences with the gestational age varying in weeks, increasing from ± 1.9 weeks at 12 gestational weeks to ± 2.5 weeks by 42 gestational weeks, while the others used mean gestational age with the abdominal circumference varying in centimeters. This latter approach has no practicality in everyday obstetrical ultrasound measurements. Therefore, the data of Hadlock et al.[26] were chosen (Table 25–3) because of their real-world applicability. The discrepancies between an equation-produced circumference and a digitized-produced circumference, while appearing to be small, cannot be resolved at the present time.

The abdominal circumference has been shown to vary with fetal gender, ethnic background, and maternal diabetes mellitus in three articles, all in graph form.[27–29] Parker et al.[28] examined 96 pregnant European women and claimed that male fetuses were statistically larger than female fetuses after 28 weeks, increasing to term. However, the only numbers given in this article were at 36 gestational weeks and revealed a difference of only 10 mm with overlap at 1 SD. Meire and Farrant[29] compared Indian to European women and found 30% of the Indian fetuses to be 2 SD below their counterparts throughout pregnancy. No numbers were given. Ogata et al.[27] evaluated the growth of the abdominal circumference from 18 to 40 weeks in 23 diabetics, classes A through C. In 13, there was normal abdominal circumference growth throughout gestation. In the other 10 (43% of the cases), "accelerated somatic growth" was noted after 28 to 32 weeks. While the biparietal diameters stayed the same in size, this increase in abdominal circumference was reflected at birth by increased subcutaneous tissues as measured by skin-fold thickness and increase in the fetal weight. Clearly, more work is needed in these areas to define the true incidence and severity of these changes.

ABDOMINAL AREA

Eight articles have measured the abdominal area with comparison to gestational age.[3, 13–15, 17, 18, 43, 44] Two have previously been described under thoracic area.[13, 14] Since these articles stated that the thoracic area was measured below the cardiac pulsations, they were most likely measured at the region of the liver.[13, 14] An additional article by Wladimiroff et al.[16] has a graph which appears to be identical to a

multiplied by the length of the fetus (the exact landmarks for obtaining the length are not stated), and the transverse and AP diameters (measured in the transaxial view from the upper abdomen at the umbilical vein). At 18 weeks, the fetal body volume was 40 cc, increasing steadily to greater than 800 cc by 40 weeks. In the same article, the fetal body volume was compared to the fetal head volume and was found after 29 weeks to increase more than the head volume. The interobserver and intraobserver errors were estimated for the body volume measurements and found to be 6.4 and 6.3 cc, respectively.

In the other two articles,[48, 49] the fetal body volume was computed from two diameters taken in the transaxial view at the level of the liver. In graph form, the body volume increased from approximately 10 cc at 12 weeks to approximately 50 cc at 18 weeks to greater than 1,400 cc at term.

Despite the theoretical probability that a body volume is a better method for evaluating overall body size, these formulas (particularly extrapolating a volume from transaxial measurements alone), have not proved accurate. Fetal body volumes are therefore not recommended.

TOTAL FETAL VOLUMES

Two articles have attempted to calculate fetal volume.[47, 50] One combined close interval static scans of the fetus, to compute a total fetal volume.[50] In comparing their in utero results to hydrostatic weight of aborted fetus or birth weight, the authors found that their formula consistently underestimated the true volume by 10%. The other article[47] used ellipsoid calculations of the head and body.

There were large differences in the volumes between the two articles. While this is an interesting concept, these two methods are so discrepant in technique and results that total fetal volumes are not recommended.

TOTAL FETAL LENGTH

Articles have been published evaluating live premature infants from approximately 24 gestational weeks until term,[11, 51–53] two in numeric form[11, 51] and the other two in graph form. All measurements were obtained with infants fully extended and measured from the crown (top of the head) to the heel. All articles gave a mean newborn length with a variation around the mean of 2 SD, revealing an overall size increase from approximately 355 mm at 26 weeks to 500 mm by term. This neonatal growth was found in one article to be linear.[52] In the other three, it was biphasic with a more rapid initial growth until approximately 36 weeks followed by a decrease until term.[11, 51, 53] Male infants were found to be equal to females in length in one article[51] with males slightly larger in the other two.[11, 53]

There have been seven ultrasound articles evaluating the length of the fetus,[1, 4, 7, 54–57] by either measuring the length of the fetal head and body,[1, 4, 7, 54] or by measuring its femoral length.[53–57] The fetus was analyzed throughout the entire second and third trimesters from 12 to 15 weeks until 40 weeks in two articles[1, 4] while the other five articles evaluated the fetus from 20 or more weeks to term. Three presented the data as numbers,[1, 7, 57] two as graphs only,[4, 54] and two in graph and equation form.[55, 56] Only three[4, 55, 57] also gave a standard deviation.

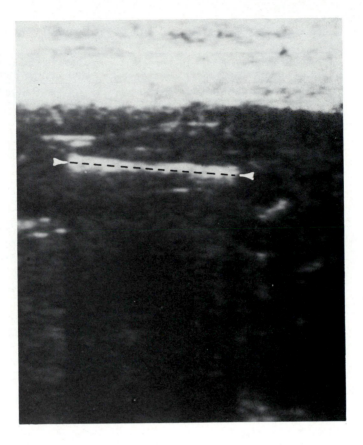

FIG 25–4.
Long-axis image of fetal femur at 30 weeks. The femoral shaft is ossified and the measurement is taken along its longest length, excluding the nonossified proximal and distal epiphyseal cartilages. Measurement denoted by *arrowheads* and *dashed line.*

Although four[1, 4, 7, 54] imaged the fetus with static scans, none specifically mentioned the points from where the measurements were obtained. Presumably, three of these[1, 7, 54] evaluated the full length of the fetus from the top of the head to the bottom of the rump, while the last article[4] only measured the length of the trunk. Nevertheless, when their numbers were compared, particularly the three evaluating the full length of the fetus, two[7, 54] had numbers similar to the full length of the premature infants. This is quite surprising since the ultrasound measurements could not have incorporated the length of the fetal extremities.

The other three articles[55–57] measured the fetal femur with real-time scanners, all within 72 hours of delivery, one in numeric form[57] and the other two as graphs.[55, 56] All found a close linear relationship to the neonatal crown-heel length, from approximately 20 weeks until term. While these articles could not be compared with the ones in the preceding paragraph, there may be a value in determining fetal length for the prediction of birth weight or of growth retardation.[57] Further work is needed to verify these data. The Vintzileos et al.[57] table is nevertheless recommended to predict fetal crown-heel length by using the femoral length measurement (Fig 25–4) since it is in numeric form and over a wider range than the other articles (Table 25–4).

TABLE 25–4.
Fetal Length Measurements—Use of Femur Length to Predict Fetal Crown-Heel
Length*

Femur Length (mm)	Predicted Fetal Crown-Heel Length (mm)		Femur Length (mm)	Predicted Fetal Crown-Heel Length (mm)	
	Predicted Mean	Range From 5th to 95th Percentile		Predicted Mean	Range From 5th to 95th Percentile
30	239	226–251	60	416	413–419
31	245	233–256	61	422	419–425
32	251	239–262	62	428	424–431
33	257	245–268	63	434	430–437
34	262	252–273	64	439	436–443
35	268	258–279	65	445	442–449
36	274	264–284	66	451	447–455
37	280	270–290	67	457	453–461
38	286	277–295	68	463	458–468
39	292	283–306	69	469	464–474
40	298	289–306	70	475	470–480
41	304	295–312	71	481	475–486
42	310	302–318	72	487	481–493
43	316	308–323	73	493	486–499
44	321	314–329	74	498	492–505
45	327	321–334	75	504	497–511
46	333	327–340	76	510	503–518
47	339	333–345	77	516	508–524
48	345	339–351	78	522	514–530
49	351	346–356	79	528	520–536
50	357	352–362	80	534	525–543
51	363	358–368	81	540	531–549
52	369	364–373	82	546	536–555
53	375	370–379	83	552	542–561
54	380	377–384	84	557	547–568
55	386	383–390	85	563	553–574
56	392	389–396	86	569	558–580
57	398	395–401	87	575	564–587
58	404	401–407	88	581	569–593
59	410	407–413	89	587	575–599
			90	593	580–606

*From Vintzileos AM, Campbell WA, Neckles S, et al: *Obstet Gynecol* 1984; 64:779–782. Used by permission.

BODY ORGAN MEASUREMENTS

Heart

Since the late 1970s, high-resolution real-time equipment, frequently with M-mode capabilities, has permitted accurate evaluation of the fetal heart. The planes of section involved in imaging the normal heart and its internal structures have been extensively studied.[58-68] Throughout the second and third trimester, preferably after 16 weeks, the success in visualizing cardiac structures varied with fetal position, fetal heart size (directly related to fetal size), and examiner experience.[65] Visualization of the great vessels, the atrial and ventricular size and function, the atrioventricular valves, and the presence and continuity of ventricular and atrial septa was greater than 90%.[60, 64] Only the semilunar valves, aortic arch, ascending and descending arota, and venae cavae were visualized less frequently—55% to 87% of the time.[60, 64, 68]

Articles have described as few as two and as many as eight planes of section to adequately evaluate the fetal heart. While detailed descriptions of these sections are beyond the scope of this book, two articles offer comparisons of ultrasound images to diagrams and/or autopsy pictures.[65, 66] Of all the views, the easiest and most routine is the four-chamber image which offers almost all significant intracardiac information and only fails in its inability to image the great vessels and their values. The procedure for the four-chamber view is as follows. The large size of the fetal liver and the unexpanded lungs causes the fetal heart to lie almost perpendicular to the fetal trunk, a different axis than in children and adults. In the transaxial plane, through the lower chest, the four-chamber view visualizes both ventricles, the interventricular septum, both atria, the foramen ovale, the mitral and tricupsid valves, and the descending thoracic aorta (Figs 25–5 and 25–6). The fetal heart is on the left side with the right ventricle positioned anteriorly and closest to the chest wall. If transaxial and oblique longitudinal views can also be obtained higher in the chest at the cardiac base, continuity of the aortic root to the left ventricle, the pulmonary artery to the right ventricle, and the aortic and pulmonic valves can be shown.[66] These views eliminate all major cardiac anomalies except for transposition of the great vessels.

Because of the rapid movement of the fetal heart, approximately 120 to 180 beats per minute[69] with frequent additional movements of the fetus, rapid-scanning real-time ultrasound (with scan rates of at least 20 to 30 frames per second) is essential for proper orientation. Since the cardiac structures are relatively small, a high-resolution transducer (at least 3.5 MHz, if not 5.0 MHz) should be used. There has been discussion in the literature as to whether real-time or M-mode should be used to obtain the cardiac measurements. Real-time requires less skill and time for proper orientation and can measure a structure at any angle. Freeze-framing capabilities, however, usually degrade the image. M-mode, on the other hand, scans and records faster but has to be perpendicular to the object imaged. It frequently requires increased time to obtain a measurement.

Real-time imaging is required initially to obtain the proper orientation before M-mode recording is obtained. If the fetus shifts position, real-time may have to be used again to reorient for M-mode. Once oriented correctly, M-mode is superior for arrhythmias, particularly the tachyarrhythmias,[68-71] and for the evaluation of valvular motion. It is also slightly better for evaluating the exact phase of the cardiac cycle, systole or diastole. For structural abnormalities, both real-time and M-mode have their advantages but real-time is favored because of increased ease of scanning. Almost all structural cardiac abnormalities detected by ultrasound in utero have been large.

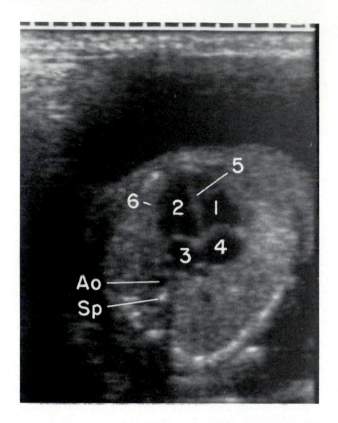

FIG 25–5.
Transaxial image of lower fetal chest in a 25-week fetus showing a four-chamber view of the heart in systole. The left side of the fetus is on the reader's left. *1* = right ventricle, closest to anterior chest wall; *2* = left ventricle; *3* = left atrium, closest to descending thoracic aorta; *4* = right atrium; *5* = interventricular septum; *6* = left ventricular wall. *Ao* = descending thoracic aorta; *Sp* = spine.

They have been visually obvious, at least 3 to 4 mm in size, and therefore measurements were not necessary. Nevertheless, structural cardiac abnormalites could be so subtle that only abnormal measurements might suggest their diagnosis.

A number of articles have been published describing different normal cardiac parameters.[2, 72–90] Unfortunately, many of these failed to measure the same structures or to use the same phase of the cardiac cycle or same anatomic plane. Levi and Erbsman,[2] using static scans from the mid–second trimester until term, evaluated the outer cardiac AP and transverse diameters, circumference, and area. Suzuke et al.[72] analyzed the heart volume with static scans from 30 weeks to term using the formula approximating the equation for a sphere, that is:

$$4/3 \; \pi \times \text{the AP dimension}/2 \times (\text{transverse dimension}/2)^2$$

They found their volumes to increase throughout gestation and to correlate well with the biparietal diameter, gestational age, and fetal weight, particularly if the fetus weighed more than 2,500 g. Although outer cardiac margins were used, the exact anatomic place where these measurements were taken was not stated. Jeanty et al.[73] also measured the outer dimensions of the heart with real-time from 12 to

40 weeks. Their measurements for transverse and longitudinal diameters and for volume were very different from those of Levi and Erbsman,[2] and deviate near term from those of Suzuke et al.[72] DeVore and Platt,[74] taking into account the phase of the cardiac cycle with M-mode, found that cardiac measurements by Jeanty et al.[73] were "random" and inaccurate in over 40% of cases because the phase of the cardiac cycle was not taken into account. DeVore and Platt[74] felt that measurement should only be made in end-diastole or end-systole.

Filkins et al.[75] evaluated the cardiothoracic ratio from 16 to 36 weeks and found that the ratio of the transverse cardiac to transverse thoracic diameters had a constant mean value of 0.50 (range 0.45–0.55) and the ratio of the AP dimensions of the heart to the thorax had a mean value of 0.52 (range 0.45–0.58). These ratios are compelling

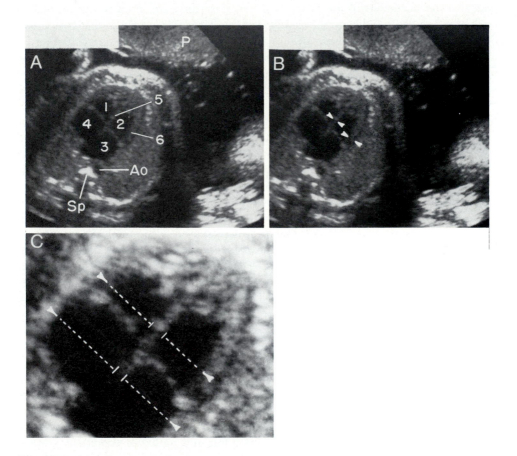

FIG 25–6.
Transaxial scan of lower fetal chest in a 20-week fetus. **A,** a four-chamber view of the heart in diastole is shown. (Note the atria are much larger than in Fig 25–5). The left side of the fetus is on the reader's right. *1* = right ventricle, closest to anterior chest wall; *2* = left ventricle; *3* = left atrium; *4* = right atrium; *5* = interventricular septum; *6* = left ventricular septum; *Ao* = descending thoracic aorta; *Sp* = spine; *P* = placenta. **B,** same image as **A** showing the thickness of the interventricular septum and left ventricular wall, denoted by *arrowheads,* measured close to the atrioventricular valves. **C,** magnified same image as **A** showing measurements of the inner dimensions of the atria and ventricles, just above and below the atrioventricular valves, denoted by *arrowheads, perpendicular* and *dotted lines.*

because of their simplicity. However, the article failed to take into account the phase of the cardiac cycle, an omission that might introduce significant error.[74] In addition, the exact points of measurement were not specified. Using both real-time and M-mode, DeVore et al.[76] measured the biventricular outer diameter in end-diastole from the four-chamber transaxial view and compared it to the thoracic circumference at the same level. The exact outer borders of the heart and chest were well defined. A graph was created with a mean and 2 SD and was helpful in defining four cases of cardiothoracic disproportion. In addition, the head, abdomen, and femur were measured and graphs were created comparing these parameters to the heart and chest. While the comparison of the heart to chest is undoubtedly valid and of clinical value, numbers were not given and therefore no table can be recommended. Wladimiroff and McGhie[77] calculated the left ventricular cardiac output and blood flow in the descending aorta by using a combination of real-time and Doppler. Exact points of measurement of the heart were not described and an assumption had to be made of an exact and constant diameter of the descending aorta so that true blood flow could be calculated. These articles will therefore not be considered further.

There have been 10 articles that have analyzed the same ventricular cardiac dimension: the left ventricular diameter, the right ventricular diameter, and their ratio.[78–86, 90] Seven of these articles using M-mode after real-time obtained the correct cardiac orientation,[79–84, 86] while the other three used real-time ultrasound exclusively.[78, 85, 90] Six articles evaluated the fetal heart from the early second trimester until term[78–80, 84, 85, 90] while the other four examined the fetal heart in the third trimester. Five of these articles[78–80, 84, 90] evaluated the maximum transverse diameter of the left ventricle and right ventricle at the atrioventricular valves in end-diastole while the remainder measured the ventricular chambers below the area of the mitral and tricuspid valves, evaluating the diameters in both end-diastole and end-systole.

There are several points which can be made from these studies. While the left and right ventricular size and wall thicknesses increased with increasing gestational age, the ratio of the right to left ventricles remained relatively constant throughout gestation, between 0.85 to 1.3[78, 79, 81, 84, 86, 90] (Figs 25–5 to 25–7). This ratio was confirmed in a postmortem study.[90] The ventricular dimensions and wall thickness increased with increasing gestational age. The close similarity between the ventricular dimensions does not suggest dominance of the right ventricle in utero.[84]

In addition, Allan et al.[80] and Voster et al.[88] evaluated the interventricular septum and found it to increase in both end-diastole and end-systole from 1.0 mm at 16 weeks to 4.0 mm at term (see Figs 25–5 and 25–6). In addition, the interventricular septum and left ventricular wall thicknesses grew equally during pregnancy so that their ratio remained approximately 1:1, confirmed in a fetal postmortem study where a ratio of 1.14 ± 0.34 was found[87] (Figs 25–6,B and 25–8). It was suggested that if the ratio increased above 1.5, it was abnormal. The exact place to measure the thickness of both was not stated. Using the adult and pediatric echocardiographic positions, however, it is recommended that the measurements be obtained close to the atrioventricular valves (see Fig 25–6,B).

Allan et al.[80] and Shime et al.[90] measured the left atrium, Allan et al.[80] and Shime et al.[90] measured the right atrium, and DeVore et al.[89] and Shime et al.[90] measured the aortic root (Figs 25–6,C, 25–9, and 25–10). All showed an increase toward term. The aortic and pulmonary arteries were also measured at the valvular regions[78] (see Fig 25–9). While they were compared to fetal weight instead of to either the biparietal diameter or gestational age, they were nevertheless found to be relatively constant

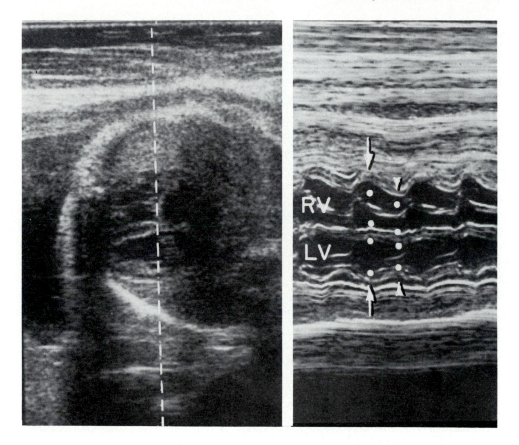

FIG 25–7.
Comparison of inner dimensions of the right and left ventricles. Split image showing a perpendicular four-chamber view of the fetal heart on the left and M-mode tracing on the right. **Left,** *dashed line* oriented through the ventricles just below the atrioventricular valves. **Right,** *dots* denote right ventricular (*RV*) and left ventricular (*LV*) inner diameters in both end-diastole (*arrows*) and end-systole (*arrowheads*). Note that they remain approximately 1:1 in both systole and diastole.

throughout gestation with the diameter of the pulmonary and aortic valves increasing from 6 to 8 mm and from 5 to 7 mm, respectively. This 1:1 ratio of the valves has been found to persist after birth.[78] Lastly, the ratio of the right to left atrium was 1:1[90] (see Figs 25–6 and 25–10).

While no tables cover the entire second and third trimester, a table is given so that the reader will have approximate values that can be expected in utero[90] (Table 25–5). In addition, several ratios appear to be of significant value throughout the second and third trimesters, each approximately 1:1 (Table 25–6): the transverse diameter of the right to left ventricle (0.85:1.3), the interventricular septum to left ventricular wall thickness (1:1) right to left atrium (1:1), and aortic to pulmonary arteries at the valvular region (1:1). In addition, the interventricular septal thickness should not be greater than 1.0 mm at 16 weeks, increasing to 4.0 mm at term. These ratios and the interventricular septal thickness seem easy to measure since they appear to also remain constant regardless of the part of the cardiac cycle in which they are measured.

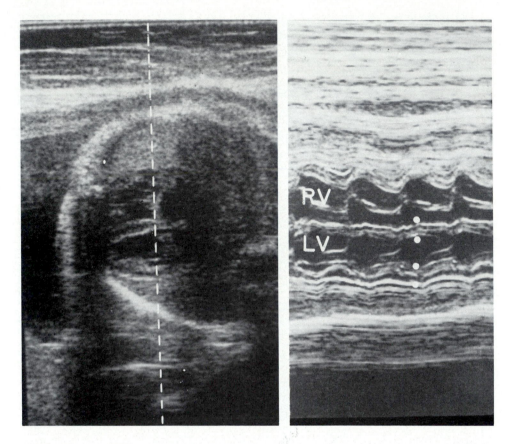

FIG 25–8.
Comparison of interventricular septum to the left ventricular wall thickness. Split image showing a perpendicular four-chamber view of the fetal heart on the left and M-mode tracing on right. **Left**, *dashed line* oriented through the ventricles just below the atrioventricular valves. **Right**, *dots* denote the thickness of the interventricular septum and left ventricular wall in diastole. Note that the ratio remains approximately 1:1 in both systole and diastole. *LV* = left ventricle; *RV* = right ventricle.

Liver

The fetal liver has been evaluated in four articles, two in the transverse[91, 92] and two in the long axis.[93, 54] In the transaxial plane of the fetus, using the left portal vein (actually the umbilical portion of the left portal vein) as a dividing line, the normal left lobe was found to be proportionately larger than in adults. A transverse ratio of the left to right lobes of the liver in utero was found to have a mean value of 1.04 with a range of 0.78 to 1.30.[91] This ratio remained constant throughout gestational life. In adults, this same ratio was performed using computed tomography (CT) and was found to be smaller, with a mean value of 0.76. While the size of the liver has been shown to decrease in asymmetric intrauterine growth retardation, as reflected by a decreased abdominal size, the ratio of the left to right lobes did not change in affected fetuses.[92] This implies that both lobes are equally decreased. Therefore, while this ratio is of academic interest, it has not been shown to have clinical value.

TABLE 25–5.
Fetal Cardiac Measurements*

	Linear Increase From 17 to 40 wk (mm)		
	17 wk	40 wk	Range From 5th to 95th Percentile
Left ventricle†	4	16	± 1.7
Right ventricle†	4	19	± 1.8
Left atrium‡	4	16	± 1.9
Right atrium‡	6	16	± 1.5
Aortic root	2.4	10	± 1.3

*From Shime J, Gresser RN, Rakowski H: *Am J Obstet Gynecol* 1986; 154:294–300. Used by permission.
†Measurements taken in end-diastole at the tips of the atrioventricular valves just prior to closure in a plane perpendicular to the interventricular septum.
‡Measurements obtained in end-systole just after atrioventricular valve closure using widest visible internal diameter in a plane perpendicular to the interatrial septum.

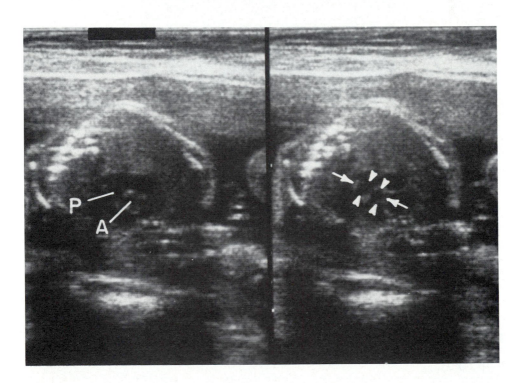

FIG 25–9.
Comparison of the aortic and pulmonary artery diameters. Transaxial image of fetal heart at 30 weeks through the cardiac base. The aorta (*A*) and pulmonary artery (*P*) are identified just at or slightly above the aortic and pulmonary valves. Measurements are obtained in any direction of the anechoic rounded structures, denoted by *arrows* and *arrowheads*.

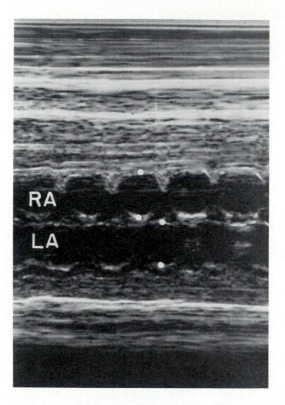

FIG 25–10.
Comparison of the inner dimensions of the right and left atria. M-mode tracing perpendicular through the right atrium (*RA*) and left atrium (*LA*). Dots show the atria in systole. Note the systoles of the atria are at slightly different times.

Two additional articles[93, 94] have measured the fetal liver in the long axis from 20 weeks to term. The long axis was detected by first locating the fetal abdominal aorta, and then moving the transducer parallel and to the right to locate the longest length of the liver.[93] The measurement was taken from the right hemidiaphragm to the liver edge (Fig 25–11). The liver length was found to increase from 27 mm to 49

TABLE 25–6.
Fetal Cardiac Ratios Throughout Second and Third Trimesters

Anatomic Areas	Ratio
Transverse inner diameters of right to left ventricle	0.85:1.3
Transverse inner diameters of right to left atrium	1:1
Thickness of interventricular septum to left ventricular wall	1:1
Inner diameters of aortic to pulmonary arteries (at base of the heart at the valvular region)	1:1

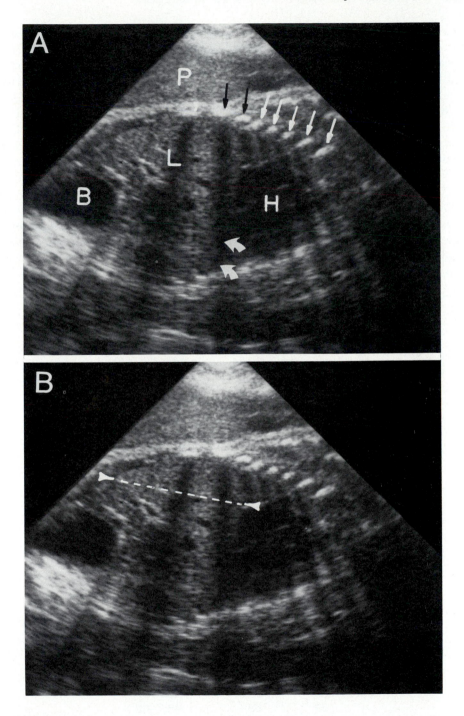

FIG 25–11.
Long-axis scan of the body in a 25-week fetus. **A,** the long axis of the liver (*L*) is identified to the right and parallel to the abdominal aorta. Note that its upper margin is partially obscured by shadowing from the ribs (*arrows*). *H* = heart; *B* = fetal bladder; *P* = placenta. *Curved arrows* denote part of the right hemidiaphragm. **B,** same image as **A** showing measurement of the liver, using the heart and/or diaphragm as its upper margin. Measurement denoted by *arrowheads* and *dashed line*.

mm with a range of 2 SD. The rate of growth of the liver was shown to increase throughout gestation and closely paralleled the increase in abdominal circumference.[93] A follow-up study by the same group[94] evaluated 16 isoimmunized fetuses and found liver size and rate of growth to be a valuable indicator of the severity of fetal hydrops. Using the amniotic fluid bilirubin values (also termed Delta OD 450) as their measure of severity, all eight severely affected fetuses had abnormal liver size and growth (>5 mm/wk). The abdominal circumference and umbilical vein diameter were also measured and found to be less sensitive. While not studied in these articles, the liver length and rate of growth would be expected to be decreased in fetuses with asymmetric growth retardation.

There may be technical factors involved in obtaining consistent measurements. While the caudal edge of the liver seems easy to identify, the dome of the right hemidiaphragm may be difficult to image routinely because of shadowing from the ribs or overlying extremities. This could significantly affect the measurements. Nevertheless, this work appears both valid and clinically useful and is therefore recommended[93] (see Fig 25–11) (Table 25–7). More work is needed, particularly

TABLE 25–7.
Fetal Liver Measurements*

Gestational Age (wk)	Long-Axis Measurement† (mm)	
	True Mean	Range From 5th to 95th Percentile
20	27.3	20.9–33.7
21	28.0	26.5–29.5
22	30.6	23.9–37.3
23	30.9	26.4–35.4
24	32.9	26.2–39.6
25	33.6	28.3–38.9
26	35.7	29.4–42.0
27	36.6	33.3–39.9
28	38.4	34.4–42.4
29	39.1	34.1–44.1
30	38.7	33.7–43.7
31	39.6	33.9–45.3
32	42.7	35.0–50.2
33	42.8	37.2–50.4
34	44.8	37.7–51.9
35	47.8	38.7–56.9
36	49.0	40.6–57.4
37	52.0	45.2–58.8
38	52.9	48.7–57.1
39	55.4	48.7–62.1
40	59.0	—
41	49.3	46.9–51.7

*From Vintzileos AM, Neckles S, Campbell WA, et al: *Obstet Gynecol* 1985; 66:477–480. Used by permission.
†Measured in longitudinal plane from top of right hemidiaphragm to tip of right lobe of liver.

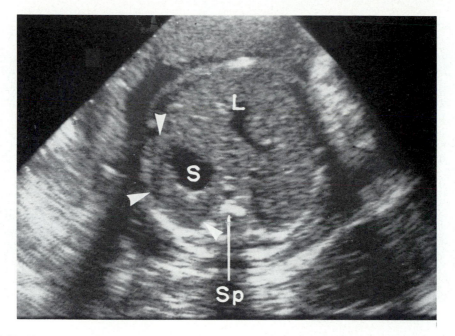

FIG 25–12.
Transaxial scan of the upper abdomen showing the hypoechoic spleen (*arrowheads*) on the left between the distended stomach (*S*), spine (*Sp*), and lateral margin of the fetal body. *L* = liver.

near term where only three patients were examined, so that standard deviations can be calculated for each mean measurement.

Spleen

A recent article[95] stated that the spleen could be routinely imaged as a hyperechoic mass in transverse and coronal views using the stomach, spine, and left hemidiaphragm as landmarks. Measurements were taken in longitudinal, coronal, and transverse dimensions, and the splenic circumferences and volumes were calculated. Mean values in numeric form and the 5th to 95th percentile ranges were given from 18 weeks to term.

While the table is interesting, it is unlikely that the spleen can be routinely imaged. First, the spleen is not hyperechoic, but hypoechoic, and frequently difficult to identify unless surrounded by ascites. Second, in the transaxial plane, the stomach, when filled, is the only consistent landmark (Fig 25–12). The long axis of the spleen, obtained by the authors in the coronal view, is even more difficult to identify and is totally dependent on fetal position.

The measurements change little from 18 weeks to term. An error of 2 to 3 mm in any dimension would cause an error of as much as 20 weeks. Nevertheless, if this work could be duplicated, it would be of value not only in determining the normal-sized spleen but also in detecting cases of enlarged spleen. The authors were able to detect splenomegaly in five of the most severely affected cases of fetal hydrops. In these cases, however, other abnormalities typical of hydrops, such as ascites, were present, which undoubtedly made splenic visualization easier.

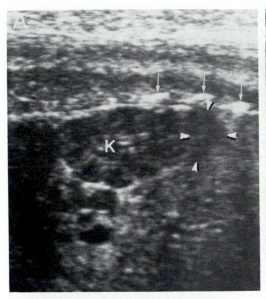
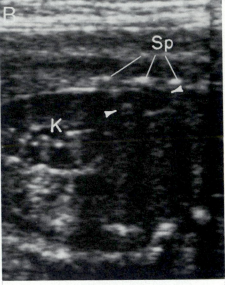
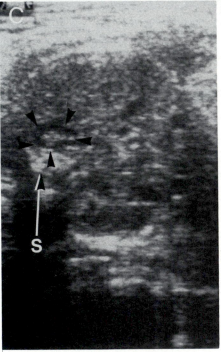

FIG 25–13.
Fetal adrenal glands, imaged in three fetuses older than 30 weeks. **A**, long-axis scan of the fetal body adjacent to the spine (*arrows*) showing the triangularly shaped adrenal gland (denoted by *arrowheads*) in long axis immediately superior to the kidney (*K*). The adrenal gland is partially obscured by shadowing from the fetal spine. **B**, long-axis scan of the fetal body showing an ovoid adrenal gland (denoted by *arrowheads*), partially obscured by shadowing from the spine (*Sp*), immediately superior to the kidney (*K*). Note the adrenal gland is about one-half the length of the kidney. **C**, transaxial scan of the fetal body showing the thin oval disclike adrenal gland (denoted by *arrowheads*) in the high retroperitoneum adjacent to the fetal spine (*S*). The other adrenal cannot be imaged because of shadowing from the spine. Note the central hyperechoic medulla and peripheral hypoechoic cortex, similar to the renal echogenicity (see **A**). The transverse shapes of the kidney and adrenal gland are dissimilar, round versus ovoid, respectively.

Adrenal Glands

The fetal adrenal glands were evaluated in three articles.[96–98] While they can be identified as early as 21 gestational weeks, the adrenal glands are not routinely imaged until the third trimester (28 weeks onward). The adrenal glands are ovoid, triangular, or heart-shaped in the long axis, with one article[96] claiming to identify both adrenal limbs as oval or disc-shaped in the transverse view (Fig 25–13). The peripheral cortex is hypoechoic with the central medulla hyperechoic, an echogenicity similar to that of the adjacent kidney (Fig 25–13,C). The adrenals and kidneys should not be confused, however, because their overall shapes and sizes are different.

The adrenal glands are not always easy to image. Because of their position in the high retroperitoneum, frequently only a peek at them between the lower ribs is possible (see Fig 25–13). In addition, because of their closeness to the fetal spine, usually only the one closest to the transducer is imaged.

Nevertheless, the adrenal glands have been measured with real-time ultrasound.[97, 98] Lewis et al.[97] measured the adrenal length from 30 to 39 weeks, presenting their data as numbers. Hata et al.[98] evaluated the length, circumference, and area of the adrenal glands from 22 to 42 weeks, presenting their data in graph form. Both showed an increase in size as the fetus grew to term. In addition, Lewis et al.[97] calculated a ratio of the adrenal to renal long axis. In a comparison of these two articles,[97, 98] the fetal adrenal glands measured 14 to 16 mm at 30 weeks to 22 to 25 mm at term. The ratio of the long axis of the adrenal to the long axis of the adjacent kidney remained relatively constant, between 0.48 to 0.66 (Fig 25–13,B). In the transaxial view, it was also found that while the adrenal width was very narrow (only several millimeters in thickness), the AP dimension was similar to the kidney (see Fig 25–13,C). When the AP dimension of the adrenal was compared to the AP abdominal diameter at the same level, the ratio was approximately 0.30.[97]

At present, the ranges are too large and not enough cases have been measured to recommend a table. In addition, there are no reported cases of abnormally sized, but otherwise normal, adrenal glands detected in utero. If small adrenal glands could be imaged, however, this might be an important sign of intrauterine growth retardation. Anderson et al.,[99] evaluating the adrenal weight in stillborn or neonatal autopsy specimens from 22 weeks to term, found that the weight of normal adrenal glands was always higher than comparable adrenal weights in neonates with pre-eclampsia and antepartum hemorrhage.

Kidneys

The fetal kidneys have been measured in four articles from the early second trimester until term,[100–103] two in numeric form,[102, 103] one in graph form,[100] and one with both equations and graphs.[101] Two of these were performed with real-time ultrasound[101, 103] while the other two were imaged with static scanners.

The fetal kidneys are not routinely seen until 15 weeks.[100] After 17 weeks, they can be imaged in approximately 90% of cases, although they are usually not easily separable from the surrounding tissues (Fig 25–14,A). After 26 weeks, presumably due to an increase in hyperechoic perinephric fat, the kidney becomes easily identified[104] (Fig 25–14,B). Quite frequently, except when the fetus is in a back-up position, the kidney closest to the transducer is optimally visualized while the opposite kidney is obscured by the fetal spine.

The kidneys have the same ovoid configuration as that seen in children and adults with an echogenicity similar to the adult kidney. The periphery (cortex) is hypoechoic[100, 102] with a hyperechoic center (renal sinus)[100] (Fig 25–14,C). On occasion the cortex can be further differentiated by identifying the almost totally anechoic medulla. The renal sinus becomes hyperechoic and easily identified by the third trimester, due to deposition of fat.[101, 104]

Three renal measurements have been evaluated: the length, width, and AP di-

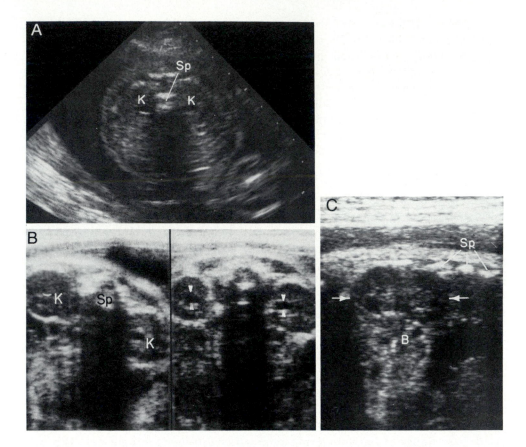

FIG 25–14.
Scans of fetal kidneys. **A,** transaxial image of the fetal body in a 20-week fetus showing the kidneys
(*K*) on both sides of the spine (*Sp*). Note how the kidneys are difficult to separate from the surrounding
tissues. **B,** transaxial dual scans of the fetal body in a 35-week fetus. In the left image, the kidneys
(*K*) are easily identified on both sides of the spine (*Sp*) because of the surrounding hyperechoic
perinephric fat. In the right image, there is an anechoic space in the middle of the hyperechoic central
collecting system (denoted by *arrowheads*), less than 10 mm in AP diameter, consistent with pyelectasis
from normal physiologic reflux. **C,** long-axis scan of the fetal kidney (denoted by *arrows*) in a 30-week
fetus. Note the hyperechoic central collecting system and hypoechoic peripheral cortex. *Sp* = spine;
B = adjacent bowel.

ameter. The renal length is measured in the coronal or sagittal plane along the long
axis of the kidney, and the AP and transverse diameters are obtained in the transaxial
view (Figs 25–15 and 25–16). This measurement of the AP dimension in the transaxial
plane is not ideal. To obtain a true AP measurement, it should be measured from
the long axis image of the kidney, perpendicular to the renal length (Fig 25–15, B).
Despite this potential shortcoming, all three measurements were analyzed by Jeanty
et al.[101] from 20 weeks to term. Two of the three measurements, the renal length
and AP dimensions, were evaluated by Lawson et al.[100] and Bertagnoli et al.[103] from
15 weeks and 24 weeks to term, respectively. Grannum et al.[102] measured the kidneys
from 16 weeks to term only in the transaxial view, calculating three measurements,
the AP diameter, transverse diameter, and circumference, and then comparing them

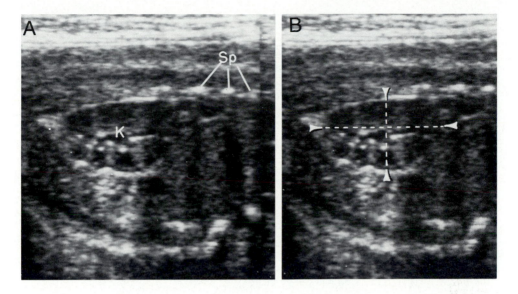

FIG 25–15.
Long-axis scan of the fetal body, adjacent to the spine (*Sp*) in a 32-week fetus. **A,** long-axis scan of the kidney (*K*) with hyperechoic central collecting system and hypoechoic peripheral cortex. **B** same image as **A** showing the length and perpendicular AP measurements, denoted by *arrowheads* and *dotted line.*

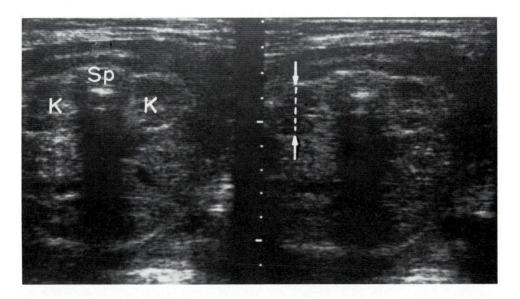

FIG 25–16.
Transaxial dual scans of fetal body. In the left image, the kidneys (*K*) are imaged on both sides of the spine (*Sp*). The right image, the same image as that on the left, shows the AP measurement, denoted by *arrowheads* and *dashed line.* The AP measurement taken from a transaxial scan is not as precise as that taken from a long-axis scan such as Fig 25–15,B.

TABLE 25–8.
Fetal Kidney Measurements*

| Gestational Age (wk) | Renal Measurements With Range of 5th to 95th Percentile (mm) (2 SD)† | | | |
| | Length | | AP Diameter | |
	Predicted Mean	2 SD	Predicted Mean	2 SD
22	—	—	11.1	8.7–13.5
23	—	—	11.5	9.1–13.9
24	24.4	22.0–26.8	11.9	9.5–14.3
25	25.0	22.6–27.4	12.4	10.0–14.8
26	25.7	23.3–28.1	13.0	10.6–15.4
27	26.4	24.0–28.8	13.5	11.1–15.9
28	27.2	24.8–29.6	14.2	11.8–16.6
29	28.0	25.6–30.4	14.8	12.4–17.2
30	28.8	26.4–31.2	15.5	13.1–17.9
31	29.6	27.2–32.0	16.3	13.9–18.7
32	30.4	28.0–32.8	17.1	14.7–19.5
33	31.3	28.9–33.7	18.0	15.6–20.4
34	32.2	29.8–34.6	18.9	16.5–21.3
35	33.1	30.8–35.4	19.9	17.5–22.3
36	34.1	31.8–36.4	20.9	18.5–23.3
37	35.1	32.8–37.4	22.0	19.6–24.4
38	36.1	33.8–38.4	23.2	20.8–25.6
39	37.1	34.8–39.4	24.4	22.0–26.8
40	38.2	35.9–40.5	25.7	23.3–28.1
41	39.3	37.0–41.6	—	—
42	40.4	38.1–42.7	—	—

*From Bertagnoli L, Lalatta F, Gallicchio R, et al: *J Clin Ultrasound* 1983; 11:349–356. Used by permission.
†Longitudinal study used.

to similar measurements of the fetal abdomen at the same level. Jeanty et al.[101] also calculated the volumes of the fetal kidneys from the prolate ellipse formula.

The data were presented as numbers in only two of the articles[102, 103] with two of the articles[101, 103] including standard deviations. The exact points for measuring the kidney were specifically stated in only one of the articles,[103] but were alluded to in the other three.[100–102] While presumably all the articles measured the kidneys accurately, Bertagnoli et al.[103] stated that the outer to outer margins were used in measuring the renal long axis and the outer to inner margins were used to obtain the AP measurement. How the inner margin could be obtained was not stated. Grannum et al.,[102] measuring the AP and transverse renal dimensions, did not measure the kidneys in the same straight AP and transverse axis as used to measure the fetal abdomen. Rather, the renal measurements were taken at an oblique angle.

Despite these differences, the fetal kidney length could be compared from three of the articles.[100, 101, 103] These three showed an increase in the renal length as the fetus increased in gestational age. The variation was very small. At 24 and 40 weeks, the mean length varied from 23 to 25 mm and from 36 to 41 mm, respectively. In the AP dimension, all four articles[100–103] could be compared and discrepancies of only 4 to 5 mm were noted throughout gestation, 11 to 14 mm at 22 weeks to 21 to 25.6 mm at term. In the transverse dimension, two articles could be compared,[101, 102] showing only a 3- to 5-mm discrepancy from 22 to 40 weeks, from 13 mm to 16.4 mm, and from 23.1 mm to 28 mm, respectively. The renal volume measurements by Jeanty et al.[101] could not be compared to any other article and did not seem to have any specific advantage in diagnosing fetal renal abnormalities.

The work by Bertagnoli et al. is recommended.[103] Specific numbers of the renal long axis and AP measurements are given with a 2-SD range. While the exact measurement points of the AP measurement are slightly in question and a predicted rather than a true mean is used, the study was performed on a large number of patients, both cross-sectionally and longitudinally. Of the two types of studies, the numbers are so close that the longitudinal study was chosen because of the possibility that it might be more accurate in serial growth of the kidneys (Table 25–8).

The kidney-to-abdomen ratios proposed by Grannum et al.[102] are also of practical value for the evaluation of changes in fetal renal size (Table 25–9). The authors stated that a ratio of the renal to abdominal circumference was constant throughout pregnancy, between 0.27 to 0.30. A similar ratio could be calculated from their data when the AP and transverse dimensions were compared (Fig 25–17). The AP diameter of the kidney divided by the AP diameter of the abdomen gave a ratio of 0.25 to 0.31 while the ratio of the transverse dimension of the kidney to abdomen was 0.27 to 0.31. As a result, any of these ratios could be used with equal accuracy. It must be emphasized, however, that in addition to these measurements, changes in renal echogenicity, particularly anechoic cystic spaces, are also signs of fetal renal disease.

Occasionally an anechoic space can be identified within the renal sinus (see Fig 25–14,B). While Lawson et al.[100] felt that this was a normal finding after 30 weeks and should not be mistaken for hydronephrosis, there is no doublt that this is pyelectasis.[105] This mild pyelectasis, while benign, is undoubtedly due to physiologic reflux in utero. It is a normal finding, present when the fetal urinary bladder is partially or totally distended. On occasion, this can be seen to resolve as the fetus spontaneously voids.

Three articles evaluated this anechoic space from 19 to 20 weeks to term and found that if the measurement of the intrarenal collecting system was 9 mm or less

TABLE 25–9.
Renal-to-Abdominal Ratio—Range Throughout Second and Third Trimester*

	Ratio
Renal-to-abdominal circumferences	0.27:0.30
Renal-to-abdominal AP diameters	0.25:0.31
Renal-to-abdominal transverse diameters	0.27:0.31

*Adapted from Grannum P, Bracken M, Silverman R, et al: *Am J Obstet Gynecol* 1980; 136:249–254.

TABLE 25–10.
Fetal Colon Diameter Measurements*

Transverse Outer Diameter (mm)		Range From 10th to 90th Percentile
Gestational Age (wk)	Predicted Mean	
26	5	1 to 9
27	5	2 to 9
28	6	3 to 10
29	7	4 to 11
30	8	4 to 11
31	8	5 to 12
32	9	6 to 13
33	10	6 to 13
34	11	7 to 14
35	11	8 to 15
36	12	9 to 16
37	13	10 to 17
38	14	11 to 18
39	15	12 to 19
40	16	13 to 20
41	17	14 to 21
42	19	15 to 22

*From Goldstein I, Lockwood C, Hobbins JC: *Obstet Gynecol* 1987; 70:682–686. Used with permission.

weeks and measured the transverse outer diameter in graph and numeric form from 26 weeks to term. Goldstein et al.[115] also analyzed the meconium echogenicity and colonic haustra, finding both increased toward term.

In analyzing the diameter of the transverse colon, Nyberg et al.[114] measured an inner and Goldstein et al.[115] an outer diameter. Both showed a steady increase from the mid-second trimester to term. Nyberg et al.[114] found an average diameter of 5 mm at 22 weeks to 14.5 mm at term, while Goldstein et al.[115] showed an average diameter of 5 mm at 26 weeks to 19 mm at term. The walls of the colon are thin and do not appear to be a major reason for the discrepancy near term. Although no reason can be found for the deviation, both articles state very similar maximum diameters at 40 weeks, 18 mm[114] versus 22 mm.[115] In addition, Goldstein et al.[115] presented their numbers in tabular form with a 10th to 90th percentile range. Their table of the transverse colon outer diameter is therefore recommended (see Fig 25–19) (Table 25–10). It has been shown by Harris and co-workers[117] that in 12 proven cases of anorectal atresia, the abnormal diameter could be detected in utero in the five cases where the colon could be measured. When these abnormal diameters were compared to Table 25–10, the diameters were above the 90th percentile in all cases, thus proving the usefulness of this measurement.

EXTREMITY MEASUREMENTS

In the late 1960s and early 1970s, measurements of fetal long bones were performed from abdominal radiographs of pregnant women[118–120] with additional com-

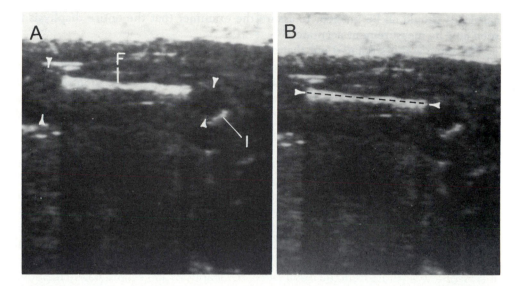

FIG 25–20.
Ultrasound scan of the long axis of a femur (*F*). **A**, the hyperechoic linear structure is the ossified shaft (diaphysis). The hypoechoic ends of the femur, denoted by *arrowheads*, are rounded structures. On the left is the distal epiphyseal cartilage and on the right the proximal epiphyseal cartilage adjacent to the ilium (*I*). **B**, same image as **A** showing the measurement of the shaft, denoted by *arrowheads* and *dashed line*.

parison to radiographs of premature newborn children.[121] While there was difficulty with magnification and orientation, the bones detected on the radiographs correlated well with gestational age.[118, 121] Since 1980, with the advent of high-resolution real-time ultrasound, numerous articles have been published analyzing the length of the fetal long bones. Three of these compared ultrasound to radiographs on aborted fetuses and found good correlation,[122–124] with one demonstrating a correlation coefficient of .998.[123] Although there was a high degree of accuracy using radiographs and ultrasound, ultrasound is preferable. There is no ionizing radiation, and real-time ultrasound allows movement of the transducer to assure that the longest extremity lengths are routinely imaged. The femur, humerus, ulna, radius, radius-ulna complex, tibia, fibula, and tibia-fibula complex have been measured. The femur is the most commonly measured bone, however, since it is the longest tubular bone and the easiest to image consistently.

The technique for obtaining the femoral length is as follows: After the long axis of the fetus is identified, the transducer is turned 90 degrees to produce a cross-sectional image of the fetal trunk. The transducer is moved down the fetus toward the rump, maintaining the 90-degree angle until the lower spine and iliac crest are identified. Since the femur is usually flexed at approximately 30 to 45 degrees, the transducer is rotated until a full femoral length is imaged. The hyperechoic linear structure represents the ossified portion of the femoral diaphysis and corresponds to the femoral length measurement from the greater trochanter to the femoral condyles[125] (Fig 25–20). The greater trochanter and the condyles do not ossify in utero but can be imaged as rounded hypoechoic masses at each end of the diaphysis, termed the epiphyseal cartilages (Fig 25–20,A). They should not be included in the femoral length measurement. Ideally, the hyperechoic diaphysis and hypoechoic

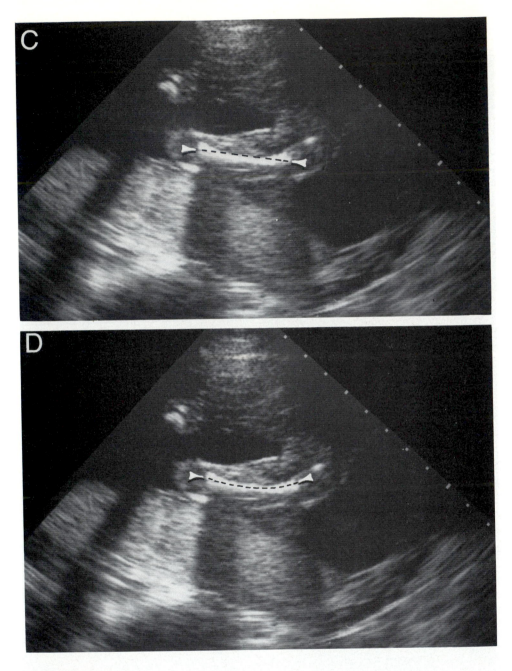

FIG 25–22 continued.

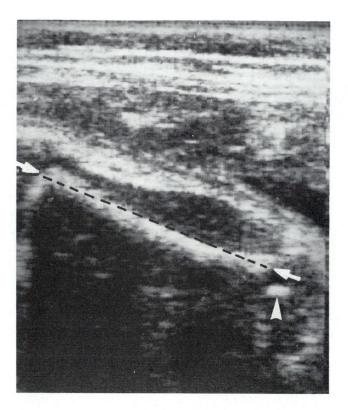

FIG 25–23.
Long axis of a femur at 37 weeks. The measurement of the hyperechoic diaphysis (denoted by *arrows* and *dashed line*) is performed from one end to the other, disregarding the separate hyperechoic distal femoral epiphysis (*arrowhead*).

humerus is obtained (Fig 25–24). Just as with the femur, only the humeral shaft (diaphysis) is ossified. The shaft is therefore measured, disregarding the nonossified ends. The forearm (radius and ulna) and distal leg (tibia and fibula) are the most difficult to image due to the paucity of adjacent landmarks and to the often rapid movements of the fetus and extremities (Figs 25–25 and 25–26). While only the diaphyseal shafts are ossified and thus measured, the bones are not the same length. In the leg, the tibia is longer than the fibula and in the forearm the ulna is longer than the radius. To make certain that the correct bone is measured, both should be imaged. The fibula is lateral to the tibia and is a little thinner.[130] The ulna always appears longer than the radius proximally, while distally they meet at the same level.

Unless the fetus is in a face-up or face-down orientation, all the fetal extremities are often not imaged. More commonly, the fetus is in an oblique or lateral lie so that only the limbs closest to the transducer are identified while the limbs further away are partially obscured by the fetal body and spine. Nevertheless, at least one femur can be measured in almost every case. Since it is rare to have differently sized femurs in the same fetus, one femur accurately represents the length of both. This femoral length serves two purposes, as a predictor of gestational age and as an indicator of skeletal dysplasias and asymmetric intrauterine growth retardation. Rarely, one femur is either fractured or hypoplastic, the latter occurring secondary to maternal diabetes mellitus.

TABLE 25–11.

Fetal Long Bone Measurements*

Gestational Age (wk)	True Mean and Range From 5th to 95th Percentile (mm) (2 SD)					
	BPD		Femur		Humerus	
	True Mean	2 SD	True Mean	2 SD	True Mean	2 SD
13	23	20–26	11	9–13	10	8–12
14	27	24–30	13	11–15	12	10–14
15	30	29–31	15	13–17	14	12–16
16	33	31–35	19	16–22	17	15–19
17	37	34–40	22	19–25	20	16–24
18	42	37–47	25	22–28	23	20–26
19	44	40–48	28	25–31	26	23–29
20	47	43–51	31	28–34	29	26–32
21	50	45–55	35	31–39	32	28–36
22	55	50–60	36	33–39	33	30–36
23	58	53–63	40	36–44	37	34–40
24	61	56–66	42	39–45	38	34–42
25	64	59–69	46	43–49	42	38–46
26	68	63–73	48	44–52	43	40–46
27	70	67–73	49	46–52	45	43–47
28	73	68–78	53	48–58	47	43–51
29	76	71–81	53	48–58	48	44–52
30	77	71–83	56	53–59	50	45–55
31	82	75–89	60	54–66	53	49–57
32	85	79–91	61	55–68	54	50–58
33	86	82–90	64	59–69	56	51–61
34	89	84–94	66	60–72	58	53–63
35	89	82–96	67	61–73	59	53–65
36	91	84–98	70	63–77	60	54–66
37	93	84–102	72	68–76	61	57–65
38	95	89–101	74	68–80	64	61–67
39	95	89–101	76	68–84	65	59–71
40	99	92–107	77	73–81	66	62–70
41	97	91–103	77	73–81	66	62–70
42	100	95–105	78	71–83	68	61–75

*From Merz E, Kim-Kern M, Pehl S: *J Clin Ultrasound* 1987; 15:175–183. Used by permission.

TABLE 25–12.
Femur and Humerus Measurements*

| Bone Length (mm) | Gestational Age (wk) | | | |
| | Femur | | Humerus | |
	Predicted Mean Value	Range From 5th to 95th Percentile	Predicted Mean Value	Range From 5th to 95th Percentile
10	12.6	10.4–14.9	12.6	9.9–15.3
11	12.9	10.7–15.1	12.9	10.1–15.6
12	13.3	11.1–15.6	13.1	10.4–15.9
13	13.6	11.4–15.9	13.6	10.9–16.1
14	13.9	11.7–16.1	13.9	11.1–16.6
15	14.1	12.0–16.4	14.1	11.4–16.9
16	14.6	12.4–16.9	14.6	11.9–17.3
17	14.9	12.7–17.1	14.9	12.1–17.6
18	15.1	13.0–17.4	15.1	12.6–18.0
19	15.6	13.4–17.9	15.6	12.9–18.3
20	15.9	13.7–18.1	15.9	13.1–18.7
21	16.3	14.1–18.6	16.3	13.6–19.1
22	16.6	14.4–18.9	16.7	13.9–19.4
23	16.9	14.7–19.1	17.1	14.3–19.9
24	17.3	15.1–19.6	17.4	14.7–20.1
25	17.6	15.4–19.9	17.9	15.1–20.6
26	18.0	15.9–20.1	18.1	15.6–21.0
27	18.3	16.1–20.6	18.6	15.9–21.4
28	18.7	16.6–20.9	19.0	16.3–21.9
29	19.0	16.9–21.1	19.4	16.7–22.1
30	19.4	17.1–21.6	19.9	17.1–22.6
31	19.9	17.6–22.0	20.3	17.6–23.0
32	20.1	17.9–22.3	20.7	18.0–23.6
33	20.6	18.3–22.7	21.1	18.4–23.9
34	20.9	18.7–23.1	21.6	18.9–24.3
35	21.1	19.0–23.4	22.0	19.3–24.9
36	21.6	19.4–23.9	22.6	19.7–25.1
37	22.0	19.9–24.1	22.9	20.1–25.7
38	22.4	20.1–24.6	23.4	20.6–26.1
39	22.7	20.6–24.9	23.9	21.1–26.6
40	23.1	20.9–25.3	24.3	21.6–27.1
41	23.6	21.3–25.7	24.9	22.0–27.6
42	23.9	21.7–26.1	25.3	22.6–28.0
43	24.3	22.1–26.6	25.7	23.0–28.6
44	24.7	22.6–26.9	26.1	23.6–29.0
45	25.0	22.9–27.1	26.7	24.0–29.6
46	25.4	23.1–27.6	27.1	24.6–30.0
47	25.9	23.6–28.0	27.7	25.0–30.6

(Continued.)

TABLE 25–12 (cont.).
Femur and Humerus Measurements*

| Bone Length (mm) | Gestational Age (wk) | | | |
| | Femur | | Humerus | |
	Predicted Mean Value	Range From 5th to 95th Percentile	Predicted Mean Value	Range From 5th to 95th Percentile
48	26.1	24.0–28.4	28.1	25.6–31.0
49	26.6	24.4–28.9	28.9	26.0–31.6
50	27.0	24.9–29.1	29.3	26.6–32.0
51	27.4	25.1–29.6	29.9	27.1–32.6
52	27.9	25.6–30.0	30.3	27.6–33.1
53	28.1	26.0–30.4	30.9	28.1–33.6
54	28.6	26.4–30.9	31.4	28.7–34.1
55	29.1	26.9–31.3	32.0	29.1–34.7
56	29.6	27.2–31.7	32.6	29.9–35.3
57	29.9	27.7–32.1	33.1	30.3–35.9
58	30.3	28.1–32.6	33.6	30.9–36.4
59	30.7	28.6–32.9	34.1	31.4–36.9
60	31.1	28.9–33.3	34.9	32.0–37.6
61	31.6	29.4–33.9	35.3	32.6–38.1
62	32.0	29.9–34.1	35.9	33.1–38.7
63	32.4	30.1–34.6	36.6	33.9–39.3
64	32.9	30.7–35.1	37.1	34.4–39.9
65	33.4	31.1–35.6	37.7	35.0–40.6
66	33.7	31.6–35.9	38.3	35.6–41.1
67	34.1	32.0–36.4	38.9	36.1–41.7
68	34.6	32.4–36.9	39.6	36.9–42.3
69	35.0	32.6–37.1	40.1	37.4–42.9
70	35.6	33.3–37.7	—	—
71	35.9	33.7–38.1	—	—
72	36.4	34.1–38.6	—	—
73	36.9	34.6–39.0	—	—
74	37.3	35.1–39.6	—	—
75	37.7	35.6–39.9	—	—
76	38.1	36.0–40.4	—	—
77	38.6	36.4–40.9	—	—
78	39.1	36.9–41.3	—	—
79	39.6	37.3–41.7	—	—
80	40.0	37.9–42.1	—	—

*From Jeanty P, Rodesch F, Delbeke D, et al: *J Ultrasound Med* 1984; 3:75–79. Used by permission.

The ulna, radius, tibia, and fibula have been evaluated in five articles.[122, 124, 130, 159, 160] As with the femur and humerus, these bones also increase in size as the fetus grows. The same two articles[130, 160] are again recommended and for the same reasons (Tables 25–13 to 25–16). Jeanty et al.[160] evaluated the ulna and tibia and Merz et al.[130] measured all four bones. There are discrepancies between the two articles in ulna and tibia measurements, increasing to 4 mm at term. This error is approximately 6% and is of questionable significance. Further work is needed to establish which table is more accurate.

TABLE 25–13.
Fetal Long Bone (Radius and Ulna) Measurements*

Gestational Age (wk)	True Mean and Range From 5th to 95th Percentile (mm) (2 SD)					
	BPD		Radius		Ulna	
	True Mean	2 SD	True Mean	2 SD	True Mean	2 SD
13	23	20–26	6	4–8	8	5–11
14	27	24–30	8	6–10	10	8–12
15	30	29–31	11	10–12	12	11–13
16	33	31–35	14	11–17	16	13–19
17	37	34–40	15	12–18	17	14–20
18	42	37–47	19	17–21	22	19–25
19	44	40–48	21	18–24	24	21–27
20	47	43–51	24	22–26	27	24–30
21	50	45–55	27	23–31	30	26–34
22	55	50–60	28	23–33	31	27–35
23	58	53–63	31	27–35	35	33–37
24	61	56–66	33	29–37	36	32–40
25	64	59–69	35	32–38	39	35–43
26	68	63–73	36	32–40	40	37–43
27	70	67–73	37	34–40	41	39–43
28	73	68–78	39	35–43	44	39–49
29	76	71–81	40	35–45	45	41–49
30	77	71–83	41	35–47	47	44–50
31	82	75–89	42	39–45	49	45–53
32	85	79–91	44	38–50	50	44–56
33	86	82–90	45	40–50	52	49–55
34	89	84–94	47	42–53	54	49–59
35	89	82–96	48	42–54	54	50–58
36	91	84–98	49	44–54	55	52–58
37	93	84–102	51	48–54	56	52–60
38	95	89–101	51	46–56	58	52–64
39	95	89–101	53	48–58	60	54–66
40	99	92–107	53	50–56	60	55–65
41	97	91–103	56	52–60	63	58–68
42	100	95–105	57	52–62	65	60–70

*From Merz E, Kim-Kern M, Pehl S: *J Clin Ultrasound* 1987; 15:175–183. Used by permission.

TABLE 25–14.
Ulna Measurements*

| Ulna Length (mm) | Gestational Age (wk) | | Ulna Length (mm) | Gestational Age (wk) | |
	Predicted Mean	Range From 5th to 95th Percentile		Predicted Mean	Range From 5th to 95th Percentile
10	13.1	10.1–16.1	40	26.1	23.1–29.1
11	13.6	10.6–16.4	41	26.7	23.6–29.7
12	13.9	10.9–16.9	42	27.1	24.1–30.3
13	14.1	11.1–17.3	43	27.7	24.7–30.9
14	14.6	11.6–17.7	44	28.3	25.1–31.3
15	15.0	11.9–18.0	45	28.9	25.9–31.9
16	15.4	12.3–18.4	46	29.4	26.3–32.4
17	15.7	12.7–18.9	47	29.9	26.9–33.0
18	16.1	13.1–19.1	48	30.6	27.4–33.6
19	16.6	13.6–19.6	49	31.1	28.0–34.1
20	16.9	13.9–20.0	50	31.6	28.6–34.7
21	17.3	14.3–20.6	51	32.1	29.1–35.3
22	17.7	14.7–20.9	52	32.9	29.7–35.9
23	18.1	15.1–21.1	53	33.4	30.3–36.4
24	18.6	15.6–21.6	54	34.0	30.9–37.0
25	19.0	16.0–22.1	55	34.6	31.6–37.7
26	19.4	16.4–22.6	56	35.1	32.1–38.3
27	19.9	16.9–22.9	57	35.9	32.9–38.9
28	20.3	17.3–23.4	58	36.4	33.4–39.6
29	20.9	17.7–23.9	59	37.1	34.0–40.1
30	21.1	18.1–24.3	60	37.7	34.6–40.9
31	21.7	18.6–24.9	61	38.3	35.3–41.4
32	22.1	19.1–25.1	62	39.0	35.9–42.0
33	22.7	19.6–25.7	63	39.6	36.6–42.7
34	23.1	20.1–26.1	64	40.3	37.1–43.3
35	23.6	20.6–26.7			
36	24.1	21.1–27.1			
37	24.6	21.4–27.7			
38	25.1	22.1–28.1			
39	25.6	22.6–28.7			

*From Jeanty P, Rodesch F, Delbeke D, et al: *J Ultrasound Med* 1984; 3:75–79. Used by permission.

TABLE 25–15.
Fetal Long Bone (Tibia and Fibula) Measurements*

| | True Mean and Range From 5th to 95th Percentile (mm) (2 SD) | | | | | |
| | BPD | | Tibia | | Fibula | |
Gestational Age (wk)	True Mean	2 SD	True Mean	2 SD	True Mean	2 SD
13	23	20–26	9	7–11	8	6–10
14	27	24–30	10	8–12	9	6–12
15	30	29–31	13	11–15	12	10–14
16	33	31–35	16	13–19	15	12–18
17	37	34–40	18	15–21	17	15–19
18	42	37–47	22	19–25	21	18–24
19	44	40–48	25	22–28	23	20–26
20	47	43–51	27	25–29	26	24–28
21	50	45–55	30	26–34	29	25–33
22	55	50–60	32	29–35	31	28–34
23	58	53–63	36	34–38	34	32–36
24	61	56–66	37	34–40	36	33–39
25	64	59–69	40	37–43	39	35–43
26	68	63–73	42	39–45	40	37–43
27	70	67–73	44	41–47	42	39–45
28	73	68–78	45	41–49	44	41–47
29	76	71–81	46	43–49	45	42–48
30	77	71–83	48	43–53	47	44–50
31	82	75–89	51	48–54	49	44–54
32	85	79–91	52	48–56	51	47–55
33	86	82–90	54	49–59	53	50–56
34	89	84–94	57	52–62	55	51–59
35	89	82–96	58	54–66	56	52–60
36	91	84–98	60	54–66	56	51–61
37	93	84–102	61	57–65	60	56–64
38	95	89–101	62	59–65	60	56–64
39	95	89–101	64	57–71	61	55–67
40	99	92–107	65	62–68	62	61–63
41	97	91–103	66	62–70	63	58–68
42	100	95–105	68	63–73	67	60–74

*From Merz E, Kim-Kern M, Pehl S: *J Clin Ultrasound* 1987; 15:175–183. Used by permission.

articles.[166, 167] The foot was evaluated from 12 to 40 weeks in numeric and graph form and the growth was found to have an overall curvilinear shape, linear in the second and early third trimester with slowing near term.[166] The other two articles, also in graph and numeric form, evaluated the growth of the foot either from 12 to 28 weeks[167] or from 14 to 35 weeks.[168] The mean numbers in all three were very close, frequently no different than 1 to 2 mm. In all the articles, comparison of the foot to the head, body, and femur, in graph and equation, showed similarly close correlations. It was the conclusion of these articles that fetal foot length measurements are a reliable estimator of gestational age and can be used in normal singleton and multiple gestations and in cases of skeletal dysplasias.[166-168] While not often needed, the table by Mercer and co-workers[166] encompassing the entire second and third trimester is recommended (Table 25–17).

TABLE 25–17.

Fetal Foot Length Measurements*

Mean Gestational Age (wk)	Foot Length (mm)	
	Predicted Mean	Range From 5th to 95th Percentile (2 SD)
12	8	7–9
13	11	10–12
14	15	13–16
15	18	16–20
16	21	19–23
17	24	22–27
18	27	24–30
19	30	27–34
20	33	30–37
21	36	32–40
22	39	35–43
23	42	37–46
24	45	40–50
25	47	42–53
26	50	45–55
27	53	47–58
28	55	49–61
29	58	51–64
30	60	54–67
31	62	56–68
32	65	58–72
33	67	60–74
34	69	62–77
35	71	64–79
36	74	66–82
37	76	67–84
38	78	69–86
39	80	71–88
40	81	72–90

*From Mercer BM, Sklar S, Shariatmadar A, et al: *Am J Obstet Gynecol* 1987; 156:350–355. Used with permission.

Ossification centers can also be measured (see Fig 25–23). Not only their detection but also their size is helpful in establishing gestational age.[129, 168, 170–174] In the second trimester, two ossification centers in the foot were analyzed.[168] The calcaneus and the talus discriminated between gestations of 18 weeks or more and 22 weeks or more, respectively, especially when they measured at least 2 mm in size. In the third trimester, the distal femoral epiphysis (DFE) and proximal tibial epiphysis (PTE) were evaluated. The DFE and PTE were not identified prior to 28 and 34 weeks, respectively,[170] were 1 to 2 mm by 33 and 36 weeks, respectively,[129, 170] and were 3 mm or more by 37 and 38 weeks, respectively.[170] Tabsh[173] found somewhat larger measurements for both the DFE and PTE, 3 mm or more by 32 and 34 weeks and 5 mm or more by 34 and 36 weeks, respectively.[173] By term, Tabsh found the DFE to be 6 to 9 mm, the PTE to be 4 to 6 mm, the calcaneus to be 13 to 16 mm, and the talus to be 9 to 12 mm.[173] Exactly how the measurements were obtained is not completely clear, but presumably the ossification centers were measured along their longest axis. If the epiphyses were not identified or were delayed in their size compared to the expected fetal ages, this was found to be a sign of growth retardation, particularly symmetric intrauterine growth retardation.[172, 174]

The DFE and PTE have also been used to predict pulmonary maturity. Tabsh[173] and Gentili et al.[174] found that the lecithin-sphingomyelin ratio was 2.0 or greater (mature) in 100% of cases when the PTE was equal to 5 to 7 mm and in 95% of cases when the DFE was 5 to 7 mm. Goldstein et al.[171] found that a DFE of 3 mm or more with additional identification of the PTE in nondiabetic patients was also equal to a mature ratio in 100% of cases. In diabetics, there were no measurements that insured 100% sensitivity.

OTHER OSSEOUS STRUCTURES—CLAVICLE

Yarkoni et al. measured the length of the fetal clavicle.[175] A table in numeric form with a mean predicted value and a 2-SD range was given from 15 to 40 weeks. The clavicle was measured from the ossified ends, disregarding any curve in the bone, and found to correlate linearly with gestational age. While this is an interesting measurement, the authors failed to discuss the degree of difficulty and technical expertise needed to make this measurement. In addition, while they suggested its potential usefulness in detecting both congenital anomalies and shoulder dystocia during delivery, no abnormal cases were analyzed.

SOFT TISSUE MEASUREMENTS—ARMS, LEGS, NECK

Fetal subcutaneous fat has been observed radiographically and correlated with weight from 32 weeks to term.[176] The mean numbers for the buttocks and upper dorsal "shoulder hump" at 36 weeks and at term were 3 to 5 mm and 3 to 4 mm, respectively. It was also noted that this fat thickness decreased in cases of fetal starvation.

Fetal subcutaneous tissues have also been evaluated by fetoscopy, attempting to predict fetal weight.[177] The scalp thickness at the vertex of the head and the ratio of the thigh soft tissue thickness on the extensor surface to the cross-sectional diameter of the femur have been measured. It was found that the fetal scalp soft tissues correlated well to fetal weight. When the subcutaneous tissues were less than 3.4 mm, the fetus weighed less than 2,500 g. When more than 3.4 mm, the soft tissue thickness of the scalp was predictive of a fetus greater than 2,500 g.[176] When the ratio of the soft tissues of the thigh to the femoral diameter was analyzed, there was also a high degree of correlation to weight. If the ratio were greater than 4.2, all fetuses weighed more than 3,000 g.

Seven ultrasound articles have attempted to evaluate the soft tissues, five of the extremities,[1, 178–181] and two of the back of the neck.[178, 179] For the thigh measurements, Hoffbauer et al.[1] measured the transaxial diameter with static scans, and, while not stating exactly where the measurements were taken, found that the soft tissue diameter of the entire thigh increased linearly from 24 to 38 weeks. Vintzileos et al.[178] measured the transverse thigh and calf circumferences from 20 weeks to term. Both articles presented their data in numeric form with a 2-SD range. The measurements were taken at somewhat arbitrary places, midthigh and below the knee, and both incorporated the bone, muscle, and subcutaneous tissue in their measurements. Jeanty et al.[179] measured the midlevel of the arm and thigh, and determined the transverse and AP thicknesses. In addition, the subcutaneous thickness and the humeral and femoral length and thickness were also measured. Limb volume were computed in equation and graph form and found to correlate with gestational age. Of interest was the finding that a subcutaneous tissue thickness in the arm of greater than 6 mm and in the thigh of greater than 10 mm, in the absence of edema, was suspicious for macrosomia. Lastly, two articles from the same group[180, 181] analyzed the transverse thigh circumference from 12 weeks to term, using a "transition plane" in the femur at the junction of the upper and middle third of the thigh to take their measurements. The data were presented in numeric form, with a mean and 2 SD. The authors found a close correlation to gestational age, 13 mm at 22 weeks, increasing to 31 mm at term.[180] They also found that their numbers were larger than those of Vintzileos et al.[178] and Jeanty et al.,[179] as much as 9 mm at 23 weeks to 30 mm at term, which they attributed to different methodologies! The reason for these differences, however, cannot be ascertained from the article. Because of these marked differences, measurements are not recommended at the present time. In addition, it would be helpful to have a lower limit of skin thickness to aid in the diagnosis of growth retardation. At present, this too is not available.

Benacerraf et al.[182, 183] and a follow-up article by Perrella et al.[154] measured the skin or soft tissue thickness at the back of the neck behind the occiput in second trimester pregnancies (15–21 weeks). Benacerraf and co-workers found the normal range to be 1 to 5 mm, with only one false-positive in greater than 1,700 normal fetuses. In 10 cases of Down's syndrome, diagnosed by abnormal karyotype from the amniotic fluid, four had skin thickening greater than 5 mm. The measurements were obtained in the transaxial view, angled toward the occiput with the skin measured from the outer edge of the occiput to the skin edge. Using similar technique, Perrella et al.[154] found skin thickening of 6 mm or greater in 12 of 108 normal and in only 3 of 14 Down's syndrome fetuses for a sensitivity of only 42% and a specificity of 88%. Because of the lack of sensitivity of this measurement, nuchal skin measurements are not recommended.

REFERENCES

1. Hoffbauer H, Pachaly J, Arabin B, et al: Control of fetal development with multiple ultrasonic body measures. *Contrib Gynecol Obstet* 1979; 6:147–156.
2. Levi S, Erbsman F: Antenatal fetal growth from the nineteenth week: ultrasonic study of 12 head and chest dimensions. *Am J Obstet Gynecol* 1975; 121:262–268.
3. Weinraub Z, Schneider D, Langer R, et al: Ultrasonographic measurement of fetal growth parameters for estimation of gestational age and fetal weight. *Isr J Med Sci* 1979; 15:829–832.
4. Issel EP, Prenzlau P, Bayer H, et al: The measurement of fetal growth during pregnancy by ultrasound (B-scan). *J Perinat Med* 1975; 3:269–275.
5. Pap G, Pap L: Ultrasonic estimation of gestational age and fetal weight. *Paediatr Acad Sci Hung* 1979; 20:119–135.
6. Pap G, Szoke J, Pap L: Intrauterine growth retardation: ultrasonic diagnosis. *Acta Paediatr Hung* 1983; 24:7–15.
7. Hansmann M: A critical evaluation of the performance of ultrasonic diagnosis in present-day obstetrics. *Gynakologe* 1974; 7:26–35.
8. Nimrod C, Davies D, Iwanicki S, et al: Ultrasound prediction of pulmonary hypoplasia. *Obstet Gynecol* 1986; 68:495–498.
9. Fong K, Ohlsson A, Zalev A: Fetal thoracic circumference: a prospective cross-sectional study with real-time ultrasound. *Am J Obstet Gynecol* 1988; 158:1154–1160.
10. Chitkara U, Rosenberg J, Chervenak FA, et al: Prenatal sonographic assessment of the fetal thorax: normal values. *Am J Obstet Gynecol* 1987; 156:1069–1074.
11. Usher R, McLean F: Intrauterine growth of live-born Caucasian infants at sea level: standards obtained from measurements in 7 dimensions of infants born between 25 and 44 weeks of gestation. *Pediatrics* 1969; 74:901–910.
12. Kossoff G, Garrett WJ, Radovanovich G: Grey scale echography in obstetrics and gynaecology. *Australas Radiol* 1974; 18:63–111.
13. Wladimiroff JW, Bloemsma CA, Wallenburg HCS: Ultrasonic assessment of fetal head and body sizes in relation to normal and retarded fetal growth. *Am J Obstet Gynecol* 1978; 131:857–860.
14. Wladimiroff JW, Bloemsma CA, Wallenburg HCS: Ultrasonic assessment of fetal growth. *Acta Obstet Gynecol Scand* 1977; 56:37–42.
15. Varma TR, Taylor H, Bridges C: Ultrasound assessment of fetal growth. *Br J Obstet Gynaecol* 1979; 86:623–632.
16. Wladimiroff JW, Bloemsma CA, Wallenburg HCS: Ultrasonic diagnosis of the large-for-dates infant. *Obstet Gynecol* 1978; 52:285–288.
17. Fescina RH, Ucieda FJ, Cordano MC, et al: Ultrasonic patterns of intrauterine fetal growth in a Latin American country. *Early Hum Dev* 1982; 6:239–248.
18. Garrett W, Robinson D: Assessment of fetal size and growth rate by ultrasonic echoscopy. *Obstet Gynecol* 1979; 38:525–534.
19. Eriksen PS, Secher NJ, Weis-Bentzon M: Normal growth of the fetal biparietal diameter and the abdominal diameter in a longitudinal study. *Acta Obstet Gynecol Scand* 1985; 64:65–70.
20. Persson PH, Weldner BM: Normal range growth curves for fetal biparietal diameter, occipito-frontal diameter, mean abdominal diameters and femur length. *Acta Obstet Gynecol Scand* 1986; 65:759–761.
21. Grandjean H, Sarramon MF, De Mouzon J, et al: Detection of gestational diabetes by means of ultrasonic diagnosis of excessive fetal growth. *Am J Obstet Gynecol* 1980; 138:790–792.
22. Tamura RK, Sabbagha RE, Pan WH, et al: Ultrasonic fetal abdominal circumference: Comparison of direct versus calculated measurement. *Obstet Gynecol* 1986; 67:833–835.
23. Kurtz AB, Wapner RJ, Kurtz RJ, et al: Analysis of biparietal diameter as an accurate indicator of gestational age. *J Clin Ultrasound* 1980; 8:319–326.
24. Deter RL, Harrist RB, Hadlock FP, et al: Fetal head and abdominal circumferences: I. Evaluation of measurement errors. *J Clin Ultrasound* 1982; 10:357–363.
25. Tamura RK, Sabbagha RE: Percentile ranks of sonar fetal abdominal circumference measurements. *Am J Obstet Gynecol* 1980; 138:475–479.
26. Hadlock FP, Deter RL, Harrist RB, et al: Fetal abdominal circumference as a predictor of menstrual age. *AJR* 1982; 139:367–370.
27. Ogata ES, Sabbagha R, Metzger BE, et al: Serial ultrasonography to assess evolving fetal macrosomia: studies in 23 pregnant diabetic women. *JAMA* 1980; 243:2405–2408.

28. Parker AJ, Davies P, Mayho AM, et al: The ultrasound estimation of sex-related variations of intrauterine growth. *Am J Obstet Gynecol* 1984; 149:665–669.

29. Meire HG, Farrant P: Ultrasound demonstration of an unusual fetal growth pattern in Indians. *Br J Obstet Gynaecol* 1981; 88:260–263.

30. Athey PA, Hadlock FP: Appendix in Harshberger SE (ed): *Ultrasound in Obstetrics and Gynecology.* St Louis, CV Mosby Co, 1981, p 269.

31. Deter RL, Harrist RB, Hadlock FP, et al: Fetal head and abdominal circumferences: II. A critical reevaluation of the relationship to menstrual age. *J Clin Ultrasound* 1982; 10:365–372.

32. Deter RL, Harrist RB, Hadlock FP, et al: Longitudinal studies of fetal growth with the use of dynamic image ultrasonography. *Am J Obstet Gynecol* 1982; 143:545.

33. Deter RL, Harrist RB, Hadlock FP, et al: The use of ultrasound in the assessment of normal fetal growth: A review. *J Clin Ultrasound* 1981; 9:481–493.

34. Tamura RK, Sabbagha RE, Pan WH, et al: Ultrasonic fetal abdominal circumference: Comparison of direct versus calculated measurement. *Obstet Gynecol* 1986; 67:833–835.

35. Campbell S, Wilkin D: Ultrasonic measurement of fetal abdomen circumference in the estimation of fetal weight. *Br J Obstet Gynaecol* 1975; 82:689–697.

36. Bree RL, Mariona FG: The role of ultrasound in the evaluation of normal and abnormal fetal growth. *Semin Ultrasound* 1980; 1:264–277.

37. Hobbins JC, Grannum PAT, Berkowitz RL, et al: Ultrasound in the diagnosis of congenital anomalies. *Am J Obstet Gynecol* 1979; 134:331–345.

38. Clement D, Silverman R, Scott D, et al: Comparison of abdominal circumference measurements by real-time and B-scan techniques. *J Clin Ultrasound* 1981; 9:1–3.

39. Weiner CP, Sabbagha RE, Tamur RK, et al: Sonographic abdominal circumference: dynamic versus static imaging. *Am J Obstet Gynecol* 1981; 139:953–955.

40. Hadlock FP, Kent WR, Loyd JL, et al: An evaluation of two methods for measuring fetal heads and body circumferences. *J Ultrasound Med* 1982; 1:359–360.

41. Shields JR, Medearis AL, Bear MB: Fetal head and abdominal circumferences: Effect of profile shape on the accuracy of ellipse equations. *J Clin Ultrasound* 1987; 15:241–244.

42. Shields JR, Medearis AL, Bear MB: Fetal head and abdominal circumferences: Ellipse calculations versus planimetry. *J Clin Ultrasound* 1987; 15:237–239.

43. Wittman BK, Robinson HP, Aitchison T, et al: The value of diagnostic ultrasound as a screening test for intrauterine growth retardation: comparison of nine parameters. *Am J Obstet Gynecol* 1979; 134:30.

44. Rossavik IK, Deter RL, Hadlock FP: Mathematical modeling of fetal growth. IV. Evaluation of trunk growth using the abdominal profile area. *J Clin Ultrasound* 1987; 15:31–35.

45. Woo JSK, Liang ST, Wan CW, et al: Abdominal circumference vs abdominal area—which is better? *J Ultrasound Med* 1984; 3:101–105.

46. Selbing A, Wichman K, Ryden G: Screening for detection of intra-uterine growth retardation by means of ultrasound. *Acta Obstet Gynecol Scand* 1984; 63:543–548.

47. Martinez DA, Barton JL: Estimation of fetal body and fetal head volumes: description of technique and nomograms for 18 to 41 weeks of gestation. *Am J Obstet Gynecol* 1980; 137:78–84.

48. Rossavik IK, Deter RL: Mathematical modeling of fetal growth: I. Basic principles. *J Clin Ultrasound* 1984; 12:529–533.

49. Rossavik IK, Deter RL: Mathematical modeling of fetal growth: II. Head cube (A), abdominal cube (B) and their ratio (A/B). *J Clin Ultrasound* 1984; 12:535–545.

50. Deter RL, Harrist RB, Hadlock FP, et al: Longitudinal studies of fetal growth using volume parameters determined with ultrasound. *J Clin Ultrasound* 1984; 12:313–324.

51. Lubchenco LO, Hansmann C, Boyd E: Intrauterine growth in length and head circumference as estimated from live births at gestational ages from 26 to 42 weeks. *Pediatrics* 1966; 37:403–408.

52. Babson SG, Benda GI: Growth graphs for the clinical assessment of infants of varying gestational age. *Pediatrics* 1976; 89:814–820.

53. Wong KS, Scott KE: Fetal growth at sea level. *Biol Neonate* 1972; 20:175–188.

54. Ojala A, Ylostalo P, Jouppila P, et al: Fetal cephalometry by ultrasound in normal and complicated pregnancy. *Ann Chir Gynaecol Fenn* 1970; 59:71–75.

55. Ott WJ: Fetal femur length, neonatal crown-heel length, and screening for intrauterine growth retardation. *Obstet Gynecol* 1985; 65:460–464.

56. Hadlock FP, Deter RL, Roecker E, et al: Relation of fetal femur length to neonatal crown-heel length. *J Ultrasound Med* 1984; 3:1–3.

57. Vintzileos AM, Campbell WA, Neckles S, et al: The ultrasound femur length as a predictor of fetal length. *Obstet Gynecol* 1984; 64:779–782.

58. Yamaguchi DT, Lee FYL: Ultrasonic evaluation of the fetal heart: a report of experience and anatomic correlation. *Am J Obstet Gynecol* 1979; 134:422–430.

59. DeVore GR, Donnerstein RL, Kleinman CS, et al: Fetal echocardiography. I. Normal anatomy as determined by real-time-directed M-mode ultrasound. *Am J Obstet Gynecol* 1982; 144:249–259.

60. Shime J, Bertrand M, Hagen-Ansert S, et al: Two-dimensional and M-mode echocardiography in the human fetus. *Am J Obstet Gynecol* 1984; 148:679–685.

61. DeVore GR, Donnerstein RL, Kleinman CS, et al: Fetal echocardiography. II. The diagnosis and significance of a pericardial effusion in the fetus using real-time-directed M-mode ultrasound. *Am J Obstet Gynecol* 1982; 144:693–699.

62. Nimrod C, Nicholson S, Machin G, et al: In utero evaluation of fetal cardiac structure: a preliminary report. *Am J Obstet Gynecol* 1984; 148:516–518.

63. DeVore GR, Siassi B, Platt L: Fetal echocardiography. III. The diagnosis of cardiac arrhythmias using real-time directed M-mode ultrasound. *Am J Obstet Gynecol* 1983; 146:792–799.

64. Lange LW, Sahn DJ, Allen HD, et al: Qualitative real-time cross-sectional echocardiographic imaging of the human fetus during the second half of pregnancy. *Circulation* 1980; 62:799–806.

65. Allan LD, Tynan MJ, Campbell S, et al: Echocardiographic and anatomical correlates in the fetus. *Br Heart J* 1980; 44:444–451.

66. Axel L: Real-time sonography of fetal cardiac anatomy. *AJR* 1983; 141:283–288.

67. Allan LD, Crawford DC, Anderson RH, et al: Echocardiographic and anatomical correlations in fetal congenital heart disease. *Br Heart J* 1984; 52:542–548.

68. Sandor GGS, Farquarson D, Wittman B, et al: Fetal echocardiography: Results in high-risk patients. *Obstet Gynecol* 1986; 67:358–364.

69. Allan LD, Crawford DC, Anderson RH, et al: Evaluation and treatment of fetal arrhythmias. *Clin Cardiol* 1984; 7:467–473.

70. Kleinman CS, Donnerstein RL, Jaffe CC, et al: Fetal echocardiography. A tool for evaluation of in utero cardiac arrhythmias and monitoring of in utero therapy: analysis of 71 patients. *Am J Cardiol* 1983; 51:237–243.

71. Kleinman CS, Donnerstein RL, DeVore GR, et al: Fetal echocardiography for evaluation of in utero congestive heart failure: A technique for study of nonimmune fetal hydrops. *N Engl J Med* 1982; 306:568–575.

72. Suzuki K, Minei LJ, Schnitzer LE: Ultrasonographic measurement of fetal heart volume for estimation of birthweight. *Obstet Gynecol* 1974; 43:867–871.

73. Jeanty P, Romero R, Cantraine F, et al: Fetal cardiac dimensions: A potential tool for the diagnosis of congenital heart defects. *J Ultrasound Med* 1984; 3:359–364.

74. DeVore GR, Platt LD: The random measurement of the transverse diameter of the fetal heart: A potential source of error. *J Ultrasound Med* 1985; 4:335–341.

75. Filkins KA, Brown TF, Levine OR: Real time ultrasonic evaluation of the fetal heart. *Int J Gynaecol Obstet* 1981; 19:35–39.

76. DeVore GR, Horenstein J, Platt LD: Fetal echocardiography. VI. Assessment of cardiothoracic disproportion—A new technique for the diagnosis of thoracic hypoplasia. *Am J Obstet Gynecol* 1986; 155:1066–1071.

77. Wladimiroff JW, McGhie J: Ultrasonic assessment of cardiovascular geometry and function in the human fetus. *Br J Obstet Gynaecol* 1981; 88:870–875.

78. Sahn DJ, Lange LW, Allen HD, et al: Quantitative real-time cross-sectional echocardiography in the developing human fetus and newborn. *Circulation* 1980; 62:588–597.

79. DeVore GR, Siassi B, Platt LD: Fetal echocardiography. IV. M-mode assessment of ventricular size and contractility during the second and third trimesters of pregnancy in the normal fetus. *Am J Obstet Gynecol* 1984; 150:981–988.

80. Allan LD, Joseph MC, Boyd EGCA, et al: M-mode echocardiography in the developing human fetus. *Br Heart J* 1982; 47:573–583.

81. Wladimiroff JW, McGhie JS: M-mode ultrasonic assessment of fetal cardiovascular dynamics. *Br J Obstet Gynaecol* 1981; 88:1241–1245.

82. Kleinman CS, Donnerstein RL: Ultrasonic assessment of cardiac function in the intact human fetus. *J Am Coll Cardiol* 1985; 5:845–945.

83. Wladimiroff JW, Vosters R, Stewart PA: Fetal echocardiography: Basic and clinical considerations. *Ultrasound Med Biol* 1984; 10:315–327.

84. St John Sutton MG, Gewitz MH, Shah B, et al: Quantitative assessment of growth and function of the cardiac chambers in the normal human fetus: A prospective longitudinal echocardiographic study. *Circulation* 1984; 69:645–654.

85. Azancot A, Caudell TP, Allen HD, et al: Analysis of ventricular shape by echocardiography in normal fetuses, newborns and infants. *Circulation* 1983; 68:1201–1211.
86. Wladimiroff JW, Vosters R, McGhie JS: Normal cardiac ventricular geometry and function during the last trimester of pregnancy and early neonatal period. *Br J Obstet Gynaecol* 1982; 89:839–844.
87. Leslie J, Shen S, Thornton JC, et al: The human fetal heart in the second trimester of gestation: A gross morphometric study of normal fetuses. *Am J Obstet Gynecol* 1983; 145:312–316.
88. Vosters R, Wladimiroff JW, Versprille A: M-mode ultrasound recording of perinatal geometry and dynamics of the cardiac interventricular septum. *Eur J Obstet Gynecol Reprod Biol* 1984; 16:299–308.
89. DeVore GR, Siassi B, Platt LD: Fetal echocardiography. V. M-mode measurements of the aortic root and aortic valve in second and third-trimester normal human fetuses. *Am J Obstet Gynecol* 1985; 152:543–550.
90. Shime J, Gresser CD, Rakowski H: Quantitative two-dimensional echocardiographic assessment of fetal cardiac growth. *Am J Obstet Gynecol* 1986; 154:294–300.
91. Gross BH, Harter LP, Filly RA: Disproportionate left hepatic lobe size in the fetus: Ultrasonic demonstration. *J Ultrasound Med* 1982; 1:79–81.
92. Gross BH, Filly RA, Harter LP: Inability of relative fetal hepatic lobar size to diagnose intrauterine growth retardation. *J Ultrasound Med* 1982; 1:299–300.
93. Vintzileos AM, Neckles S, Campbell WA, et al: Fetal liver ultrasound measurements during normal pregnancy. *Obstet Gynecol* 1985; 66:477–480.
94. Vintzileos AM, Campbell WA, Storlazzi E, et al: Fetal liver ultrasound measurements in isoimmunized pregnancies. *Obstet Gynecol* 1986; 68:162–167.
95. Schmidt W, Yarkoni S, Jeanty P, et al: Sonographic measurements of the fetal spleen: clinical implications. *J Ultrasound Med* 1985; 4:667–672.
96. Rosenberg ER, Bowie JD, Andreotti RF, et al: Sonographic evaluation of fetal adrenal glands. *AJR* 1982; 139:1145–1147.
97. Lewis E, Kurtz AB, Dubbins PA, et al: Real-time ultrasonographic evaluation of normal fetal adrenal glands. *J Ultrasound Med* 1982; 1:265–270.
98. Hata K, Hata T, Kitao M: Ultrasonographic identification and measurement of the human fetal adrenal gland in utero. *Int J Gynaecol Obstet* 1985; 23:355–359.
99. Anderson ABM, Laurence KM, Davies K, et al: Fetal adrenal weight and the cause of premature delivery in human pregnancy. *J Obstet Gynaecol Br Commw* 1971; 78:481–487.
100. Lawson TL, Foley WD, Berland LL, et al: Ultrasonic evaluation of fetal kidneys: analysis of normal size and frequency of visualization as related to stage of pregnancy. *Radiology* 1981; 138:153–156.
101. Jeanty P, Dramaix-Wilmet M, Elkhazen N, et al: Measurement of fetal kidney growth on ultrasound. *Radiology* 1982; 144:159–162.
102. Grannum P, Bracken M, Silverman R, et al: Assessment of fetal kidney size in normal gestation by comparison of ratio of kidney circumference to abdominal circumference. *Am J Obstet Gynecol* 1980; 136:249–254.
103. Bertagnoli L, Lalatta F, Gallicchio R, et al: Quantitative characterization of the growth of the fetal kidney. *J Clin Ultrasound* 1983; 11:349–356.
104. Bowie JD, Rosenberg ER, Andreotti RF, et al: The changing sonographic appearance of fetal kidneys during pregnancy. *J Ultrasound Med* 1983; 2:505–507.
105. Hoddick WK, Filly RA, Mahony BS, et al: Minimal fetal renal pyelectasis. *J Ultrasound Med* 1985; 4:85–89.
106. Arger PH, Coleman BG, Mintz MC, et al: Routine fetal genitourinary tract screening. *Radiology* 1985; 156:485–489.
107. Grignon A, Filion R, Filiatrault D, et al: Urinary tract dilatation in utero: Classification and clinical applications. *Radiology* 1986; 160:645–647.
108. Blane CE, Koff SA, Bowerman RA, et al: Nonobstructive fetal hydronephrosis: sonographic recognition and therapeutic implications. *Radiology* 1983; 147:95–99.
109. Diamond DA, Sanders R, Jeffs RD: Fetal hydronephrosis: considerations regarding urological intervention. *J Urol* 1984; 131:1155–1159.
110. Campbell S, Wladimiroff JW, Dewhurst CJ: The antenatal measurement of fetal urine production. *J Obstet Gynaecol Br Commw* 1973; 80:680–686.
111. Campbell S: The assessment of fetal development by diagnostic ultrasound. *Clin Perinatol* 1974; 1:507–525.

112. Dubbins PA, Kurtz AB, Wapner RJ, et al: Renal agenesis: Spectrum of in utero findings. *J Clin Ultrasound* 1981; 9:189–193.
113. Goldstein I, Reece EA, Yarkoni S, et al: Growth of the fetal stomach in normal pregnancies. *Obstet Gynecol* 1987; 70:641–644.
114. Nyberg DA, Mack LA, Patten RM, et al: Fetal bowel. Normal sonographic findings. *J Ultrasound Med* 1987; 6:3–6.
115. Goldstein I, Lockwood C, Hobbins JC: Ultrasound assessment of fetal intestinal development in the evaluation of gestational age. *Obstet Gynecol* 1987; 70:682–686.
116. Pretorius DH, Gosink BB, Clautice-Engle T, et al: Sonographic evaluation of the fetal stomach: Significance of nonvisualization. *AJR* 1988; 151:987–989.
117. Harris RD, Nyberg DA, Mack LA, et al: Anorectal atresia: prenatal sonographic diagnosis. *AJR* 1987; 149:395–400.
118. Russell JGB: Radiological assessment of fetal maturity. *J Obstet Gynaecol Br Commw* 1969; 76:208–219.
119. Russell JGB, Mattison AE, Easson WT, et al: Skeletal dimensions as an indication of foetal maturity. *Br J Radiol* 1972; 45:667–669.
120. Owen RH: The estimation of foetal maturity. *Br J Radiol* 1971; 44:531–534.
121. Martin RH, Higginbottom J: A clinical and radiological assessment of fetal age. *J Obstet Gynaecol Brit Commw* 1971; 78:155–162.
122. Queenan JT, O'Brien GD, Campbell S: Ultrasound measurement of fetal limb bones. *Am J Obstet Gynecol* 1980; 138:297–302.
123. O'Brien GD, Queenan JT, Campbell S: Assessment of gestational age in the second trimester by real-time ultrasound measurement of the femur length. *Am J Obstet Gynecol* 1981; 139:540–545.
124. Farrant P, Meire H: Ultrasound measurement of fetal limb lengths. *Br J Radiol* 1981; 54:660–664.
125. Jeanty P, Kirkpatrick C, Dramaix-Wilmet M, et al: Ultrasonographic evaluation of fetal limb growth. *Radiology* 1981; 140:165–168.
126. Goldstein RB, Filly RA, Simpson G: Pitfalls in femur length measurements. *J Ultrasound Med* 1987; 6:203–207.
127. Abrams SL, Filly RA: Curvature of the fetal femur: A normal sonographic finding. *Radiology* 1985; 156:490.
128. Warda AH, Deter RL, Rossavik IK, et al: Fetal femur length: A critical reevaluation of the relationship to menstrual age. *Obstet Gynecol* 1985; 66:69–75.
129. Chinn DH, Bolding DB, Callen PW, et al: Ultrasonographic identification of fetal lower extremity epiphyseal ossification centers. *Radiology* 1983; 147:815–818.
130. Merz E, Kim-Kern MS, Pehl S: Ultrasonic mensuration of fetal limb bones in the second and third trimesters. *J Clin Ultrasound* 1987; 15:175–183.
131. Hadlock FP, Harrist RB, Deter RL, et al: A prospective evaluation of fetal femur length as a predictor of gestational age. *J Ultrasound Med* 1983; 2:111–112.
132. Hadlock FP, Harrist RB, Deter RL, et al: Fetal femur length as a predictor of menstrual age: sonographically measured. *AJR* 1982; 138:875–878.
133. Wolfson RN, Peisner DB, Chik LL, et al: Comparison of biparietal diameter and femur length in the third trimester: Effects of gestational age and variation in fetal growth. *J Ultrasound Med* 1986; 5:145–149.
134. Woo JSK, Wan CW, Fang A, et al: Is fetal femur length a better indicator of gestational age in the growth-retarded fetus as compared with biparietal diameter? *J Ultrasound Med* 1985; 4:139–142.
135. Yeh MN, Bracero L, Reilly KB, et al: Ultrasonic measurement of the femur length as an index of fetal gestational age. *Am J Obstet Gynecol* 1982; 144:519–522.
136. Tse CH, Lee KW: A comparison of the fetal femur length and biparietal diameter in predicting gestational age in the third trimester. *Aust NZ J Obstet Gynaecol* 1984; 24:186–188.
137. Hohler CW, Quetel TA: Fetal femur length: Equations for computer calculation of gestational age from ultrasound measurements. *Am J Obstet Gynecol* 1982; 143:479.
138. Oman SD, Wax Y: Estimating fetal age by ultrasound measurements: an example of multivariate calibration. *Biometrics* 1984; 40:947–960.
139. Yagel S, Adoni A, Oman S, et al: A statistical examination of the accuracy of combining femoral length and biparietal diameter as an index of fetal gestational age. *Br J Obstet Gynaecol* 1986; 93:109–115.
140. Abramowicz J, Jaffe R: Comparison between lateral and axial ultrasonic measurements of the fetal femur. *Am J Obstet Gynecol* 1988; 159:921–922.

141. Winter J, Kimme-Smith C, King W: Measurement accuracy of sonographic sector scanners. *AJR* 1985; 144:645–648.

142. Gamba JL, Bowie JD, Dodson WC, et al: Accuracy of ultrasound in fetal femur length determination. Ultrasound phantom study. *Invest Radiol* 1985; 20:316–323.

143. Pretorius DH, Nelson TR, Manco-Johnson ML: Fetal age estimation by ultrasound: the impact of measurement error. *Radiology* 1984; 152:763–766.

144. Jeanty P, Beck GJ, Chervenak FA, et al: A comparison of sector and linear array scanners for the measurement of the fetal femur. *J Ultrasound Med* 1985; 4:525–530.

145. Mahoney MJ, Hobbins JC: Prenatal diagnosis of chondroectodermal dysplasia (Ellis-van Creveld syndrome) with fetoscopy and ultrasound. *N Engl J Med* 1977; 297:258–260.

146. Hobbins JC, Bracken MB, Mahoney MJ: Diagnosis of fetal skeletal dysplasias with ultrasound. *Am J Obstet Gynecol* 1982; 142:306–312.

147. Filly RA, Golbus MS, Carey JC, et al: Short-limbed dwarfism: Ultrasonographic diagnosis by mensuration of fetal femoral length. *Radiology* 1981; 138:653–656.

148. Kurtz AB, Wapner RJ: Ultrasonographic diagnosis of second-trimester skeletal dysplasias: a prospective analysis in a high-risk population. *J Ultrasound Med* 1983; 2:99–106.

149. O'Brien FD, Queenan JT: Ultrasound fetal femur length in relation to intrauterine growth retardation. Part II. *Am J Obstet Gynecol* 1982; 144:35–39.

150. Kurtz AB, Filly RA, Wapner RJ, et al: In utero analysis of heterozygous achondroplasia: Variable time of onset as detected by femur length measurements. *J Ultrasound Med* 1986; 5:137–140.

151. Roopnarinesingh S, Ramseqak S: Decreased birth weight and femur length in fetuses of patients with the sickle-cell trait. *Obstet Gynecol* 1986; 68:46–48.

152. Benacerraf BR, Gelman R, Frigoletto FD Jr: Sonographic identification of second-trimester fetuses with Down's syndrome. *N Engl J Med* 1987; 317:1371–1376.

153. Lockwood C, Benacerraf BR, Krinsky A, et al: A sonographic screening method for Down syndrome. *Am J Obstet Gynecol* 1987; 157:803–808.

154. Perrella R, Duerinckx AJ, Grant EG, et al: Second-trimester sonographic diagnosis of Down syndrome: role of femur-length shortening and nuchal-fold thickening. *AJR* 1988; 151:981–985.

155. Brumfield CG, Hauth JC, Cloud GA, et al: Sonographic measurements and ratios in fetuses with Down syndrome. *Obstet Gynecol* 1989; 73:644–646.

156. Ruvolo KA, Filly RA, Callen PW: Evaluation of fetal femur length for prediction of gestational age in a racially mixed obstetric population. *J Ultrasound Med* 1987; 6:417–419.

157. Quinlan RW, Brumfield C, Martin M, et al: Ultrasonic measurement of femur length as a predictor of fetal gestational age. *J Reprod Med* 1982; 27:392–394.

158. Jeanty P, Dramaix-Wilmet M, Van Kerkem J, et al: Ultrasonic evaluation of fetal limb growth. *Radiology* 1982; 143:751–754.

159. Jeanty P: Fetal limb biometry. *Radiology* 1983; 147:601–602.

160. Jeanty P, Rodesch F, Delbeke D, et al: Estimation of gestatonal age from measurements of fetal long bones. *J Ultrasound Med* 1984; 3:75–79.

161. O'Brien GD, Queenan JT: Growth of the ultrasound fetal femur length during normal pregnancy. Part I. *Am J Obstet Gynecol* 1981; 141:833–837.

162. Shalev E, Feldman E, Weiner E, et al: Assessment of gestational age by ultrasonic measurement of the femur length. *Acta Obstet Gynecol Scand* 1985; 64:71–74.

163. Haines CJ, Langlois Slep, Jones WR: Ultrasonic measurement of fetal femoral length in singleton and twin pregnancies. *Am J Obstet Gynecol* 1986; 155:838–841.

164. Seeds JW, Cefalo RC: Realtionship of fetal limb lengths to both biparietal diameter and gestational age. *Obstet Gynecol* 1982; 60:680–685.

165. Hohler CW, Quetel TA: Comparison of ultrasound femur length and biparietal diameter in late pregnancy. *Am J Obstet Gynecol* 1981; 141:759–762.

166. Mercer BM, Sklar S, Shariatmadar A, et al: Fetal foot length as a predictor of gestational age. *Am J Obstet Gynecol* 1987; 156:350–355.

167. Platt LD, Medearis AL, DeVore GR, et al: Fetal foot length: relationship to menstrual age and fetal measurements in the second trimester. *Obstet Gynecol* 1988; 71:526–531.

168. Goldstein I, Reece A, Hobbins JC: Sonographic appearance of the fetal heel ossification centers and foot length measurements provide independent markers for gestational age estimation. *Am J Obstet Gynecol* 1988; 159:923–926.

169. Shalev E, Weiner E, Zuckerman H, et al: Reliability of sonographic measurement of the fetal foot. *J Ultrasound Med* 1989; 8:259–262.

170. Goldstein I, Lockwood C, Belanger K, et al: Ultrasonographic assessment of gestational age with the distal femoral and proximal tibial ossification centers in the thrid trimester. *Am J Obstet Gynecol* 1988; 158:127–130.

171. Goldstein I, Lockwood CJ, Reece EA, et al: Sonographic assessment of the distal femoral and proximal tibial ossification centers in the prediction of pulmonic maturity in normal women and women with diabetes. *Am J Obstet Gynecol* 1988; 159:72–76.

172. Zilianti M, Fernandez S, Azuaga A, et al: Ultrasound evaluation of the distal femoral epiphyseal ossification center as a screening test for intrauterine growth retardation. *Obstet Gynecol* 1987; 70:361–364.

173. Tabsh KMA: Correlation of ultrasonic epiphyseal centers and the lecithin:sphingomyelin ratio. *Obstet Gynecol* 1984; 64:92–96.

174. Gentili P, Trasimeni A, Giorlandino C: Fetal ossification centers as predictors of gestational age in normal and abnormal pregnancies. *J Ultrasound Med* 1984; 3:193–197.

175. Yarkoni S, Schmidt W, Jeanty P, et al: Clavicular measurement: A new biometric parameter for fetal evaluation. *J Ultrasound Med* 1985; 4:467–470.

176. Russell JGB, Lewis GJ: Radiological assessment of fetal growth retardation. *Clin Radiol* 1981; 32:567–569.

177. Ogita S, Kamei T, Sugawa T: Estimation of fetal weight by fetography. *Am J Obstet Gynecol* 1977; 127:37–42.

178. Vintzileos AM, Neckles S, Campbell WA, et al: Ultrasound fetal thigh-calf circumferences and gestational age—independent fetal ratios in normal pregnancy. *J Ultrasound Med* 1985; 4:287–292.

179. Jeanty P, Romero R, Hobbins JC: Fetal limb volume: A new parameter to assess fetal growth and nutrition. *J Ultrasound Med* 1985; 4:273–282.

180. Deter RL, Warda A, Rossavik IK, et al: Fetal thigh circumference: A critical evaluation of its relationsip to menstrual age. *J Clin Ultrasound* 1986; 14:105–110.

181. Warda A, Deter RL, Duncan G, et al: Evaluation of fetal thigh circumference measurements: A comparative ultrasound and anatomical study. *J Clin Ultrasound* 1986; 14:99–103.

182. Benacerraf BR, Frigoletto FD Jr, Laboda LA: Sonographic diagnosis of Down syndrome in the second trimester. *Am J Obstet Gynecol* 1985; 153:49–52.

183. Benacerraf BR, Barss VA, Laboda LA: A sonographic sign for the detection in the second trimester of the fetus with Down's syndrome. *Am J Obstet Gynecol* 1985; 151:1078–1079.

Chapter 26

Combined Fetal Head and Body Measurements

Alfred B. Kurtz, M.D.

Barry B. Goldberg, M.D.

In the neonatal literature, parameters have been combined in an attempt to better evaluate the newborn infant. One of the most popular is Rohrer's ponderal index, a weight-length ratio used to obtain a three-dimensional newborn volume.[1] This index is equal to 100 times the weight in grams divided by the length in centimeters cubed.

This same type of analysis can be performed in utero. By combining or comparing fetal parameters during one examination or by evaluating these parameters serially during gestation, attempts have been made to better understand and predict fetal growth.

MEASUREMENT COMPARISONS

Head to Abdomen

The head and body grow symmetrically through most of fetal life. Any large discrepancy often implies abnormality. If the fetal body is significantly smaller than the normal fetal head, particularly after 30 weeks, this strongly suggests asymmetric growth retardation.[2, 3] Conversely, if the fetal head is significantly smaller than the normal fetal body, this suggests microcephaly or anencephaly.[4] There is always one central problem in the comparison of any two dissimilar parameters: Which is normal and which is abnormal? It is therefore necessary to have a third independent variable, either another fetal measurement such as femoral length or an outside parameter such as an accurate last menstrual period. Using this third variable, it can often be determined which of the two original measurements was normal. Then the abnormal parameter can be further evaluated.

In analyzing the ratio of the head to body, linear, circumference, and area measurements have been compared. For linear measurements, the biparietal diameter and abdominal diameter at the appropriate anatomic positions were evaluated in five articles.[5-9] Gottesfeld[5] found that linear measurements of the biparietal diameter should be within ±5 mm of the average body diameter. Sarti et al.[7] examined the anteroposterior (AP) and transverse body diameters, the average body diameter, and the longitudinal body diameter, comparing each to the biparietal diameter from 12 to 26 weeks. In chart form, the best correlation was with the average and transverse body diameters. The abdominal growth during this interval of fetal life was slightly less than the biparietal diameter and was found to be linear with a slope of 0.96, approximately 1:1. Sarti et al.[7] then examined five cases of abnormal head-to-body ratios. In three, the head was smaller and either microcephaly or anencephaly was detected. In the other two with the body smaller, growth retardation and triploidy were found.

The findings of Eriksen and co-workers[10] agreed with the work of Sarti et al.[7] While no ratio table of biparietal-to-abdominal diameters is available, a ratio of mean biparietal and average body diameters can be computed at each stage of gestation from their table (Table 26–1). The ratio is approximately 1:1 throughout the second trimester, 1.12 at 13 weeks decreasing to 0.97 by 28 weeks.[10] In the third trimester, however, the body progressively enlarges in relation to the fetal head so that the ratio decreases to 0.94, 0.90, and 0.85 at 33, 37, and 40 weeks, respectively. Fescina et al.[6] computed the biparietal-to-abdominal diameter ratio in numeric form from 15 to 40 weeks. While the authors did not state how these measurements were obtained, the progression from a higher to a lower ratio was also found. Their range was wider than that found by Eriksen et al.,[10] a mean of 1.20 at 15 weeks decreasing to 0.84 at term. At a range of 2 SD, the variation was even wider.

Gross et al.[8] compared the transverse and Elliott et al.[9] the average body diameter to the biparietal diameter. Both approached their evaluation in unusual ways. Gross et al.[8] analyzed their data from 26 weeks to term and obtained an increase in body size, similar to that of Eriksen et al.,[10] as the pregnancy progressed to term. Using an equation of transverse body diameter (TBD) minus biparietal diameter (BPD), a number was obtained from 26 weeks to term which attempted to distinguish normal from growth-retarded fetuses. When the BPD was equal to or less than 70 mm (a mean gestational age of up to 27.5 weeks), the TBD minus BPD was equal to or greater than −3. When the BPD was 70 to 75 mm (mean gestational ages of 27.5–29.5 weeks), the TBD was equal to or greater than the BPD. When the BPD was 76 to 80 mm (mean gestational ages of 30.0–31.6 weeks), the TBD minus BPD was equal to or greater than 2, and when the BPD was greater than 80 mm (mean gestational age >31.6 weeks), the TBD minus BPD was equal to or greater than 4. Using these ratios, Gross et al.[8] detected asymmetric growth retardation with a sensitivity of 68%, a specificity of 69%, an accuracy of positive diagnosis of 42%, and an accuracy of negative diagnosis of 87%. They cautioned not to compress the fetal body during scanning since this could distort the TBD measurement. Elliott et al.[9] used their comparison differently, that is, to establish a number which would distinguish normal from large (macrosomic) fetuses. They used an average "chest" diameter minus the biparietal diameter from 35 weeks to term. In actuality, the "chest" was measured at the liver and will be considered an abdominal measurement. If the average abdominal diameter minus BPD were equal to or greater than 1.4 cm, the fetal body was so large that shoulder dystocia occurred in four of 15 macrosomic infants from diabetic mothers. The work by both groups[8, 9] appears to be of limited value in the evaluation of small and large fetuses. Both methods are somewhat cumbersome and do not offer increased detection rates. The work by Elliott et al.[9] is especially questionable since an adequate analysis of shoulder dystocia would have to include a measurement of the upper chest or shoulders, not just the abdomen.

TABLE 26–1.
Comparison of Biparietal Diameter to Abdominal Diameter*

Gestational Age (wk)	Predicted Mean Biparietal Diameter (mm)	Predicted Mean Average Abdominal Diameter (mm)
13	25.6	22.7
14	28.5	26.4
15	31.5	30.1
16	34.6	33.7
17	37.7	37.3
18	40.9	40.9
19	44.1	44.5
20	47.4	48.0
21	50.6	51.4
22	53.9	54.9
23	57.1	58.3
24	60.4	61.7
25	63.5	65.0
26	66.6	68.4
27	70.0	71.7
28	72.6	74.9
29	75.4	78.2
30	78.1	81.4
31	80.7	84.6
32	83.1	87.7
33	85.4	90.8
34	87.5	93.9
35	89.4	97.0
36	91.1	100.1
37	92.6	103.1
38	93.8	106.1
39	94.8	109.0
40	95.5	112.0

*From Eriksen PS, Sechor NJ, Weis-Bentzon M: *Acta Obstet Gynecol Scand* 1985; 64:65–70. Used by permission.

The discrepancies in this direct comparison of the mean biparietal diameter and average body diameter, without a consistent approach, are too great to recommend a table. However, these two mean numbers can be compared in another way, by analyzing the number of standard deviations between them. Since the biparietal and average body diameters are almost the same number throughout the second and into the early third trimester, a deviation of one from the other of 2 to 3 SD would strongly suggest that one of the two measurements is abnormal. For the biparietal diameter, one article found 2 SD to be 1.4 mm,[11] two articles calculated 2 SD as approximately 3 mm,[7, 8] and two articles determined 2 SD to be 5 mm or greater.[12–14] While these numbers are somewhat discrepant, our experience agrees with those that found each standard deviation to be 3 mm.[14] Therefore, if the biparietal diameter and average body diameter are within 6 mm (2 SD) of each other throughout the second and into the early third trimester (from 13–34 weeks) (see Table 26–1), the two are most likely normal. If, however, there is a deviation of at least 6 mm (2 SD) and definitely 9 mm (3 SD), abnormalities should be carefully sought.

This approach can be used to evaluate both an abnormally small body (most commonly seen in asymmetric growth retardation) and an abnormally small head (microcephaly). While this approach has not been adequately evaluated in the detection of growth retardation, microcephaly has been analyzed.[5, 14, 15] Chervenak et al.,[14] in the first of two studies, found that microcephaly could be diagnosed if the biparietal diameter were more than 3 SD below the norm. In a follow-up prospective study,[15] they found that to eliminate all false-negative diagnoses the occipitofrontal diameter, head circumference, and head–abdominal circumference ratio also had to be decreased by 4, 5, and 3 SD, respectively.[15] Furthermore, to eliminate all false-positive diagnoses, the ratio of femur length to head circumference had to be taken into account.[15] While this approach is undoubtedly accurate, it seems cumbersome and would not have to be used in most cases of microcephaly since, in addition to an abnormally small head, the internal brain structures are usually also grossly abnormal.[5]

The circumferences of the head and abdomen have also been compared using the same anatomic landmarks that were used for the biparietal diameter and abdominal diameter. Six articles compared the ratio of the head to abdominal circumference.[6, 14, 16–19] All were calculated throughout the second and third trimester, three giving numbers with the 5th and 95th percentile confidence limits,[6, 14, 17] and three in graph form.[16, 18, 19] The results were similar to those found for the linear ratio of biparietal diameter and average abdominal diameter. In the early second trimester, all articles showed the head circumference to be greater than the abdominal circumference so that the head-to-body ratio was slightly greater than 1. As the abdomen increased in size in the mid- to late third trimester, this ratio then decreased. At term, Fescina et al.,[6] Campbell and Thoms,[17] and Deter et al.[16] found a reversal in the ratio to less than 1, while the other three[14, 18, 19] showed the ratio to decrease but to still remain greater than 1. Campbell and Thoms[17] stated further that the ratio, which slowly decreased between 17 and 29 weeks, had a sharper decline to 40 weeks. Of all the circumference ratio articles, Campbell and Thoms' work[17] most closely parallels the linear head-to-abdomen ratio analysis of Eriksen et al.[10] and is therefore recommended (Fig 26–1) (Table 26–2).

In the evaluation of in utero growth retardation, Campbell and Thoms[17] found that if the ratio of the head to abdominal circumference were abnormally high, indicative of a small fetal body, it was strongly suggestive of asymmetric growth retardation. In a prospective study using the table of Campbell and Thoms, Crane and Kopta[20] evaluated 47 fetuses. When the head–abdominal circumference ratio was normal, all fetuses were found to be normal. However, when the head–abdominal circumference ratio was abnormally high, all the fetuses had asymmetric growth retardation. They therefore concluded that the head-to-body ratio was a sensitive indicator of asymmetric growth retardation and particularly useful as an initial determination of growth retardation when only one examination had been performed.

An additional method of evaluating the head and abdominal circumferences is to compare the two by using the number of standard deviations between them. As stated for the linear dimensions of the biparietal diameter and average body diameter,

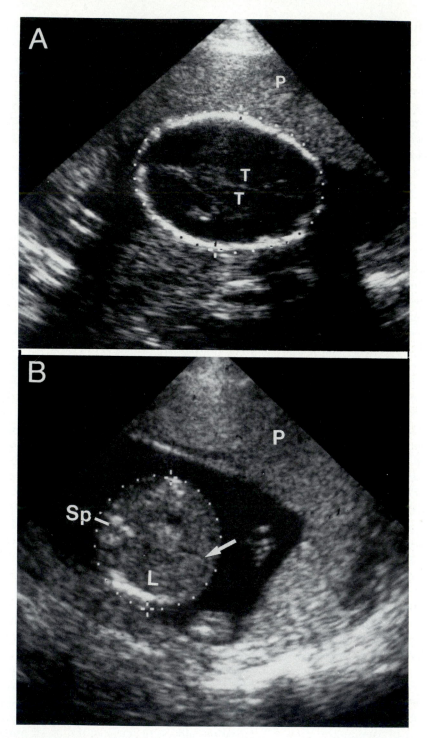

FIG 26–1.
Circumference measurements of the fetal head and abdomen. **A,** transaxial image of the head at the thalami *(T)*. With either the thalami or midbrain in the midline, the circumference is traced around the outer margin of the head with a digitizer or map reader *(dotted line)* or can be calculated from an equation. **B,** transaxial image of the upper abdomen at the region of the liver *(L)*. The umbilical portion of the left portal vein *(arrow)* is situated within the liver in the midline. The circumference is traced with a digitizer or map reader *(dotted line)* or can be calculated from an equation. *P* = placenta; *Sp* = spine.

TABLE 26–2.
Head–Abdominal Circumference Ratio*

| Gestational Age (wk) | Ratio of Head Circumference–Abdominal Circumference | |
	Mean	Range From 5th to 95th Percentile
13–14	1.23	1.14–1.31
15–16	1.22	1.05–1.39
17–18	1.18	1.07–1.29
19–20	1.18	1.09–1.39
21–22	1.15	1.06–1.25
23–24	1.13	1.05–1.21
25–26	1.13	1.04–1.22
27–28	1.13	1.05–1.21
29–30	1.10	0.99–1.21
31–32	1.07	0.96–1.17
33–34	1.04	0.96–1.11
35–36	1.02	0.93–1.11
37–38	0.98	0.92–1.05
39–40	0.97	0.87–1.06
41–42	0.96	0.93–1.00

*From Campbell S, Thoms A: *Br J Obstet Gynaecol* 1977; 84:165–174. Used by permission.

any variation of 2 and definitely of 3 SD is strongly suggestive of an abnormality. Athey and Hadlock[21] stated that 1 SD for a head circumference was 9.5 mm and 1 SD for an abdominal circumference was 11.4 mm. The average of the two is approximately 10 mm per standard deviation. Therefore, if the head and abdomen circumference measurements deviate from their expected values at any gestational age by 20 mm (2 SD) and certainly by 30 mm (3 SD), this is indicative of abnormality.

In the evaluation of the ratio of the head to body, the question remains whether linear (diameters) or circumference measurements are more accurate. Persson and Marsal[22] evaluated the circumference ratios of the head and abdomen and compared them to the linear ratios of the biparietal and average body diameters. They found that the circumference ratios were wide and that differentiation could not be made between average and small-for-gestational-age babies. This finding had also been suggested by Deter et al.[23] when they found great variability in the head to abdominal circumferences. Persson and Marsal[22] felt that linear ratios might be more accurate since the ratio of the biparietal to average abdominal diameter was significantly better in differentiating small from average gestational age fetuses and was able to detect 72% of average and 75% of small-for-gestational-age fetuses. They found that the biparietal diameter–average abdominal diameter ratio for small-for-gestational-age fetuses was never greater than 1:1, while for average-gestational-age fetuses it was always greater than or equal to 1. Unfortunately, while a table of linear ratios would be desirable and might offer some clinical advantage over circumference ratios, none is recommended at present.

Four articles compared the head to the abdominal areas,[6, 11, 13, 24] two in numeric form[6, 13] and two in graph form.[11, 24] All showed a decrease in the ratio from the second trimester to term, similar to linear and circumference ratios. Wladimiroff et al.[11, 13] obtained the head area by squaring the biparietal diameter and obtained the fetal body area with a digitizer. Their landmarks for the body measurement included visualization of the liver so that although they termed this a chest area, it will be considered instead an abdominal area. Fescina et al.[6] used two formulas, one for the head and another for the body, to obtain their areas. Varma et al.[24] used a planimeter to obtain both the head and abdomen areas. In two articles, the overall accuracy reported in the detection of asymmetric growth retardation was 76%[13] and 85%.[24] While these numbers are encouraging, they are not significantly better than those reported for linear and circumference ratios. In addition, since the use of a digitizer or formula to obtain the head and abdominal areas is not as well established as the linear or circumference techniques, there appears at present to be no benefit to the use of area ratios.

Lastly, a ratio of the head to abdominal volume has been proposed.[25] The volumes were computed solely from transverse images rather than by using a long-axis measurement. Nevertheless, the data in number form reveal a decreasing ratio of 2.1 at 12 weeks to 0.9 at term, with a 2-SD range. Although the decreasing ratio has also been observed with the linear and circumference ratios, the mean and range values are much larger for these volume measurements. Therefore, the linear and circumference ratios are recommended.

Femur to Head

Hohler and Quetel[26] evaluated the femoral length to the biparietal diameter and found a ratio from 23 weeks to term of 79 ± 8 at the 90% confidence limits. Chervenak et al.[14] and Hadlock et al.[19] calculated the femur length–head circumference ratio from either 15 weeks[19] or 20 weeks[14] to term. They both used head circumferences instead of biparietal diameters so that an unusually shaped head would not affect the ratio. Their numbers were in close agreement, a mean number of 18 at 20 weeks, increasing linearly to 23 at term, all with 2 SD.

These ratios may have clinical value in the detection of short-limbed dwarfism and in cases of microcephaly where the internal intracranial anatomy is normal. While more clinical evaluation is necessary, the ratios of femur length to biparietal diameter[26] and femur length to head circumference[19] are recommended (Figs 26–2 and 26–3) (Tables 26–3 and 26–4).

Articles have been published using a comparison of the biparietal diameter to the femur length.[27–30] All found that in cases of Down syndrome (trisomy 21) the femur length was decreased in relation to the biparietal diameter. In two of these studies,[28, 30] the ratio of the two was felt to be the best predictor of this shortening, better than using any other parameter or combination of parameters of the head, body, and femur.[30]

Both Lockwood et al.[28] and Brumfield et al.[30] analyzed the biparietal diameter–femur length ratio. This is the inverse of Table 26–3 where a ratio of femur length to biparietal diameter was used. An inverse of the numbers in Table 26–3, 1 divided by the number, gives a mean of 1.27 with range of 1.16 to 1.39 (10th to 90th percentile). Lockwood et al.[28] evaluated this ratio from two institutions and found statistical differences in the normal femur length measurements at the two centers. This gave different ratio values for normals, both considerably different from the

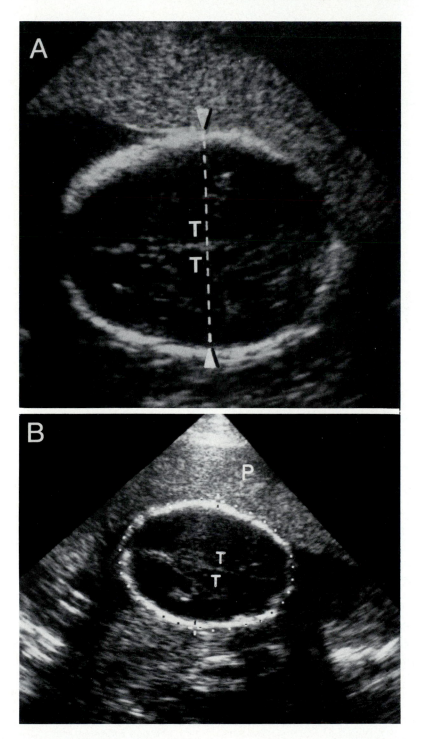

FIG 26–2.
Biparietal diameter and circumference measurements of the head. Both are taken from the transaxial image with the thalami *(T)* or midbrain in the midline. **A,** biparietal diameter measurement, denoted by *arrowheads* and *dashed line,* taken leading edge (outer margin) to leading edge (inner margin). **B,** head circumference measurement, denoted by a *dotted line,* is traced around the outer margin of the head with a digitizer or map reader. It can also be calculated by using an equation. *P* = placenta.

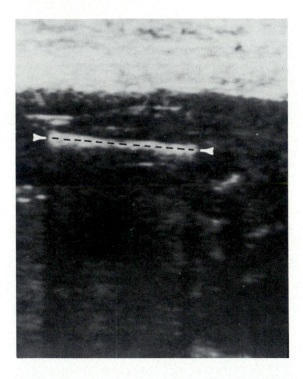

FIG 26–3.
Femur length measurement. The long axis of the femoral shaft is measured, denoted by *arrowheads* and *dashed line*, disregarding the hypoechoic nonossified epiphyseal cartilages.

normal values stated above. Nevertheless, at 1.5 SD below the control group, 55 Down syndrome fetuses were evaluated. Solely by the use of this ratio, 40% of cases were detected at Yale University Perinatal Unit with a false-positive rate of 7%, and 60% of cases were detected by the Diagnostic Ultrasound Associates in Boston with a false-positive rate of 4.6%.[28] Brumfield et al.[30] found that using a biparietal diameter–femur ratio equal to or greater than 1.8 on 15 cases of Down syndrome, the elevated number detected the syndrome with a sensitivity of 40%, a specificity of 97.8%, and a false-positive rate of 2.2%.

While these results appear encouraging, caution must be exhibited in the use of this ratio as the sole method of detecting Down syndrome. In any statistical analysis, a cutoff limit is needed. If, as in the article by Lockwood et al.,[28] 1.5 SD is used, then 87% or 87/100 normal cases are within, and 13% or 13/100 normal cases are outside these limits. Of the 13/100 cases, 6.5 cases will be above and 6.5 cases below

TABLE 26–3.
Femur Length (FL)–Biparietal Diameter (BPD)
Ratio (Range 23–40 wk)*

Ratio	Mean	Range From 10th to 90th Percentile
FL/BPD × 100	79	72–86

*Data from Hohler CW, Quetel TA: *Am J Obstet Gynecol* 1981; 141:759–762.

these limits. The 6.5 normal cases per 100 below 1.5 SD must be balanced against the chance of detecting Down syndrome in a low-risk population, at a risk rate of 1/800–1000 cases. This group of women would not ordinarily obtain an amniocentesis for chromosomal analysis unless something in the ultrasound study suggested Down syndrome. For every 800 cases studied, we would correctly predict one case of Down syndrome and incorrectly suggest that 52 normal cases (8 × 6.5/100) might also have Down syndrome. This is not an acceptable rate of Down syndrome detection, particularly since all of these cases would need an amniocentesis or chorionic villus sampling, both with a small but not negligible loss rate.

TABLE 26–4.
Femur Length (FL)–Head Circumference (HC) Ratio*

Predicted Mean Gestational Age (wk)	FL/HC Ratio	
	Predicted Mean	Range 16%–84% (1 SD)
15	16.2	15.3–17.1
16	14.9	13.3–16.5
17	16.1	14.6–17.6
18	16.9	15.8–18.0
19	17.2	16.1–18.3
20	18.3	16.8–19.8
21	18.1	15.9–20.3
22	19.3	18.4–20.2
23	20.0	19.2–20.8
24	19.8	18.7–20.9
25	19.5	18.7–20.3
26	19.5	18.6–20.4
27	19.5	18.6–20.4
28	19.7	18.8–20.6
29	20.2	19.6–20.8
30	20.3	19.2–21.4
31	20.3	19.3–21.3
32	20.2	19.1–21.3
33	20.7	19.9–21.5
34	20.6	19.4–21.8
35	21.2	20.1–22.3
36	21.1	20.1–22.1
37	21.7	20.8–22.6
38	21.8	20.9–22.7
39	22.0	20.6–23.4
40	21.6	20.7–22.5
41	22.4	21.6–23.2
42	22.0	20.1–23.9

*From Hadlock FP, Harrist RB, Shah Y, et al: *J Ultrasound Med* 1984; 3:439–442. Used by permission.

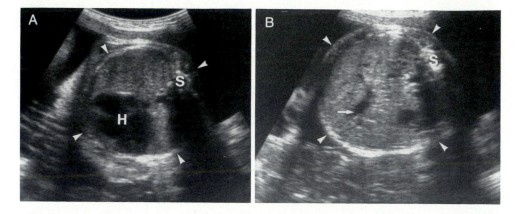

FIG 26–4.
Transaxial chest and abdominal measurements in the same fetus at 32 gestational weeks. *Arrowheads* outline the outer margins of the body. **A,** chest image taken in lower thorax at the region of the four-chambered view of the heart *(H).* **B,** upper abdominal image at the region of the liver and umbilical portion of left portal vein *(arrow).* The circumference can be obtained by tracing outer margins with a digitizer or map reader or by calculation from an equation. *S* = spine.

If we further analyze the work by Brumfield et al.,[30] a similar conclusion can be drawn. The sensitivity rate of 40% is unacceptably low for the detection of Down syndrome. Sensitivity is defined as true-positives divided by true-positives plus false-negatives. A rate of 40% misses 60% of the cases and is almost as poor a result as simply guessing. In addition, this group claimed a specificity rate of 97.8%. Since specificity is defined as true-negatives divided by true-negatives plus false-positives, a very high specificity rate is not surprising and would be expected since almost all cases will be normal (true-negative).

Therefore, while there is no doubt that the literature[27–30] supports a shortening of the femur, it is not short enough to consistently detect Down syndrome. Perhaps if the biparietal diameter–femur length ratio can be combined with other parameters, then the sensitivity for Down syndrome detection could be increased to an acceptable level.

Chest to Abdomen

Six articles compared the circumference of the chest to the circumference of the abdomen.[31–36] This ratio was evaluated from early second trimester until term with a mean value and a 2-SD range. All articles measured the lower thorax at the level of the four-chambered heart view and the abdomen at the liver (the standard abdominal level) and obtained the circumferences by either planimeter tracing or using the equation for the circumference of a circle (Fig 26–4). Two articles showed an increase in both parameters in graph form as the pregnancy progressed toward term.[31, 32] Three others stated that the chest-to-abdomen ratio was age-independent, unchanged throughout the second and third trimester.[33–35]

The comparison of the chest to abdomen is potentially important because it can be used to establish an abnormally small thorax, a finding seen in certain types of fetal skeletal dysplasias and also frequently a predictor of pulmonary hypoplasia. Three of the articles[32, 35, 36] base their ratio on a scientific abstract presented at the

TABLE 26–5.
Thoracic–Abdominal
Circumference Ratio (Age-
Independent)

Mean	Range (2 SD)
0.94	0.84–1.04*
0.89	0.77–1.01†
0.91	0.86–0.96‡
0.90 (av)	.77–1.04

*Data from Callan NA, Colmorgen GHC, Weiner S: *Am J Obstet Gynecol* 1985; 151:756–757.
†Data from Chitkara U, Rosenberg J, Chervenak FA, et al: *Am J Obstet Gynecol* 1987; 156:1069–1074.
‡Data from Fong K, Ohlsson A, Zalev A: *Am J Obstet Gynecol* 1988; 158:1154–1160.

31st Annual Meeting of the Society for Gynecologic Investigation in 1984, without further scientific review, with Callan et al.[35] then reporting the ratio 1 year later as 0.94 ±0.05 (2 SD). Skiptunas and Weiner[32] showed a graph and its use in the detection of a small thorax, giving credit to the graph by Callan and co-workers and misquoting the ratio mean number as 0.85. Unfortunately Callan et al.[35] did not have this graph. Lastly, Johnson and co-workers[36] referenced the work by Callan et al.[35] and used the ratio in their analysis of patients at risk for pulmonary hypoplasia.

Despite these irregularities, the ratio and 2-SD ranges are in close agreement among the three articles[33–35] including the work by Callan et al.[35] Table 26–5 takes an average of the mean numbers and a range of 2 SD. The lower limit is the more important number because it can be used to detect a chest that is too small. It is possible, however, that the lowest number of 0.77 from the study by Chitkara et al.[33] may be too low.

The use of this ratio to evaluate patients at risk for developing pulmonary hypoplasia was performed by Fong et al.[34] using a lower limit of 0.86 and by Johnson and co-workers[36] using a lower limit of 0.89 (only 1 SD, rather than 2). Fong et al.[34] evaluated 18 patients with prolonged oligohydramnios or ruptured membranes. The nine that survived had a normal ratio and no significant pulmonary problems. Of the nine that died, eight had an abnormally low ratio with seven of the eight having significant pulmonary problems. Similarly Johnson et al.[36] found that in a high-risk group of 16 children that died with a low chest-to-abdomen ratio detected in utero, 14 had a significant contribution from pulmonary hypoplasia. Therefore, although the causes of pulmonary hypoplasia are many, not just secondary to a small chest circumference, this ratio could be of clinical significance. More work is needed to establish the lower limit of normal.

Femur to Abdomen

Bracero et al.[37] evaluated a ratio of the mean abdominal diameter to the femur length, attempting to detect large-for-gestational-age (LGA or macrosomic) fetuses in a group of diabetic and nondiabetic patients. The LGA fetuses of diabetic mothers could be separated from the others if the ratio were greater than 1.385. They identified 19 of 24 large fetuses and incorrectly included four of 20 normal fetuses. The sensitivity, specificity, positive predictive, and negative predictive values in the prediction of large fetuses were good, 79%, 80%, 83%, and 76%, respectively. In addition, by combining these results with an abdominal–biparietal diameter ratio of greater than 1.065, they were able to lower their false-negative rate to 8%.

While these results sound encouraging in the detection of LGA fetuses from diabetic mothers, the authors stated that they measured the abdomen at the level of the umbilical vein, measured an outer to inner diameter, and implied that a mean diameter was obtained from only one measurement perpendicular to the spine. There are problems with this study. First, does the umbilical vein imply the correct level of the high abdomen where the umbilical portion of the left portal vein (within the liver) is located, or a lower abdominal level where the umbilical vein enters the abdomen? Second, there is no reproducible way of obtaining an abdominal inner measurement. Third, many abdominal shapes are ovoid so that an average of two diameters is more accurate in determining a mean diameter. As a result, these data cannot be recommended.

Femur length has been more extensively compared to abdominal circumference. Hadlock et al.[38] evaluated the femoral length–abdominal circumference ratio from 21 weeks to term and found a ratio independent of gestational age, 22 ±2 at 2 SD. When the ratio was greater than 23.5, they felt that it predicted asymmetric growth retardation in 19 (63%) of 30 affected fetuses.[38] This is not at all impressive since in the same article there were much higher detection rates (true-positives) with many fewer false-negatives with the use of the abdominal circumference, the ratio of the head circumference to abdominal circumference, and even the estimated weight. In addition, this ratio did not detect any cases not diagnosed by the other measurements.

Ott,[39] Vintzileos et al.,[40] Brown et al.,[41] and Benson et al.[42] also evaluated the femoral length–abdominal circumference ratio. They too found the ratio to be independent of gestational age. Their mean numbers and standard deviations, however, were somewhat different for the detection of growth retarded fetuses, 22.33 ±1.86,[39] 22.3 ±2.4,[40] 24.2 ±1.6,[41] and 23.7 ±1.4.[42] Therefore the 23.5 value did not consistently discriminate between normal and growth-retarded fetuses.

In four studies,[41–44] small-for-gestational-age fetuses overlapped with the normal range and showed much less of a discriminatory value than that originally reported by Hadlock et al.[38] In fact, Benson et al.[42] found such an overlap between normal (22.4 ±1.7) and growth-retarded (23.7 ±1.4) fetuses that this ratio had no clinical value in the prediction of growth retardation. In addition, Brown et al.[41] found the abdominal circumference much more predictive of small-for-gestational-age (SGA) than the femur length–abdominal circumference ratio. Divon et al.[43] evaluated this ratio against the rate of growth of the abdominal circumference and amniotic fluid and found that an abdominal circumference rate of growth of less than 10 mm in 14 days or a femur length–abdominal circumference greater than 23.5 identified most SGA fetuses, the abdominal rate of growth being more sensitive. By combining the two, only 15% of SGA fetuses were missed. Lastly, Hays and Patterson[44] analyzed the same ratio, comparing it to the neonatal skin-fold thickness, birth weight, and ponderal index. While they summarized their data by stating that the ratio was significantly related to these three newborn variables, at best their data showed a weak correlation. It is therefore felt that the femur length–abdominal circumference ratio offers nothing except another calculation in the diagnosis of growth retardation. The ratio may even be misleading since in the original work[38] many false-negatives (missed diagnoses) occurred.

Hadlock et al.[45] employed the same formula to evaluate macrosomic or LGA fetuses. Using a cutoff of 20.5 or less, they were able to predict 32 (63%) of 51 large-for-date fetuses. As with growth retardation, this formula appears to be no more accurate than the other measurements. When comparing the normal to the LGA fetus, the biparietal diameter and abdominal circumference were, on average, larger by 4 mm and 38 mm, respectively, for the LGA fetus so that a simple evaluation of the biparietal diameters and abdominal circumferences should make the diagnosis without the use of this ratio.

There was also an overlap of this ratio with that found in three other articles.[41, 42, 48] One of these, Benson et al.,[46] specifically analyzed the femur length–abdominal circumference ratio in normal fetuses and macrosomic fetuses from diabetic mothers. The ratios were 20.4 ± 1.6 and 19.5 ± 1.4, respectively, with considerable overlap and no cutoff value to give a high specificity or sensitivity. Even the positive predictive value was poor, 36% to 43%, and only slightly greater than the 26% for the control group. The only possible flaw in this study (discussed by the author and felt to be insignificant) was that some of the ultrasound femoral measurements were obtained using mechanical sector scanners. Therefore the 20.5 value does not consistently discriminate between normal and macrosomic fetuses.

Other Comparisons

The following is a list of other ratios that have been reported in the literature but without further confirmation or proven clinical utility:

Biparietal diameter to transverse thoracic diameter[47]
Biparietal diameter to thoracic circumference[31]
Head circumference to thoracic circumference[31]
Tibial length to calf circumference[48]
Femur length to thigh circumference[48]
Tibial length to abdominal circumference[40]
Femur and tibial length to abdominal circumference[40]
Thoracic circumference to femoral length[31, 44]
Abdominal circumference to diastolic biventricular outer dimension[49]
Abdominal circumference to diastolic biventricular inner dimension[49]
Abdominal circumference to diastolic right internal dimension[49]
Abdominal circumference to diastolic left internal dimension[49]
Abdominal circumference to tricuspid valve opening excursion[49]
Abdominal circumference to mitral valve opening excursion[49]
Abdominal circumference to right wall thickness[49]
Abdominal circumference to left wall thickness[49]
Abdominal circumference to interventricular septal thickness[49]
Femur length to end-diastolic right ventricular dimension[50]
Femur length to end-diastolic left ventricular dimension[50]
Femur length to end-diastolic biventricular outer dimension[50]
Femur length to end-diastolic biventricular inner dimension[50]
Femur length to tricuspid valve opening excursion[50]
Femur length to mitral valve opening excursion[50]
Femur length to right ventricular thickness[50]
Femur length to left ventricular thickness[50]

Femur length to interventricular septal thickness[50]
Fractional spine length to abdominal circumference[51]
Fetal ponderal index = weight divided by femur length cubed[52]
Cardiac circumference to biparietal diameter[53]
Cardiac circumference to abdominal circumference[53]
Cardiac circumference to femur length[53]
Cardiac circumference to fetal weight[53]
Femur length to foot length[54]
Lung span to hemithorax[55]

MULTIPLE PARAMETERS

Fetal measurements have also been added, subtracted, and multiplied together in an attempt to increase the accuracy of fetal growth and age.

Fetal Age

The combination of fetal parameters was performed in an attempt to increase the accuracy of fetal age dating.[56–60] Oman and Wax[56] claimed that a quadratic equation containing both biparietal diameter and femoral length was more accurate than either measurement alone, approximately a 1-week variation throughout the second and third trimesters. These results are unusually good and as yet have not been duplicated.

Hadlock et al. analyzed this concept in three articles,[57–59] two retrospectively[57, 58] and the third prospectively.[59] All three found the biparietal diameter to be increasingly inaccurate toward term, to greater than ±3 weeks after 30 weeks. Because of this, they combined the mean values for biparietal diameter, head circumference, abdominal circumference, and femoral length. This combination decreased the inaccuracy at all stages of gestation, especially after 30 weeks. From 30 to 36 weeks and from 36 to 42 weeks, the variation was only ±2.44 and ±2.3 weeks, respectively.[58] Hadlock et al.[58] felt that this combination of mean numbers decreased a maximum error that could be created by a discrepancy in any one or two measurements. Ott,[60] using the same four parameters, substantiated this observation. He found that the simple arithmetic average of four gave the lowest systematic and random errors.

Despite these encouraging results, there are several aspects of the multiple parameter concept which need further investigation. The inaccuracy of their biparietal diameter measurements, particularly near term, are large. Not all previous authors have found similar inaccuracies in the biparietal diameter in the third trimester.[61–63] Others have not found the biparietal diameter to be the most inaccurate (as these articles have stated) of all single parameters. In fact, two[64, 65] found the biparietal diameter to be the single most reliable indicator of gestational age.

In the three articles,[57–59] the entire study group for the second and third trimester was not greater than 360 women,[58] and it was much smaller in the other two.[57, 59] It is possible that the large standard error near term was due to the relatively small number of patients. In addition, despite the finding that the biparietal diameter was clearly the most inaccurate, a cephalic index was not performed to determine which head shapes were so abnormal that biparietal diameters should not have been used.

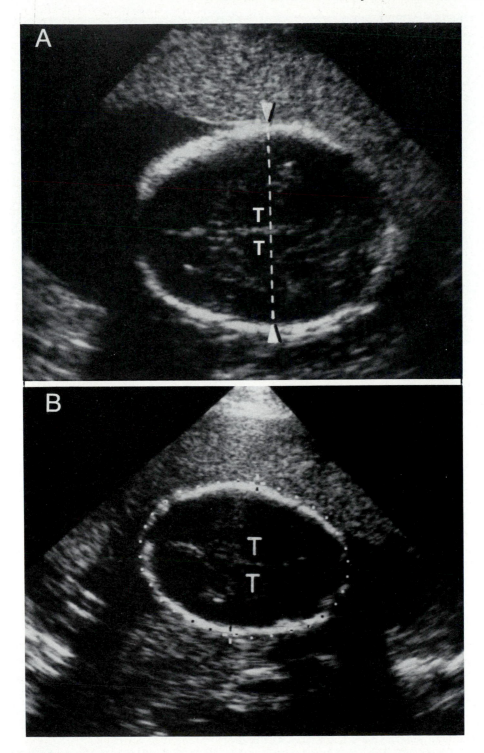

FIG 26–5.
Biparietal diameter and circumference measurements of the head. Both are taken from the transaxial image with the thalami *(T)* or midbrain in the midline. **A,** biparietal diameter measurement, denoted by *arrowheads* and *dashed line,* taken leading edge (outer margin) to leading edge (inner margin). **B,** head circumference measurement, denoted by a *dotted line,* is traced around the outer margin of the head with a digitizer or map reader. It can also be calculated by using an equation.

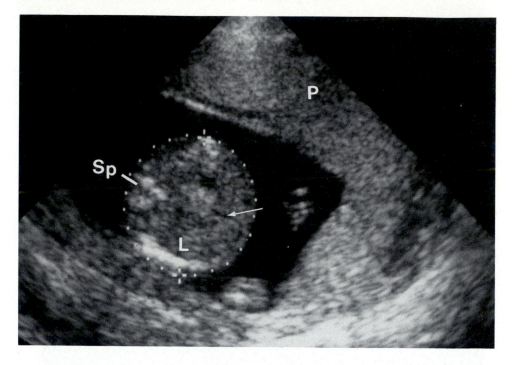

FIG 26–6.
Circumference measurement of the fetal abdomen. Transaxial image of the upper abdomen at the region of the liver *(L)*. The umbilical portion of the left portal vein *(arrow)* is situated within the liver in the midline. The circumference is traced with a digitizer or map reader *(dotted line)* or can be calculated from an equation. *P* = placenta; *Sp* = spine.

Furthermore, all circumferences for the head and body were taken using a linear array transducer. In the third trimester, many heads and bodies cannot be fitted onto one image so that the margins have to be estimated in order to calculate a circumference. This could lead to significant errors.

Despite all of these misgivings, this work does appear to have clinical usefulness in eliminating a maximum error when one, or possibly two, measurements are discrepant from the others. Therefore, a table by Hadlock et al.[58] is recommended (Figs 26–5 to 26–7, Table 26–6).

Product of the Crown-Rump Length and Trunk Area

Five articles[66–70] have evaluated the product of the crown-rump length and trunk area, one from 16 weeks to term[66] and the others from 33 weeks to term. All were shown in graph form, with the measurement points obtained from static scans using a method described by Wittman et al.[67] The crown-rump length was obtained in longitudinal axis from the top of the head to the bottom of the bladder and the trunk area from an upper abdominal transaxial image. All showed an increase in the product of the fetal length times trunk area as the fetus enlarged to term.

Parker et al.[66] claimed that this product correlated well with fetal weight. In three others,[68–70] in utero growth retardation was detected in up to 94% of cases. This measurement is time-consuming and requires static scans. It may, however, offer

TABLE 26–6.

Multiple Fetal Parameters in the Assessment of Gestational Age*†

Mean Gestational Age (wk)	Mean Biparietal Diameter (mm)	Mean Head Circumference (mm)	Mean Abdominal Circumference (mm)	Mean Femur Length (mm)
12.0	17	68	46	7
12.5	19	75	53	9
13.0	21	82	60	11
13.5	23	89	67	12
14.0	25	97	73	14
14.5	27	104	80	16
15.0	29	110	86	17
15.5	31	117	93	19
16.0	32	124	99	20
16.5	34	131	106	22
17.0	36	138	112	24
17.5	38	144	119	25
18.0	39	151	125	27
18.5	41	158	131	28
19.0	43	164	137	30
19.5	45	170	144	31
20.0	46	177	150	33
20.5	48	183	156	34
21.0	40	189	162	35
21.5	51	195	168	37
22.0	53	201	174	38
22.5	55	207	179	40
23.0	56	213	185	41
23.5	58	219	191	42
24.0	59	224	197	44
24.5	61	230	202	45
25.0	62	235	208	46
25.5	64	241	213	47
26.0	65	246	219	49
26.5	67	251	224	50
27.0	68	256	230	51
27.5	69	261	235	52
28.0	71	266	240	54
28.5	72	271	246	55
29.0	73	275	251	56
29.5	75	280	256	57
30.0	76	284	261	58
30.5	77	288	266	59
31.0	78	293	271	60
31.5	79	297	276	61

(Continued.)

TABLE 26–6 (cont.).
Multiple Fetal Parameters in the Assessment of Gestational Age*†

Mean Gestational Age (wk)	Mean Biparietal Diameter (mm)	Mean Head Circumference (mm)	Mean Abdominal Circumference (mm)	Mean Femur Length (mm)
32.0	81	301	281	62
32.5	82	304	286	63
33.0	83	308	291	64
33.5	84	312	295	65
34.0	85	315	300	66
34.5	86	318	305	67
35.0	87	322	309	68
35.5	88	325	314	69
36.0	89	328	318	70
36.5	89	330	323	71
37.0	90	333	327	72
37.5	91	335	332	73
38.0	92	338	336	74
38.5	92	340	340	74
39.0	93	342	344	75
39.5	94	344	348	76
40.0	94	346	353	77

*From Hadlock, FP, Deter RL, Harrist RB, et al: *Radiology* 1984; 152:497–501. Used by permission.
†Instructions: Take the mean measurements for the four parameters–biparietal diameter, head circumference, abdominal circumference, femur length. Find mean gestational ages of each, add them together, and divide by 4.

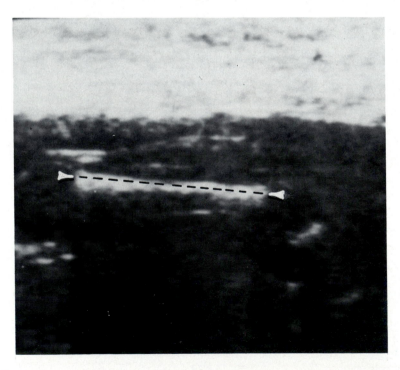

FIG 26–7.
Femur length measurement. The long axis of the hyperechoic femoral shaft is measured, denoted by *arrowheads* and *dashed line,* disregarding the hypoechoic nonossified epiphyseal cartilages.

information that other measurements do not. More work is needed, including the availability of numbers, before this product can be recommended.

INTERVAL GROWTH

Interval growth of the fetus can be analyzed when serial ultrasound examinations are performed during pregnancy. Since the early 1970s, this concept has been used to determine the appropriate growth of the fetal head.[71, 72] The biparietal diameter was found to have an expected growth at each stage of gestation in millimeters per week.[71] This growth decreased linearly from the early second trimester until term.[71] When normal, 83% of fetuses were found to be normal at birth; when slow, 68% were small-for-dates.[72] Interval growth was carried one step further by noting that most normal fetal biparietal diameters could be separated into one of three percentile rankings: large (above the 75th percentile), average (25th to 75th percentile), and small (below the 25th percentile).[73] When 142 fetuses were evaluated, the biparietal diameter maintained the same percentile from 20 to 40 weeks in 128 cases (90%), and all were normal at birth. Of the remaining 14 fetuses, 11 showed a drop from the initial percentile rank to the next lower and five of these had low birth weight. The remaining three showed an increase in percentile rank to the next higher rank and all were normal at birth. Therefore, from these studies, it was determined that (1) the fetal head is expected to grow at a certain rate in millimeters per week throughout the second and third trimester, decreasing linearly from the early second trimester until term, and (2) most fetuses maintain a certain percentile growth throughout the pregnancy.[71–73] It would be expected (and discussed later in this section), based on the close relationship between the head, body, and extremity growth, that the same concept could be used to evaluate interval growth of other body parts.[6]

Since at least two examinations are needed to evaluate interval growth, it was initially suggested that the two be performed at specific times in the gestation, one prior to 26 weeks and the other between 30 and 33 weeks.[74–76] In two articles by the same group,[75, 76] it was stated that these two measurements, termed the growth-adjusted sonographic age (GASA), could do three things: (1) determine the fetal growth in the correct percentile ranking, (2) detect growth retardation, and (3) date the fetus to within ±1 to 3 days. An additional study found that any two biparietal diameter measurements taken between 19 and 30 weeks, with at least a 3-week interval between examinations, was as accurate as GASA in predicting the fetal age.[77] More recently, however, the accuracy of GASA has come into question. It has been shown that either a first trimester crown-rump length or a biparietal diameter measured up to 24 weeks is as accurate as GASA and that this accuracy was not ±1 to 3 days, as initially reported, but rather ±5 to 7 days.[78, 79] In addition, an accurate menstrual history is as correct as the first and second trimester measurement in establishing fetal age.[78, 79]

Despite the inability of GASA or of any two readings between 19 and 30 weeks to narrow the estimated date of confinement to less than 5 to 7 days, the concept of interval growth is very important since it allows assessment of fetal growth.[80, 81] There have been discrepancies among articles as to both the correct growth in millimeters per week at each stage of gestation and the shape of the growth curve. Two articles determined that the interval growth of the fetus had two slopes, initially fast at 3.0

to 3.2 mm/week until 31 to 33 weeks, then decreasing to 1.8 mm/week until term.[82, 83] Hohler et al.[83] reviewed an additional five studies and agreed that between 34 and 40 weeks the mean growth rate of the biparietal diameter was between 1.35 to 1.91 mm/week. Another study, however, contradicted both the slope of the curve and the mean fetal growth near term by finding that the normal growth was linear at 2.6 mm/week from 18 to 38 weeks.[84] An additional article determined that the biparietal diameter growth rate was triphasic, 3 mm/week in the first trimester, 3.5 mm/week in the second trimester, and 2 mm/week throughout the third trimester.[85] Lastly, an article in graph and equation form,[86] without giving numbers, found a growth from 12 weeks to term to be slightly curvilinear. For simplicity, because of the discrepancies among studies, it will be assumed that the growth of the biparietal diameter decelerates linearly in the second and third trimesters.

Eight articles have been published giving specific numbers for the biparietal diameter in millimeters per week of growth,[6, 12, 13, 71, 87–90] seven throughout the second and third trimesters,[6, 12, 71, 87–90] and the last from 24 weeks to term.[13] All showed a somewhat linear decrease in the biparietal diameter growth throughout the second and third trimester with four of the articles having a biphasic configuration, initially fast until 30 to 34 weeks and then slower to term.[12, 71, 87, 88] At 20 weeks, the interval growth from seven articles[12, 71, 73, 87–90] ranged from 2.63 to 3.4 mm, decreasing in all eight articles from 2.3 to 2.63 mm by 30 weeks, and from 0.98 to 1.71 mm at term. In addition to the mean values, six gave percentile ratings, two at the 10th and 90th percentiles,[12, 87] two at the 5th and 95th percentiles (2 SD),[6, 71] two at the 1st and 99th percentiles (3 SD).[89, 90]

The determination of which table to use was based on sample size, statistical analysis and range around the mean. While Levi and Smets[12] and Campbell et al.[72] were both acceptable, the sample size of Levi and Smets[12] was much larger and is therefore recommended (Fig 26–8, Table 26–7). An example of how to use Table 26–7 is as follows: A pregnant woman is examined twice. On the first study the fetus is found to have a biparietal diameter measuring 50 mm. Ten weeks later, the woman is reexamined and a biparietal diameter of 80 mm is obtained. The interval change between the two examinations is 80 mm minus 50 mm, or 30 mm. The average rate of growth in millimeters per week is 30 mm divided by 10 weeks, or 3 mm/week. Since the growth decelerates linearly from the early second to late third trimester, the mean point of growth is halfway between the two numbers. In this case, the halfway point between 50 and 80 mm is 65 mm. Along the 65-mm line, a 3 mm/week growth is found to be normal at an 80% growth rate.

The use of interval growth has been carefully evaluated in only one article.[89] Five types of fetal growth patterns were described in an attempt to determine the probability that growth retardation would occur. Although the series of 121 patients with serial measurements was relatively small, a normal interval growth or a growth which initially started low and then rose into the normal range was found in 95 fetuses. At birth, 92 (97%) were normal with the other three growth-retarded. In a much smaller subgroup of nine patients, the growth was initially normal and then fell below normal. While this pattern would theoretically seem to portend growth retardation, only one of these nine fetuses was growth-retarded at birth. The two most diagnostic patterns for growth retardation were found to be a single subnormal growth or a uniformly low profile with growth never rising above the lower 10th percentile. In these patterns, eight of 17 fetuses (47%) had growth retardation at birth.

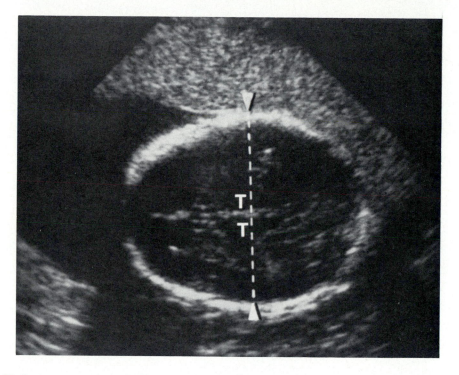

FIG 26–8.
The biparietal diameter measurement is taken in transaxial view with the thalamus *(T)* or midbrain in the midline. The measurement, denoted by *arrowheads* and *dashed line,* is taken leading edge (outer margin) to leading edge (inner margin).

Interval growth has also been analyzed in the first trimester. In 53 normal gestations, Nyberg et al.[91] found that between 4.5 and 11 gestational weeks the average gestational sac size grew at a constant rate, at a mean of 1.13 mm/day (range 0.71–1.75 mm/day). Evaluating an additional 30 abnormal gestations, 24 demonstrated a slower mean growth of 0.70 mm/day (range 0.14–1.71 mm/day). The authors therefore concluded that a gestational sac growth rate less than or equal to 0.6 mm/day is evidence of abnormal growth.[91] Crown-rump length has been evaluated in graph and equation form,[86] but no conclusion of the type of curve or rate of growth could be determined because the sample size was too small. Further work on both gestational sac and crown-rump length is needed. The work on the gestational sac is particularly interesting since the sac can be imaged approximately 2 weeks earlier than the embryo. To avoid potential measurement errors, which can be as large as 1 to 2 mm for each study, or 2 to 4 mm for two studies, a growth of at least 4 mm is needed. Using the authors' criterion of a minimum growth of 0.6 mm/day, 7 days between studies is therefore needed to be certain of adequate growth.

Interval growth has also been used to evaluate other fetal parameters. In the head, the interval growth of the fronto-occipital diameter, the head circumference, and the head area have been tabulated numerically[6] with the fronto-occipital diameter and head circumference also analyzed in graphs and equations.[86, 92] In the body, the weekly growth of the chest area was analyzed in one article[13] and the abdominal AP and transverse diameters, circumference, and area in three.[6, 43, 92] In one,[43] it was found that within 2 weeks of delivery, the abdominal circumference should grow at

TABLE 26–7.
Biparietal Diameter Growth Rate*

| Gestational Age (wk) | Mean Biparietal Diameter (mm)[†] | Predicted Interval Growth (mm/wk)[‡] | | | | |
| | | Percentiles | | | | |
		10th	20th	50th	80th	90th
15	32	—	—	3.88	—	—
16	36	—	—	3.20	—	—
17	39	—	2.86	3.20	3.44	—
18	41	—	2.85	3.05	3.85	—
19	44	—	2.80	3.25	3.90	—
20	48	2.56	2.69	3.15	3.33	3.63
21	50	2.56	2.70	3.10	3.70	3.89
22	54	2.50	2.78	3.09	3.43	3.90
23	57	2.31	2.58	2.85	3.31	3.49
24	59	2.32	2.56	2.85	3.20	3.47
25	63	2.41	2.55	2.74	3.06	3.36
26	66	2.26	2.34	2.58	3.01	3.21
27	68	2.16	2.33	2.57	2.97	3.22
28	71	2.12	2.25	2.47	2.76	3.06
29	75	2.06	2.17	2.42	2.68	2.93
30	78	1.86	2.00	2.30	2.64	2.90
31	80	1.69	1.87	2.16	2.42	2.68
32	82	1.56	1.78	2.02	2.37	2.61
33	84	1.17	1.45	1.92	2.32	2.56
34	85	1.15	1.39	1.85	2.23	2.60
35	87	0.95	1.21	1.67	1.95	2.25
36	89	0.90	1.10	1.56	1.95	2.44
37	90	0.76	0.91	1.40	1.91	2.25
38	92	0.69	0.89	1.45	1.92	2.36
39	93	0.43	0.85	1.38	1.94	2.88
40	94	0.57	0.87	1.38	2.35	2.91
41	94	0.63	0.87	1.57	2.86	2.93
42	95	0.62	0.87	1.38	1.91	1.95
43	95	—	—	—	—	—

*From Levi S, Smets P: *Acta Obstet Gynecol Scand* 1973; 52:193–198. Used by permission.
[†]Data from Table I in Levi and Smets.
[‡]Data from Table II in Levi and Smets.

greater than or equal to 10 mm/14 days, a number close to the growth of the biparietal diameter near term. In addition, Fescina et al.[6] found that the incremental growth of the abdominal diameters, both AP and transverse, was also similar to that of the biparietal diameter. This finding suggests that the use of the table of interval growth of the biparietal diameter could possibly be used in the evaluation of incremental growth of the abdominal diameter. In symmetric growth retardation, where both the fetal head and body are equally affected,[80, 81] one would expect both to have similar decreases in interval growth. In asymmetric growth retardation,[80, 81] however, the initial finding would be a decrease in the interval growth of the body with the fetal head remaining relatively normal. Only in the late stages of severe asymmetric growth retardation would the growth of both the head and body be equally affected.

The interval growth of the femoral length has also been examined, first in a clinical-radiographic study[93] and then by ultrasound.[92, 94] The clinical-radiographic study, performed on newborn children from 30 to 43 weeks, showed the length of the thigh to grow at a linear rate of 3 mm/week.[93] In utero radiographs were then evaluated and the gestational age predicted by the measurement of the femur to within 2 weeks.[92] The in utero ultrasound study found different results.[94] At 14 weeks, the femoral length grew at 3.15 mm/week, slowly decreasing to 1.55 mm/week at term. This type of growth would be more consistent with the ultrasound in utero growth of the biparietal diameter and body diameter.[6, 12] The growth of all the long bones can be affected, as can the fetal head and body, by various negative maternal effects, such as smoking.[92]

At present, not enough data are available for recommendation of interval growth of any fetal parameter other than the biparietal diameter (see Table 26–7).

FETAL WEIGHT

The weight of live infants born between 20 and 48 gestational weeks has been extensively studied in the pediatric and obstetrical literature.[95–114] All except one series weighed more than 10,000 infants, with the one exception[95] analyzing fewer than 4,000. In addition, aborted fetuses from 8 to 26 weeks[100, 105, 106] were weighed in much smaller series, 170 to 1,800 fetuses. The combination of these studies permitted an understanding of fetal weight throughout gestational life. Almost all of the articles showed an S-shaped fetal weight growth curve with the fastest linear growth occurring in the second and early third trimester and a slower curvilinear growth at both ends. The numbers were found to group closely together. At 25 weeks, five studies[97, 100, 102, 103, 106] were within 150 g, while from 30 weeks until term 10 studies[95–104] were within 250 g. These articles showed a slight difference in weight between blacks and whites and between males and females, with whites and males slightly heavier at term. The same linear growth and weight difference was confirmed in an ultrasound study in the second and early third trimester where gestational age was established by an early second trimester biparietal diameter measurement.[107] While it could be suggested that some of the preterm infants evaluated in these studies might have been growth-retarded with decreased weight and an abnormal growth curve, all of the series had large numbers and used care in establishing gestational age. The weights and growth curves are therefore undoubtedly valid for normal fetuses.

Knowing the weight of a fetus at time of birth is important, particularly in very large and very small fetuses. It has been estimated that after 36 gestational weeks, poor perinatal outcome occurs in 3.9% of fetuses and tends to occur at the extremes of birth weight.[108] In low-birth-weight infants, defined as below 2,500 g,[109] and in very-low-birth-weight infants, defined as below 1,500 g,[110] morbidity and mortality increase. Although it is difficult to separate all of the complications of the low- from the very-low-birth-weight infants, major neurodevelopmental handicaps including cerebral palsy, seizure disorders, and congenital anomalies have been noted, particularly in the very-low-birth-weight infants. Lower respiratory tract difficulties are seen in low-birth-weight infants with 8% of very-low-birth-weight infants having chronic pulmonary changes usually secondary to treatment after birth. Large fetuses, termed macrosomic and defined as greater than 4,000 g at birth, have other problems,[111-113] particularly related to difficulty during delivery. These include perinatal asphyxia and trauma, with trauma further divided into brachial palsy, fractured clavicle, and shoulder dystocia. The incidence of shoulder dystocia appears to be higher with increased fetal weight and to be more of a problem in diabetic than in nondiabetic fetuses, presumably due to a different distribution of weight to the upper extremities in diabetic fetuses.[112, 113]

Fetal weight is not an absolute predictor of the outcome of a pregnancy. Nevertheless, in one series, the newborn outcome was normal in 98% of babies born between the 10th and 90th percentile.[108] As a result, attempts have been made to accurately determine fetal weight prior to delivery. Initially, studies were performed with radiographs of the pregnant uterus.[114, 115] At first the volume of the fetal head was measured with an error of 1 lb (455 g) or less in 60% of cases.[114] Later, the skull (both the biparietal diameter and the fronto-occipital diameter) and the uterine lengths were added together, giving an accuracy of ±10% in 72% of patients. Obviously, because of difficulty in obtaining the correct plane of section and because of the use of ionizing radiation, this radiographic approach was only of academic interest and not routinely used in pregnant women. With the advent of ultrasound, however, the possibility of obtaining accurate fetal weights became more feasible.

To date, there have been 57 published analyses of fetal weight. Furthermore, 27 of these 57 articles and an additional 12 studies compared and reevaluated these fetal weight articles. The studies of fetal weight can be subdivided by the type of measurements used to obtain the weight. Eleven, in some of the earliest work from 1967 to 1978, measured only the fetal head. Six, from 1975 through 1979, analyzed only the fetal body, whereas 26 articles, most from 1976 to the present, used a combined head and body measurement to obtain fetal weight. More recently, nine articles, from 1984 to the present, incorporated the femur with measurements of the fetal body and fetal head to obtain fetal weight. Lastly, in five articles, fetal volumes have been calculated to estimate fetal weight.

Despite these approaches, some quite novel, the overall accuracy of fetal weight has not significantly increased. Almost all articles claimed an accuracy in fetal weight detection of between ±10% to 15%. While some in the initial study stated much better accuracies, as low as ±2% to 3%, later works could not substantiate these claims.

The 11 articles that obtained fetal weight by using the biparietal diameter[116-126] presented their results as equations with two also giving numbers.[120, 124] Six calculated a standard deviation.[116-118, 120, 121, 123] The mean error varied but in general was ±12% to 16%. While all the reasons for the inaccuracies are not known, the errors seem to be caused primarily by changes in either head shape[127] or failure to take into account the fetal body.[128] It was found, for instance, that in women with premature rupture of the membranes, the biparietal diameter measurement, even when incorporated with the abdominal circumference, underestimated actual birth weight by 12.4%.[127] Since the head shape can be significantly distorted by lack of amniotic fluid, it is likely that the alternate use of the head circumference measurement would have been more accurate. It has also been noted that different body shapes markedly changed fetal weight, despite close grouping of biparietal diameter measurements.[128]

When the biparietal diameters measured between 95 and 99 mm, for example, three babies weighed from 2,200 to 4,830!

The fetal body was used to establish fetal weight in six articles,[129–134] three with standard deviations.[130, 132, 134] Four of the articles used abdominal circumference,[130–133] one used abdominal area,[129] and the last used a combination of abdominal circumference and fetal body length.[134] Four of the articles published their values in equation form with one[130] presenting numbers and one[133] using a graph. Abdominal areas were suggested as the appropriate body measurement in cases where an ellipse formula could not provide an adequate approximation of the fetal abdomen.[135] The overall accuracies of these articles were ±10% to 20%, including the article that used abdominal area measurements. Higginbottom et al.[133] initially claimed in an evaluation of 50 fetuses to have an accuracy of ±2% to 3% in 94% of cases. While these results were impressive, their work was disputed by Finikiotis et al.[136] who compared the results of Higginbottom and co-workers to an additional 115 fetuses and found an accuracy of only ±10%, with many less accurate, in 56% of all births.

The largest group of fetal weight articles evaluated a combination of head and body parameters. There were 26 articles published,[137–162] 16 presenting their results in equation form. Of the remaining 10, five gave numbers[138–142] and five showed only graphs.[137, 143–145, 161] The type of head and body parameters varied from study to study. The majority (13 articles) used a combination of biparietal diameter and abdominal circumference.[140–142, 144–148, 155, 157, 158, 160, 161] Seven used a combination of biparietal diameter and thoracic diameter, either transverse or AP.[138, 139, 143, 149–152] The remaining six articles used the following: biparietal diameter and thoracic circumference,[137] head and thoracic areas,[153] head and abdominal areas,[154] biparietal and abdominal diameters,[162] biparietal diameter, fronto-occipital diameter, and abdominal diameter,[159] and biparietal diameter, thoracic diameter, and abdominal area.[156] All except four[139, 143, 145, 159] gave standard deviations.

To prove that combined head and body measurements were more accurate than either a head or body measurement alone, Thompson and co-workers[137, 143] calculated a decreased standard deviation error when this combined approach was employed. Thompson and Makowski[143] found the standard deviation for the combined measurements to be ±290 g as opposed to ±350 g and 364 g for the biparietal and AP chest diameters, respectively. Despite this finding, the use of combined head and body parameters did not significantly affect the predictive accuracy of fetal weight. In general, the mean standard deviation was still ±10% to 15%. Several authors, however, claimed greater accuracy. Birnholz[159] and Jordaan[158] felt that they could predict the fetal weight to within ±2% to 3%. This high accuracy could not be substantiated. Sampson et al.,[160] using his own and Birnholz's equation, found the latter to be ±8% if the fetus weighed less than 2500 g and at least ±10% if the fetus weighed greater than 2500 g. Weiner et al.[163] evaluated Jordaan's work and found accuracies approached only ±15% in over half the cases.

Some observers had suggested that the reason for persistent inaccuracies in fetal weight was the failure to take into account the length of the fetus. Since it had been shown that the fetal femur length closely correlated with the neonatal crown-heel length,[164, 165] nine articles[165–172] added femoral length measurements to the head and body parameters in the hope that greater fetal weight accuracy would occur. All the articles presented their data in equation form with three giving additional numbers.[166, 171, 172] The articles used a combination of from two to four parameters, all with standard deviations. Campbell et al.[167] and Warsof et al.[172] used the femoral length and abdominal circumference. Hadlock et al.[166, 168] combined the femur length and abdominal circumference with the head circumference while Hill et al.,[169] Woo et al.,[170, 171] and Benson et al.[173] combined these two parameters with the biparietal diameter measurement. Lastly, Roberts et al.[165] combined the femoral length and abdominal circumference with two parameters, the biparietal diameter and head circumference. The accuracy of the studies ranged from ±6.8% to 13%. Hadlock et al.[166, 168] claimed an accuracy of ±7.5% but with only a modest statistical significance of $P \leq .05$. Two studies confirmed this small increase in accuracy when the femoral length was combined with other parameters to estimate fetal weight.[165, 169] Four other studies, however, did not. One found no statistical difference[170] and the other three,[165, 172, 174] reexamining the work of Hadlock and co-workers, determined an accuracy of, at best, ±10%.

Lastly, five articles[175–179] formulated a fetal volume to determine fetal weight, all using different approaches. Picker and Saunders[175] took a biparietal diameter and a long-axis measurement of the fetus, using the formula for a cylinder. Morrison and McLennan[176] performed transverse parallel scans at 2-cm intervals, adding up all of the areas to equal a volume. Thompson and Manning[177] took volume measurements of the fetal head using a combination of biparietal diameter and fronto-occipital diameter and the volume of the fetal body and extremities using the formula for a cylinder. Brinkley et al.,[178] using a computer system, combined 19 fetal measured variables. Rossavik et al.[179] used an equation with the head and body cubed. All of the articles except one[179] gave equations with standard deviations. While the accuracy ranged from ±7% to 14%, none of this work has been duplicated and therefore will not be considered further.

There are two types of variations which can occur in the evaluation of fetal weight: the variation within a study (intrapopulation) that causes approximately a ±10% to 15% error, and the variation between studies (interpopulation). While not a great deal is known about either, it has been suggested that the intrapopulation variation may be caused by a number of factors.[158] It may be due to variance in sampling error if the sample is not representative of the general population. It may be due to variations in fetal anthropometry or dysmorphic growth, the latter a consequence of different growth patterns for the head (the growth of the brain) and for the body (somatic growth). None of these, however, fully explains the variation of approximately 10% to 15% which exists within all studies. Even the use of femoral length does not increase this accuracy. It is possible, however, that the femur length is not truly representative of the length of the fetus and that another measurement of the fetal long axis is needed.

The interpopulation variation is even less understood.[158] This type of variation can be best appreciated by Table 26–8. Using previous tables, the idealized numbers at 25, 30, 35, and 40 gestational weeks were calculated for biparietal diameter, head circumference, body diameter, abdominal circumference, and femoral length. In addition, the fronto-occipital diameter was calculated using an ideal cephalic index of 0.78. Newborn weights at each gestational age were included for comparison. At 25 weeks, there was greater than a 130-g variation between the studies, increasing to over 1,100 g at term! In addition, studies that had given low fetal weights early in gestation gave high fetal weights near term and vice versa.

As a result, the choice of which weight tables to recommend is difficult. It would be useful, however, to have more than one table, using different parameters. There are occasions when a certain parameter cannot be adequately measured so that a

TABLE 26–8.
Comparison of Fetal Weight

Gestational Age (wk)	Ideal Fetal Measurements (mm)*					
	BPD	FOD	HC	AD	AC	FL
25	63	80	225	65	205	45
30	76	96	275	79	260	57
35	87	110	315	95	310	69
40	95	120	350	110	360	80

Gestational Age (wk)	References (Parameters Measured)					Average Newborn Weight (4 articles) (g)
	Campbell & Wilkin[130] (AC)	Shepard et al.[140] (BPD, AC)	Jordaan[158] (HC, AC)	Birnholz[159] (BPD, FOD, AC)	Hadlock et al.[166] (HC, AC, FL)	
	Fetal Weights (g)					
25	900	790	915	928	766	808
30	1,690	1,533	1,790	1,438	1,485	1,446
35	2,690	2,554	2,767	2,264	2,546	2,530
40	3,640	3,791	3,728	2,850	3,947	3,346

*BPD = biparietal diameter; FOD = fronto-occipital diameter; HC = head circumference; AD = abdominal diameter; AC = abdominal circumference; FL = femur length.

TABLE 26–9.
Estimated Fetal Weight (g) Based on Biparietal Diameter (BPD) and Abdominal Circumference (AC)*†

BPD (mm)	AC (mm)												
	155	160	165	170	175	180	185	190	195	200	205	210	215
31	224	234	244	255	267	279	291	304	318	332	346	362	378
32	231	241	251	263	274	286	299	312	326	340	355	371	388
33	237	248	259	270	282	294	307	321	335	349	365	381	397
34	244	255	266	278	290	302	316	329	344	359	374	391	408
35	251	262	274	285	298	311	324	338	353	368	384	401	418
36	259	270	281	294	306	319	333	347	362	378	394	411	429
37	266	278	290	302	315	328	342	357	372	388	404	422	440
38	274	286	298	310	324	337	352	366	382	398	415	432	451
39	282	294	306	319	333	347	361	376	392	409	426	444	462
40	290	303	315	328	342	356	371	386	403	419	437	455	474
41	299	311	324	338	352	366	381	397	413	430	448	467	486
42	308	320	333	347	361	376	392	408	424	442	460	479	498
43	317	330	343	357	371	387	402	419	436	453	472	491	511
44	326	339	353	367	382	397	413	430	447	465	484	504	524
45	335	349	363	377	393	408	425	442	459	478	497	517	538
46	345	359	373	386	404	420	436	454	472	490	510	530	551
47	355	369	384	399	415	431	448	466	484	503	524	544	565
48	366	380	395	410	426	443	460	478	497	517	537	558	580
49	376	391	406	422	438	455	473	491	510	530	551	572	594
50	387	402	418	434	451	468	486	505	524	544	565	587	610
51	399	414	430	446	463	481	499	518	538	559	580	602	625
52	410	426	442	459	476	494	513	532	552	573	595	618	641
53	422	438	455	472	489	508	527	547	567	589	611	634	657
54	435	451	468	485	503	522	541	561	582	604	627	650	674
55	447	464	481	499	517	536	556	577	598	620	643	667	691
56	461	477	495	513	532	551	571	592	614	636	660	684	709
57	474	491	509	527	547	566	587	608	630	653	677	701	727
58	488	505	524	542	562	582	603	625	647	670	695	719	745
59	502	520	539	558	578	598	619	642	664	688	713	738	764
60	517	535	554	573	594	615	636	659	682	706	731	757	784
61	532	550	570	590	610	632	654	677	700	725	750	777	804
62	547	566	586	606	627	649	672	695	719	744	770	797	824

63	563	583	603	624	645	667	690	714	738	764	790	817	845
64	580	600	620	641	663	686	709	733	758	784	811	838	867
65	597	617	638	659	682	705	728	753	778	805	832	860	889
66	614	635	656	678	701	724	748	773	799	826	853	882	911
67	632	653	675	697	720	744	769	794	820	848	876	905	935
68	651	672	694	717	740	765	790	816	842	870	898	928	958
69	670	691	714	737	761	786	811	838	865	893	922	952	983
70	689	711	734	758	782	807	833	860	888	916	946	976	1003
71	709	732	755	779	804	830	856	883	912	941	971	1002	1033
72	730	763	777	801	827	853	880	907	936	965	996	1027	1060
73	751	775	799	824	850	876	904	932	961	991	1022	1054	1087
74	773	797	822	847	874	901	928	957	987	1017	1049	1081	1114
75	796	820	845	871	898	925	954	983	1013	1044	1076	1109	1143
76	819	844	870	896	923	951	980	1009	1040	1072	1104	1137	1172
77	843	868	894	921	949	977	1007	1037	1068	1100	1133	1167	1202
78	868	894	920	947	975	1004	1034	1065	1096	1129	1162	1197	1232
79	893	919	946	974	1003	1032	1062	1094	1126	1159	1193	1228	1264
80	919	946	973	1002	1031	1061	1091	1123	1156	1189	1224	1259	1296
81	946	973	1001	1030	1060	1090	1121	1153	1187	1221	1256	1292	1329
82	974	1001	1030	1059	1089	1120	1152	1185	1218	1253	1288	1325	1363
83	1002	1030	1059	1089	1120	1151	1183	1217	1251	1286	1322	1359	1397
84	1032	1060	1090	1120	1151	1183	1216	1249	1284	1320	1356	1394	1433
85	1062	1091	1121	1151	1183	1216	1249	1283	1318	1355	1392	1430	1469
86	1093	1122	1153	1184	1216	1249	1283	1318	1354	1390	1428	1467	1507
87	1125	1155	1186	1218	1250	1284	1318	1353	1390	1427	1465	1505	1545
88	1157	1188	1220	1252	1285	1319	1354	1390	1427	1465	1504	1543	1584
89	1191	1222	1254	1287	1321	1356	1391	1428	1465	1503	1543	1583	1625
90	1226	1258	1290	1324	1358	1393	1429	1456	1504	1543	1583	1624	1666
91	1262	1294	1327	1361	1396	1432	1468	1506	1544	1584	1624	1666	1708
92	1299	1332	1365	1400	1435	1471	1508	1546	1586	1626	1667	1709	1752
93	1337	1370	1404	1439	1475	1512	1550	1588	1628	1668	1710	1753	1796
94	1376	1410	1444	1480	1516	1554	1592	1631	1671	1712	1755	1798	1842
95	1416	1450	1486	1522	1559	1597	1635	1675	1716	1758	1800	1844	1889
96	1457	1492	1528	1565	1602	1641	1680	1720	1762	1804	1847	1892	1937
97	1500	1535	1572	1609	1647	1686	1726	1767	1809	1852	1895	1940	1986
98	1544	1580	1617	1654	1693	1733	1773	1815	1857	1900	1945	1990	2037
99	1589	1625	1663	1701	1740	1781	1822	1864	1907	1951	1996	2042	2089
100	1635	1672	1710	1749	1789	1830	1871	1914	1958	2002	2048	2094	2142

(*Continued.*)

TABLE 26–9 (cont.).
Estimated Fetal Weight (g) Based on Biparietal Diameter (BPD) and Abdominal Circumference (AC)*†

BPD (mm)	AC (mm)												
	220	225	230	235	240	245	250	255	260	265	270	275	280
31	395	412	431	450	470	491	513	536	559	584	610	638	666
32	405	423	441	461	481	502	525	548	572	597	624	651	680
33	415	433	452	472	493	514	537	560	585	611	638	666	693
34	425	444	463	483	504	526	549	573	598	624	652	680	710
35	436	455	475	495	517	539	562	587	612	638	666	695	725
36	447	466	486	507	529	552	575	600	626	653	681	710	740
37	458	478	498	519	542	565	589	614	640	667	696	725	756
38	470	490	510	532	554	578	602	628	654	682	711	741	772
39	482	502	523	545	568	592	616	642	669	697	727	757	789
40	494	514	536	558	581	606	631	657	684	713	743	773	806
41	506	527	549	572	595	620	645	672	700	729	759	790	828
42	519	540	562	585	609	634	660	688	716	745	776	807	841
43	532	554	576	600	624	649	676	703	732	762	793	825	859
44	545	567	590	614	639	665	692	719	749	779	810	843	877
45	559	581	605	629	654	680	708	736	765	796	828	861	896
46	573	596	620	644	670	696	724	753	783	814	846	880	915
47	588	611	635	660	686	713	741	770	801	832	865	899	934
48	602	626	650	676	702	730	758	788	819	851	884	919	954
49	617	641	666	692	719	747	776	806	837	870	903	938	975
50	633	657	683	709	736	765	794	824	856	889	923	959	996
51	649	674	699	726	754	783	812	843	876	909	944	980	1017
52	665	690	717	744	772	801	831	863	895	929	964	1001	1039
53	682	708	734	762	790	820	851	883	916	950	986	1023	1061
54	699	725	752	780	809	839	870	903	936	971	1007	1045	1084
55	717	743	771	799	828	859	891	924	958	993	1030	1068	1107
56	735	762	789	818	848	879	911	945	979	1015	1052	1091	1131
57	753	780	809	838	869	900	933	966	1001	1038	1075	1114	1155
58	772	800	829	858	889	921	954	989	1024	1061	1099	1139	1180
59	792	820	849	879	911	943	977	1011	1047	1085	1123	1163	1205
60	811	840	870	900	932	965	999	1035	1071	1109	1148	1189	1231
61	832	861	891	922	955	988	1023	1058	1095	1134	1173	1214	1257
62	853	882	913	945	977	1011	1046	1083	1120	1159	1199	1241	1284
63	874	904	935	967	1001	1035	1071	1107	1145	1185	1226	1268	1311
64	866	927	958	991	1025	1059	1096	1133	1171	1211	1253	1295	1339

65	919	950	962	1015	1049	1084	1121	1159	1198	1238	1280	1323	1368
66	942	973	1006	1039	1074	1110	1147	1185	1225	1266	1308	1352	1397
67	965	997	1030	1065	1100	1136	1174	1213	1253	1294	1337	1381	1427
68	990	1022	1056	1090	1126	1163	1201	1241	1281	1323	1367	1411	1458
69	1015	1048	1082	1117	1153	1190	1229	1269	1310	1353	1397	1442	1489
70	1040	1074	1108	1144	1181	1219	1258	1298	1340	1383	1427	1473	1521
71	1066	1100	1135	1171	1209	1247	1287	1328	1370	1414	1459	1505	1553
72	1093	1128	1163	1200	1238	1277	1317	1358	1401	1445	1491	1538	1586
73	1121	1156	1192	1229	1267	1307	1348	1390	1433	1478	1524	1571	1620
74	1149	1184	1221	1259	1297	1338	1379	1421	1465	1511	1557	1605	1655
75	1178	1214	1251	1289	1328	1369	1411	1454	1499	1544	1592	1640	1690
76	1207	1244	1281	1320	1360	1401	1444	1487	1533	1579	1627	1676	1727
77	1238	1275	1313	1352	1393	1434	1477	1522	1567	1614	1663	1712	1764
78	1269	1306	1345	1385	1426	1468	1512	1557	1603	1650	1699	1749	1801
79	1301	1339	1378	1418	1460	1503	1547	1592	1639	1687	1737	1787	1840
80	1333	1372	1412	1453	1495	1538	1583	1629	1676	1725	1775	1826	1879
81	1367	1406	1446	1488	1531	1575	1620	1666	1714	1763	1814	1866	1919
82	1401	1441	1482	1524	1567	1612	1657	1704	1753	1803	1854	1906	1960
83	1436	1477	1518	1561	1605	1650	1696	1744	1793	1843	1895	1948	2002
84	1473	1513	1555	1599	1643	1689	1735	1784	1833	1884	1936	1990	2045
85	1510	1551	1594	1637	1682	1728	1776	1825	1875	1926	1979	2033	2089
86	1548	1589	1633	1677	1722	1769	1817	1866	1917	1969	2022	2077	2134
87	1586	1629	1673	1717	1764	1811	1859	1909	1960	2013	2067	2122	2179
88	1626	1669	1714	1759	1806	1854	1903	1953	2005	2058	2113	2169	2226
89	1667	1711	1756	1802	1849	1897	1947	1998	2050	2104	2159	2216	2274
90	1709	1753	1799	1845	1893	1942	1992	2044	2097	2151	2207	2264	2322
91	1752	1797	1843	1890	1938	1988	2039	2091	2144	2199	2255	2313	2372
92	1796	1841	1888	1936	1984	2035	2086	2139	2193	2248	2305	2363	2423
93	1841	1887	1934	1982	2032	2083	2135	2188	2242	2298	2356	2414	2475
94	1887	1934	1982	2030	2080	2132	2184	2238	2293	2350	2407	2467	2527
95	1935	1982	2030	2080	2130	2182	2235	2289	2345	2402	2460	2520	2582
96	1984	2031	2080	2130	2181	2233	2287	2342	2398	2456	2515	2575	2637
97	2033	2082	2131	2181	2233	2286	2340	2396	2452	2510	2570	2631	2693
98	2085	2133	2183	2234	2286	2340	2395	2451	2508	2567	2627	2688	2751
99	2137	2186	2237	2288	2341	2395	2450	2507	2565	2624	2684	2746	2810
100	2191	2241	2292	2344	2397	2452	2507	2564	2623	2682	2743	2806	2870

(Continued.)

TABLE 26–9 (cont.).
Estimated Fetal Weight (g) Based on Biparietal Diameter (BPD) and Abdominal Circumference (AC)*†

BPD (mm)	AC (mm)												
	285	290	295	300	305	310	315	320	325	330	335	340	345
31	696	726	759	793	828	865	903	943	985	1029	1075	1123	1173
32	710	742	774	809	844	882	921	961	1004	1048	1094	1143	1193
33	725	757	790	825	861	899	938	979	1022	1067	1114	1163	1214
34	740	773	806	841	878	916	956	998	1041	1087	1134	1183	1235
35	756	789	823	858	896	934	975	1017	1061	1107	1154	1204	1256
36	772	805	840	876	913	953	993	1036	1080	1127	1175	1226	1278
37	788	822	857	893	931	971	1012	1056	1101	1147	1196	1247	1300
38	805	839	874	911	950	990	1032	1076	1121	1168	1218	1269	1323
39	822	856	892	930	969	1009	1052	1096	1142	1190	1240	1292	1346
40	839	874	911	949	988	1029	1072	1117	1163	1212	1262	1315	1369
41	857	892	929	968	1008	1049	1093	1138	1185	1234	1285	1338	1393
42	875	911	948	987	1028	1070	1114	1159	1207	1256	1308	1361	1417
43	893	930	968	1007	1048	1091	1135	1181	1229	1279	1331	1385	1442
44	912	949	987	1027	1069	1112	1157	1204	1252	1303	1355	1410	1467
45	932	969	1008	1048	1090	1134	1179	1226	1275	1326	1380	1435	1492
46	951	989	1028	1069	1112	1156	1202	1249	1299	1351	1404	1460	1518
47	971	1010	1049	1091	1134	1178	1225	1273	1323	1375	1430	1486	1545
48	992	1031	1071	1113	1156	1201	1248	1297	1348	1401	1455	1512	1571
49	1013	1052	1093	1135	1179	1225	1272	1322	1373	1426	1482	1539	1599
50	1034	1074	1115	1158	1203	1249	1297	1347	1399	1452	1508	1566	1626
51	1056	1096	1138	1181	1226	1273	1322	1372	1425	1479	1535	1594	1655
52	1078	1119	1161	1205	1251	1298	1347	1398	1451	1506	1563	1622	1683
53	1101	1142	1185	1229	1276	1323	1373	1425	1478	1533	1591	1651	1713
54	1124	1166	1209	1254	1301	1349	1399	1452	1506	1562	1620	1680	1742
55	1148	1190	1234	1279	1327	1376	1426	1479	1534	1590	1649	1710	1773
56	1172	1215	1259	1305	1353	1402	1454	1507	1562	1619	1678	1740	1803
57	1197	1240	1285	1332	1380	1430	1482	1535	1591	1649	1709	1770	1835
58	1222	1266	1311	1358	1407	1458	1510	1564	1621	1679	1739	1802	1866
59	1248	1292	1338	1386	1435	1486	1539	1594	1651	1710	1770	1834	1899
60	1274	1319	1366	1414	1464	1515	1569	1624	1682	1741	1802	1866	1932
61	1301	1346	1393	1442	1493	1545	1599	1655	1713	1773	1835	1899	1965
62	1328	1374	1422	1471	1522	1575	1630	1686	1745	1805	1868	1932	1999
63	1356	1403	1451	1501	1552	1606	1661	1718	1777	1838	1901	1967	2034

											1970	2037	2105
66	1444	1492	1542	1594	1647	1702	1759	1817	1878	1941	2006	2073	2142
67	1474	1523	1574	1626	1679	1735	1792	1852	1913	1976	2042	2109	2179
68	1505	1555	1606	1658	1713	1769	1827	1887	1949	2012	2078	2147	2217
69	1537	1587	1639	1692	1747	1803	1862	1922	1985	2049	2116	2184	2255
70	1570	1620	1672	1726	1781	1839	1898	1959	2022	2087	2154	2223	2295
71	1603	1654	1706	1761	1817	1875	1934	1996	2059	2125	2193	2262	2334
72	1636	1688	1741	1796	1853	1911	1971	2044	2098	2164	2232	2302	2375
73	1671	1723	1777	1832	1890	1948	2009	2072	2137	2203	2272	2343	2416
74	1706	1759	1813	1869	1927	1987	2048	2111	2176	2244	2313	2384	2458
75	1742	1795	1850	1907	1965	2025	2087	2151	2217	2265	2354	2426	2501
76	1779	1833	1888	1945	2004	2065	2127	2192	2258	2326	2397	2469	2544
77	1816	1871	1927	1985	2044	2105	2168	2233	2300	2369	2440	2513	2588
78	1855	1910	1966	2025	2085	2146	2210	2275	2343	2412	2484	2557	2633
79	1894	1949	2006	2065	2126	2188	2252	2318	2386	2456	2528	2603	2679
80	1934	1990	2048	2107	2168	2231	2296	2362	2431	2501	2574	2649	2725
81	1975	2031	2089	2149	2211	2275	2340	2407	2476	2547	2620	2695	2773
82	2016	2073	2132	2193	2255	2319	2385	2462	2522	2594	2667	2743	2821
83	2059	2116	2176	2237	2300	2364	2431	2499	2569	2641	2715	2791	2870
84	2102	2160	2220	2282	2345	2410	2477	2546	2617	2689	2764	2841	2920
85	2146	2205	2266	2328	2392	2457	2525	2594	2665	2739	2814	2891	2970
86	2192	2251	2312	2375	2439	2505	2573	2643	2715	2789	2864	2942	3022
87	2238	2298	2359	2423	2488	2554	2623	2693	2765	2840	2916	2994	3074
88	2285	2346	2408	2472	2537	2604	2673	2744	2817	2892	2968	3074	3128
89	2333	2394	2457	2521	2587	2655	2725	2796	2869	2944	3021	3101	3182
90	2382	2444	2507	2572	2639	2707	2777	2849	2923	2998	3076	3155	3237
91	2433	2495	2559	2624	2691	2760	2830	2903	2977	3053	3131	3211	3293
92	2484	2547	2611	2677	2744	2814	2885	2958	3032	3109	3187	3268	3350
93	2536	2599	2664	2731	2799	2869	2940	3014	3089	3166	3245	3326	3409
94	2590	2653	2719	2786	2854	2925	2997	3070	3146	3224	3303	3384	3468
95	2644	2709	2774	2842	2911	2982	3054	3129	3205	3283	3362	3444	3528
96	2700	2765	2831	2899	2969	3040	3113	3188	3264	3343	3423	3505	3589
97	2757	2822	2889	2958	3028	3099	3173	3248	3325	3404	3484	3567	3651
98	2815	2881	2948	3017	3088	3160	3234	3309	3387	3466	3547	3630	3715
99	2874	2941	3009	3078	3149	3222	3296	3372	3450	3529	3611	3694	3779
100	2935	3002	3070	3140	3211	3285	3359	3436	3514	3594	3676	3759	3845

(Continued.)

TABLE 26–9 (cont.).
Estimated Fetal Weight (g) Based on Biparietal Diameter (BPD) and Abdominal Circumference (AC)*†

BPD (mm)	AC (mm) 350	355	360	365	370	375	380	385	390	395	400
31	1225	1279	1336	1396	1458	1523	1591	1661	1735	1812	1893
32	1246	1301	1258	1418	1481	1546	1615	1686	1761	1838	1920
33	1267	1323	1381	1441	1504	1570	1639	1711	1786	1865	1946
34	1289	1345	1403	1464	1528	1595	1664	1737	1812	1891	1973
35	1311	1367	1426	1488	1552	1619	1689	1762	1839	1918	2001
36	1333	1390	1450	1512	1577	1645	1715	1789	1865	1945	2029
37	1356	1413	1474	1536	1602	1670	1741	1815	1893	1973	2057
38	1379	1437	1498	1561	1627	1696	1768	1842	1920	2001	2086
39	1402	1461	1523	1586	1653	1722	1794	1870	1948	2030	2115
40	1426	1486	1548	1612	1679	1749	1822	1898	1977	2059	2145
41	1451	1511	1573	1638	1706	1776	1849	1926	2005	2088	2174
42	1475	1536	1599	1664	1733	1804	1878	1954	2035	2118	2205
43	1500	1562	1625	1691	1760	1832	1906	1984	2064	2148	2236
44	1526	1588	1652	1718	1788	1860	1935	2013	2094	2179	2267
45	1552	1614	1679	1746	1816	1889	1964	2043	2125	2210	2298
46	1579	1641	1706	1774	1845	1918	1994	2073	2156	2241	2330
47	1605	1669	1734	1803	1874	1948	2024	2104	2187	2273	2363
48	1633	1697	1763	1832	1904	1976	2055	2136	2219	2306	2396
49	1661	1725	1792	1861	1934	2009	2086	2167	2251	2339	2429
50	1689	1754	1821	1891	1964	2040	2118	2200	2284	2372	2463
51	1718	1783	1851	1922	1995	2071	2150	2232	2317	2406	2498
52	1747	1813	1882	1953	2027	2103	2183	2266	2351	2440	2532
53	1777	1843	1913	1984	2059	2136	2216	2299	2386	2475	2568
54	1807	1874	1944	2016	2091	2169	2250	2333	2420	2510	2604
55	1838	1906	1976	2049	2124	2203	2284	2368	2456	2546	2640
56	1869	1938	2008	2082	2158	2237	2319	2403	2491	2582	2677
57	1901	1970	2041	2115	2192	2272	2354	2439	2528	2619	2714
58	1934	2003	2075	2150	2227	2307	2390	2475	2564	2657	2752
59	1966	2037	2109	2184	2262	2342	2426	2512	2602	2694	2790
60	2000	2071	2144	2219	2298	2379	2463	2550	2640	2733	2829
61	2034	2105	2179	2255	2334	2416	2500	2588	2678	2772	2869
62	2069	2140	2215	2291	2371	2453	2538	2626	2717	2811	2909
63	2104	2176	2251	2328	2408	2491	2577	2665	2757	2851	2949

65	2176	2250	2326	2404	2485	2569	2656	2745	2838	2933	3032
66	2213	2287	2364	2443	2524	2609	2696	2786	2879	2975	3075
67	2251	2326	2403	2482	2564	2649	2737	2827	2921	3018	3117
68	2290	2365	2442	2522	2605	2690	2778	2869	2964	3061	3161
69	2329	2404	2482	2563	2646	2732	2821	2912	3007	3104	3205
70	2368	2444	2523	2604	2688	2774	2863	2955	3050	3149	3250
71	2409	2485	2564	2646	2730	2817	2907	2999	3095	3193	3295
72	2450	2527	2607	2689	2773	2861	2951	3044	3140	3239	3341
73	2491	2569	2649	2732	2817	2905	2996	3089	3186	3285	3386
74	2534	2612	2693	2776	2862	2950	3041	3135	3232	3332	3435
75	2577	2656	2737	2821	2907	2996	3088	3182	3279	3380	3483
76	2621	2700	2782	2866	2953	3042	3134	3229	3327	3428	3531
77	2666	2746	2828	2912	3000	3090	3128	3277	3376	3477	3581
78	2711	2792	2874	2959	3047	3137	3230	3326	3425	3526	3631
79	2757	2838	2921	3007	3095	3186	3279	3376	3475	3576	3681
80	2804	2886	2969	3056	3144	3235	3329	3426	3525	3627	3733
81	2852	2934	3018	3105	3194	3286	3380	3477	3577	3679	3785
82	2901	2983	3068	3155	3244	3336	3431	3529	3629	3732	3838
83	2950	3033	3118	3206	3296	3388	3483	3581	3682	3785	3891
84	3001	3084	3169	3257	3348	3441	3536	3634	3735	3839	3945
85	3052	3135	3221	3310	3401	3494	3590	3688	3790	3894	4000
86	3104	3188	3274	3363	3454	3548	3644	3743	3845	3949	4056
87	3157	3241	3328	3417	3509	3603	3700	3799	3901	4005	4113
88	3210	3295	3383	3472	3565	3659	3756	3855	3958	4063	4170
89	3265	3351	3438	3528	3621	3716	3813	3913	4015	4120	4228
90	3321	3407	3495	3585	3678	3773	3871	3971	4074	4179	4287
91	3377	3464	3552	3643	3736	3832	3930	4030	4133	4239	4347
92	3435	3522	3611	3702	3795	3891	3989	4090	4193	4299	4408
93	3494	3581	3670	3761	3855	3951	4050	4151	4254	4361	4469
94	3553	3641	3738	3822	3916	4013	4111	4213	4316	4423	4532
95	3614	3701	3791	3884	3978	4075	4174	4275	4379	4486	4595
96	3675	3763	3854	3946	4041	4138	4237	4339	4443	4550	4659
97	3738	3826	3917	4010	4105	4202	4302	4404	4508	4615	4724
98	3802	3890	3981	4074	4170	4267	4367	4469	4573	4680	4790
99	3866	3956	4047	4140	4236	4333	4433	4536	4640	4747	4857
100	3932	4022	4113	4207	4303	4400	4501	4603	4708	4815	4924

*From Shepard MJ, Richards VA, Berkowitz RL, et al: *Am J Obstet Gynecol* 1982; 147:47–54. Used by permission.

†Estimated fetal weights: Log (birth weight) = $-1.7492 + 0.166\,(BPD) + 0.046\,(AC) - 0.00264\,(AC \times BPD)$.

TABLE 26–10.

Estimated Fetal Weight Based on Abdominal Circumference: Relationship Between Fetal Abdominal Circumference Measurements From 210 to 400 mm and Birth Weight Percentiles*

Abdominal Circumference (mm)	Estimated Birth Weight Percentiles (g)		
	5	50	95
210	780	900	1,040
220	900	1,030	1,190
230	1,030	1,180	1,360
240	1,170	1,340	1,540
250	1,320	1,510	1,730
260	1,470	1,690	1,940
270	1,640	1,880	2,150
280	1,810	2,090	2,380
290	1,990	2,280	2,610
300	2,170	2,490	2,850
310	2,350	2,690	3,080
320	2,530	2,900	3,320
330	2,710	3,100	3,550
340	2,880	3,290	3,760
350	3,030	3,470	3,970
360	3,180	3,640	4,160
370	3,310	3,790	4,330
380	3,420	3,920	4,490
390	3,510	4,020	4,610
400	3,570	4,100	4,720

*From Campbell S, Wilkin D: *Br J Obstet Gynaecol* 1975; 82:689–697. Used by permission.

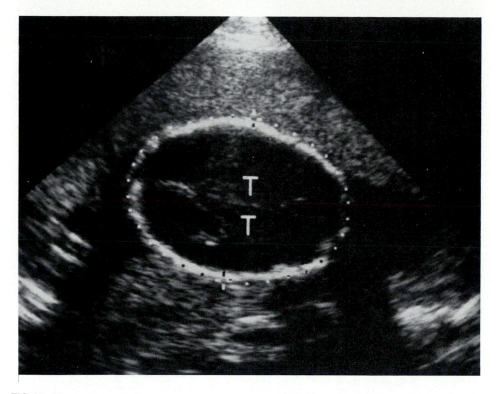

FIG 26–11.
Head circumference. Transaxial image of the head at the thalami *(T)*. With either the thalami or midbrain in the midline, the circumference is traced around the outer margin of the head with a digitizer or map reader *(dotted line)* or can be calculated from an equation.

TABLE 26–11.
Equation With Three Variables to Compute Fetal Weight*†

$$\text{Log}_{10}\,\text{BW} = 1.5662 - 0.0108\,(\text{HC}) + 0.0468\,(\text{AC}) \\ + 0.171\,(\text{FL}) + 0.00034\,(\text{HC})^2 - \\ 0.003685\,(\text{AC} \times \text{FL})$$

*From Hadlock FP, Harrist RB, Carpenter RJ, et al: *Radiology* 1984; 150:535–540. Used by permission.
†BW = body weight in grams; HC = head circumference; AC = abdominal circumference; FL = femur length. HC, AC, and FL given in centimeters.

TABLE 26–12.
Estimated Fetal Weight (g) Based on Abdominal Circumference (AC) and Femur Length (FL)*

FL (mm)	AC (mm)																				
	200	205	210	215	220	225	230	235	240	245	250	255	260	265	270	275	280	285	290	295	300
40	663	691	720	751	783	816	851	887	925	964	1006	1048	1093	1139	1188	1239	1291	1346	1403	1463	1525
41	680	709	738	769	802	836	871	907	946	986	1027	1070	1115	1162	1211	1262	1315	1371	1429	1489	1551
42	697	726	757	788	821	855	891	928	967	1007	1049	1093	1138	1186	1235	1287	1340	1396	1454	1515	1578
43	715	745	776	808	841	875	912	949	988	1029	1071	1116	1162	1209	1259	1311	1365	1422	1480	1541	1605
44	734	764	795	827	861	896	933	971	1010	1051	1094	1139	1185	1234	1284	1336	1391	1448	1507	1568	1632
45	753	783	815	847	882	917	954	993	1033	1074	1118	1163	1210	1259	1309	1362	1417	1474	1534	1596	1660
46	772	803	835	868	903	939	976	1015	1056	1098	1142	1187	1235	1284	1335	1388	1444	1501	1561	1623	1688
47	792	823	856	889	924	961	999	1038	1079	1122	1166	1212	1260	1310	1361	1415	1471	1529	1589	1652	1717
48	812	844	877	911	947	984	1022	1062	1103	1146	1191	1237	1286	1336	1388	1442	1498	1557	1618	1681	1746
49	833	865	899	933	969	1007	1046	1086	1128	1171	1216	1263	1312	1363	1415	1470	1527	1585	1647	1710	1776
50	855	887	921	956	993	1031	1070	1111	1153	1197	1243	1290	1339	1390	1443	1498	1555	1615	1676	1740	1806
51	877	910	944	980	1016	1055	1095	1136	1179	1223	1269	1317	1367	1418	1471	1527	1584	1644	1706	1770	1837
52	899	933	967	1004	1041	1080	1120	1162	1205	1250	1296	1344	1395	1447	1500	1556	1614	1674	1737	1801	1868
53	922	956	992	1028	1066	1105	1146	1188	1232	1277	1324	1373	1423	1476	1530	1586	1645	1705	1768	1833	1900
54	946	981	1016	1053	1091	1131	1172	1215	1259	1305	1352	1401	1452	1505	1560	1617	1675	1736	1799	1865	1933
55	971	1005	1041	1079	1118	1158	1199	1242	1287	1333	1381	1431	1482	1535	1591	1648	1707	1768	1832	1897	1966
56	995	1031	1067	1105	1144	1185	1227	1271	1316	1362	1411	1461	1513	1566	1622	1679	1739	1801	1864	1931	1999
57	1021	1057	1094	1132	1172	1213	1255	1299	1345	1392	1441	1491	1544	1598	1654	1712	1772	1834	1898	1964	2033
58	1047	1084	1121	1160	1200	1242	1285	1329	1375	1422	1472	1523	1575	1630	1686	1744	1805	1867	1932	1999	2068
59	1074	1111	1149	1188	1229	1271	1314	1359	1406	1454	1503	1555	1608	1663	1719	1778	1839	1902	1966	2034	2103
60	1102	1139	1178	1217	1258	1301	1345	1390	1437	1485	1535	1587	1641	1696	1753	1812	1873	1936	2002	2069	2139

61	1130	1168	1207	1247	1289	1331	1376	1421	1469	1518	1568	1620	1674	1730	1788	1847	1908	1972	2038	2105	2175
62	1160	1198	1237	1278	1319	1363	1408	1454	1501	1551	1602	1654	1709	1765	1823	1882	1944	2008	2074	2142	2212
63	1189	1228	1268	1309	1351	1395	1440	1487	1535	1585	1636	1689	1744	1800	1858	1919	1981	2045	2111	2180	2250
64	1220	1259	1299	1341	1384	1428	1473	1520	1569	1619	1671	1724	1779	1836	1895	1956	2018	2082	2149	2218	2289
65	1251	1291	1332	1373	1417	1461	1507	1555	1604	1655	1707	1760	1816	1873	1932	1993	2056	2121	2188	2256	2328
66	1284	1324	1365	1407	1451	1496	1542	1590	1640	1691	1743	1797	1853	1911	1970	2031	2094	2160	2227	2296	2367
67	1317	1357	1399	1441	1486	1531	1578	1626	1676	1728	1780	1835	1891	1949	2009	2070	2134	2199	2267	2336	2408
68	1351	1391	1433	1477	1521	1567	1615	1663	1713	1765	1819	1873	1930	1988	2048	2110	2174	2240	2307	2377	2449
69	1385	1427	1469	1513	1558	1604	1652	1701	1752	1804	1857	1913	1970	2028	2089	2151	2215	2281	2348	2418	2490
70	1421	1463	1506	1550	1595	1642	1690	1740	1791	1843	1897	1953	2010	2069	2130	2192	2256	2322	2391	2461	2533
71	1458	1500	1543	1588	1633	1681	1729	1779	1830	1883	1938	1994	2051	2110	2171	2234	2299	2365	2433	2504	2576
72	1495	1538	1581	1626	1673	1720	1769	1819	1871	1924	1979	2035	2093	2153	2214	2277	2342	2408	2477	2547	2620
73	1534	1577	1621	1666	1713	1761	1810	1861	1913	1966	2021	2078	2136	2196	2258	2321	2386	2453	2521	2592	2665
74	1573	1616	1661	1707	1754	1802	1852	1903	1955	2009	2065	2122	2180	2240	2302	2365	2431	2498	2566	2637	2710
75	1614	1657	1702	1749	1796	1845	1895	1946	1999	2053	2109	2166	2225	2285	2347	2411	2476	2543	2612	2683	2756
76	1655	1699	1745	1791	1839	1888	1939	1990	2043	2098	2154	2211	2270	2331	2393	2457	2523	2590	2659	2730	2803
77	1698	1742	1788	1835	1883	1933	1983	2035	2089	2144	2200	2258	2317	2378	2440	2504	2570	2638	2707	2778	2851
78	1741	1786	1833	1880	1928	1978	2029	2082	2135	2191	2247	2305	2365	2426	2488	2553	2618	2686	2755	2827	2899
79	1786	1832	1878	1926	1975	2025	2076	2129	2183	2238	2295	2353	2413	2474	2537	2602	2668	2735	2805	2876	2949
80	1832	1878	1925	1973	2022	2073	2124	2177	2232	2287	2344	2403	2463	2524	2587	2652	2718	2785	2855	2926	2999
81	1879	1926	1973	2021	2071	2121	2173	2227	2281	2337	2394	2453	2513	2575	2638	2702	2769	2837	2906	2977	3050
82	1928	1974	2022	2070	2120	2171	2224	2277	2332	2388	2446	2504	2565	2626	2690	2754	2821	2889	2958	3029	3102
83	1978	2024	2072	2121	2171	2223	2275	2329	2384	2440	2498	2557	2617	2679	2743	2807	2874	2942	3011	3082	3155

(Continued.)

TABLE 26-12 (cont.).
Estimated Fetal Weight (g) Based on Abdominal Circumference (AC) and Femur Length (FL)*†

FL (mm)	\	\	\	\	\	\	\	\	AC (mm)	\	\	\	\	\	\	\	\	\	\	\
	305	310	315	320	325	330	335	340	345	350	355	360	365	370	375	380	385	390	395	400
40	1590	1658	1729	1802	1879	1959	2042	2129	2220	2314	2413	2515	2622	2734	2850	2972	3098	3230	3367	3511
41	1617	1685	1756	1830	1907	1987	2071	2158	2249	2344	2442	2545	2652	2764	2880	3002	3128	3260	3397	3540
42	1644	1712	1783	1858	1935	2016	2100	2187	2279	2373	2472	2575	2683	2794	2911	3032	3159	3290	3427	3570
43	1671	1740	1812	1886	1964	2054	2129	2217	2308	2404	2503	2606	2713	2825	2942	3063	3189	3321	3458	3600
44	1699	1768	1840	1915	1993	2075	2159	2247	2339	2434	2533	2637	2744	2856	2973	3094	3220	3352	3488	3630
45	1727	1797	1869	1944	2023	2105	2189	2278	2370	2465	2565	2668	2776	2888	3004	3125	3251	3383	3519	3661
46	1756	1826	1898	1974	2053	2135	2220	2309	2401	2497	2596	2700	2807	2919	3036	3157	3283	3414	3550	3692
47	1785	1855	1928	2004	2084	2166	2251	2340	2432	2528	2628	2732	2840	2952	3068	3189	3315	3446	3582	3723
48	1814	1885	1959	2035	2115	2197	2283	2372	2464	2560	2660	2764	2872	2984	3100	3221	3347	3478	3613	3754
49	1845	1916	1990	2066	2146	2229	2315	2404	2497	2593	2693	2797	2905	3017	3133	3254	3380	3510	3645	3786
50	1875	1947	2021	2098	2178	2261	2347	2437	2530	2626	2726	2830	2938	3050	3166	3287	3412	3542	3677	3818
51	1906	1978	2053	2130	2210	2294	2380	2470	2563	2659	2760	2864	2972	3084	3200	3320	3445	3575	3710	3850
52	1938	2010	2085	2163	2243	2327	2413	2503	2597	2693	2794	2898	3006	3117	3234	3354	3479	3608	3743	3882
53	1970	2043	2118	2196	2277	2360	2447	2537	2631	2728	2828	2932	3040	3152	3268	3388	3513	3642	3776	3915
54	2003	2076	2151	2229	2311	2395	2482	2572	2665	2762	2863	2967	3075	3186	3302	3422	3547	3676	3809	3948
55	2036	2109	2185	2264	2345	2429	2516	2607	2700	2797	2898	3002	3110	3221	3337	3457	3581	3710	3843	3981
56	2070	2143	2220	2298	2380	2464	2552	2642	2736	2833	2933	3038	3145	3257	3372	3492	3616	3744	3877	4015
57	2104	2178	2254	2333	2415	2500	2587	2678	2772	2869	2970	3074	3181	3293	3408	3527	3651	3779	3911	4048
58	2139	2213	2290	2369	2451	2536	2624	2714	2808	2905	3006	3110	3218	3329	3444	3563	3686	3814	3946	4082
59	2175	2249	2326	2405	2488	2573	2660	2751	2845	2942	3043	3147	3254	3366	3480	3599	3722	3849	3981	4117
60	2211	2286	2363	2442	2525	2610	2698	2789	2883	2980	3080	3184	3292	3403	3517	3636	3758	3885	4016	4151

61	2248	2323	2400	2480	2562	2647	2736	2827	2921	3018	3118	3222	3329	3440	3554	3673	3795	3921	4052	4186
62	2285	2360	2438	2518	2600	2686	2774	2865	2959	3056	3157	3260	3367	3478	3592	3710	3832	3957	4087	4222
63	2323	2398	2476	2556	2639	2725	2813	2904	2998	3095	3195	3299	3406	3516	3630	3747	3869	3994	4124	4257
64	2362	2437	2515	2595	2678	2764	2852	2943	3037	3134	3235	3338	3445	3555	3668	3785	3906	4031	4160	4293
65	2401	2477	2555	2635	2718	2804	2892	2983	3077	3174	3274	3378	3484	3594	3707	3824	3944	4069	4197	4329
66	2441	2517	2595	2675	2759	2844	2933	3024	3118	3215	3315	3418	3524	3633	3746	3863	3983	4106	4234	4366
67	2481	2557	2636	2716	2800	2885	2974	3065	3159	3256	3355	3458	3564	3673	3786	3902	4021	4144	4271	4402
68	2523	2599	2677	2758	2841	2927	3016	3107	3200	3297	3397	3499	3605	3714	3862	3941	4060	4183	4309	4439
69	2564	2641	2719	2800	2884	2969	3058	3149	3242	3339	3438	3541	3646	3754	3866	3981	4100	4222	4347	4477
70	2607	2683	2762	2843	2927	3012	3101	3192	3285	3381	3481	3583	3688	3796	3907	4022	4140	4261	4386	4514
71	2650	2727	2806	2887	2970	3056	3144	3235	3328	3424	3523	3625	3730	3838	3948	4062	4180	4300	4425	4552
72	2694	2771	2850	2931	3014	3100	3188	3279	3372	3468	3567	3668	3772	3880	3990	4104	4220	4340	4464	4591
73	2739	2816	2895	2976	3059	3145	3233	3323	3416	3512	3610	3712	3816	3922	4032	4145	4261	4381	4503	4629
74	2785	2861	2940	3021	3105	3190	3278	3369	3461	3557	3655	3756	3859	3966	4075	4187	4303	4421	4543	4668
75	2831	2908	2987	3068	3151	3236	3324	3414	3507	3602	3700	3800	3903	4009	4118	4230	4344	4462	4583	4708
76	2878	2955	3034	3115	3198	3283	3371	3461	3553	3648	3745	3845	3948	4053	4161	4272	4387	4504	4624	4747
77	2926	3003	3081	3162	3245	3331	3418	3508	3600	3694	3791	3891	3993	4098	4205	4316	4429	4545	4665	4787
78	2974	3051	3130	3211	3294	3379	3466	3555	3647	3741	3838	3937	4039	4143	4250	4360	4472	4588	4706	4827
79	3024	3100	3179	3260	3343	3427	3514	3604	3695	3789	3885	3984	4085	4188	4295	4404	4515	4630	4748	4868
80	3074	3151	3229	3310	3392	3477	3564	3653	3744	3837	3933	4031	4131	4234	4340	4448	4559	4673	4790	4909
81	3125	3202	3280	3360	3443	3527	3614	3702	3793	3886	3981	4079	4179	4281	4386	4493	4604	4716	4832	4950
82	3177	3253	3332	3412	3494	3578	3664	3752	3843	3935	4030	4127	4226	4328	4432	4539	4648	4760	4875	4992
83	3230	3306	3384	3464	3546	3630	3716	3803	3893	3985	4080	4176	4275	4376	4479	4585	4693	4804	4918	5034

*From Hadlock FP, Harrist RB, Carpenter RJ, et al: *Radiology* 1984; 150:535–540. Used by permission.

†Based on regression, model: Log_{10} body weight = 1.3598 + 0.051 (AC) + 0.1844 (FL) − 0.0037 (AC × FL).

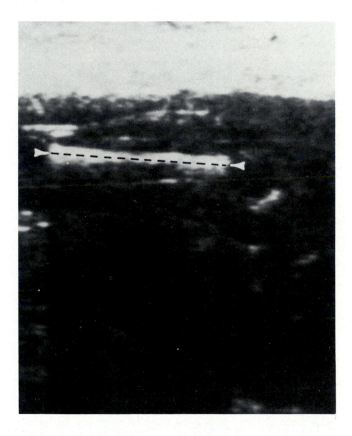

FIG 26–12.
Femoral length measurement. The long axis of the hyperechoic femoral shaft is measured, denoted by *arrowheads* and *dashed line,* disregarding the hypoechoic nonossified epiphyseal cartilages.

REFERENCES

1. Lubchenco LO, Hansmann C, Boyd E: Intrauterine growth in length and head circumference as estimated from live births at gestational ages from 26 to 42 weeks. *Pediatrics* 1966; 37:403–408.
2. Campbell S: The assessment of fetal development by diagnostic ultrasound. *Clin Perinatol* 1974; 1:507–525.
3. Hobbins JC, Berkowitz RL: Ultrasonography in the diagnosis of intrauterine growth retardation. *Clin Obstet Gynecol* 1977; 20:957–968.
4. Kurtz AB, Wapner RJ, Rubin CS, et al: Ultrasound criteria for in utero diagnosis of microcephaly. *J Clin Ultrasound* 1980; 8:11–16.
5. Gottesfeld KR: Ultrasound in obstetrics and gynecology. *Semin Roentgenol* 1975; 10:305–313.
6. Fescina RH, Ucieda FJ, Cordano MC, et al: Ultrasonic patterns of intrauterine fetal growth in a Latin American country. *Early Hum Dev* 1982; 6:239–248.
7. Sarti DA, Crandall BF, Winter J, et al: Correlation of biparietal and fetal body diameters: 12–26 weeks gestation. *AJR* 1981; 137:87–91.
8. Gross BH, Callen PW, Filly RA: The relationship of fetal transverse body diameter and biparietal diameter in the diagnosis of intrauterine growth retardation. *J Ultrasound Med* 1982; 1:361–365.
9. Elliott JP, Garite TJ, Freeman RK, et al: Ultrasonic prediction of fetal macrosomia in diabetic patients. *Obstet Gynecol* 1982; 60:159–162.
10. Eriksen PS, Secher NJ, Weis-Bentzon M: Normal growth of the fetal biparietal diameter and the abdominal diameter in a longitudinal study. *Acta Obstet Gynecol Scand* 1985; 64:65–70.

11. Wladimiroff JW, Bloemsma CA, Wallenburg HCS: Ultrasonic assessment of fetal growth. *Acta Obstet Gynecol Scand* 1977; 56:37–42.
12. Levi S, Smets P: Intra-uterine fetal growth studied by ultrasonic biparietal measurements: The percentiles of biparietal distribution. *Acta Obstet Gynecol Scand* 1973; 52:193–198.
13. Wladimiroff JW, Bloemsma CA, Wallenburg HCS: Ultrasonic assessment of fetal head and body sizes in relation to normal and retarded fetal growth. *Am J Obstet Gynecol* 1978; 131:857–860.
14. Chervenak FA, Jeanty P, Cantraine F, et al: The diagnosis of fetal microcephaly. *Am. J Obstet Gynecol* 1984; 149:512.
15. Chervenak FA, Rosenberg J, Brightman RC, et al: A prospective study of the accuracy of ultrasound in predicting fetal microcephaly. *Obstet Gynecol* 1987; 69:908–910.
16. Deter RL, Harrist RB, Hadlock FP, et al: The use of ultrasound in the assessment of normal fetal growth: A review. *J Clin Ultrasound* 1981; 9:481–493.
17. Campbell S, Thoms A: Ultrasound measurement of the fetal head to abdomen circumference ratio in the assessment of growth retardation. *Br J Obstet Gynaecol* 1977; 84:165–174.
18. Kurjak A, Breyer B: Estimation of fetal weight by ultrasonic abdominometry. *Am J Obstet Gynecol* 1976; 125:962–965.
19. Hadlock FP, Harrist RB, Shah Y, et al: The femur length/head circumference relation in obstetric sonography. *J Ultrasound Med* 1984; 3:439–442.
20. Crane JP, Kopta MM: Prediction of intrauterine growth retardation via ultrasonically measured head/abdominal circumference ratios. *Obstet Gynecol* 1979; 54:597–601.
21. Athey PA, Hadlock FP, Appendix in Harshberger SE (ed): *Ultrasound in Obstetrics and Gynecology.* St. Louis, CV Mosby Co, 1981, p 269.
22. Persson PH, Marsal K: Monitoring of fetuses with retarded BPD growth. *Acta Obstet Gynecol Scand* 1978; 78:49–55.
23. Deter RL, Harrist RB, Hadlock FP, et al: Longitudinal studies of fetal growth with the use of dynamic image ultrasonography. *Am J Obstet Gynecol* 1982; 143:545–554.
24. Varma TR, Taylor H, Bridges C: Ultrasound assessment of fetal growth. *Br J Obstet Gynaecol* 1979; 86:623–632.
25. Rossavik IK, Deter RL: Mathematical modeling of fetal growth: II. Head cube (A), abdominal cube (B) and their ratio (A/B). *J Clin Ultrasound* 1984; 12:535–545.
26. Hohler CW, Quetel TA: Comparison of ultrasound femur length and biparietal diameter in late pregnancy. *Am J Obstet Gynecol* 1981; 141:759–762.
27. Benacerraf BR, Gelman R, Frigoletto FD Jr: Sonographic identification of second-trimester fetuses with Down's syndrome. *N Engl J Med* 1987; 317:1371–1376.
28. Lockwood C, Benacerraf B, Krinsky A, et al: A sonographic screening method for Down syndrome. *Am J Obstet Gynecol* 1987; 157:803–808.
29. Perrella R, Duerinckx AJ, Grant EG, et al: Second-trimester sonographic diagnosis of Down syndrome: Role of femur-length shortening and nuchal-fold thickening. *AJR* 1988; 151:1981–1985.
30. Brumfield CG, Hauth JC, Cloud GA, et al: Sonographic measurements and ratios in fetuses with Down syndrome. *Obstet Gynecol* 1989; 73:644–646.
31. DeVore GR, Horenstein J, Platt LD: Fetal echocardiography VI. Assessment of cardiothoracic disproportion—A new technique for the diagnosis of thoracic hypoplasia. *Am J Obstet Gynecol* 1986; 155:1066–1071.
32. Skiptunas SM, Weiner S: Early prenatal diagnosis of asphyxiating thoracic dysplasia (Jeune's syndrome). Value of fetal thoracic measurement. *J Ultrasound Med* 1987; 6:41–43.
33. Chitkara U, Rosenberg J, Chervenak FA, et al: Prenatal sonographic assessment of the fetal thorax: normal values. *Am J Obstet Gynecol* 1987; 156:1069–1074.
34. Fong K, Ohlsson A, Zalev A: Fetal thoracic circumference: a prospective cross-sectional study with real-time ultrasound. *Am J Obstet Gynecol* 1988; 158:1154–1160.
35. Callan NA, Colmorgen GHC, Weiner S: Lung hypoplasia and prolonged preterm ruptured membranes: A case report with implications for possible prenatal ultrasonic diagnosis. *Am J Obstet Gynecol* 1985; 151:756–757.
36. Johnson A, Callan NA, Bhutani VK, et al: Ultrasonic ratio of fetal thoracic to abdominal circumference: An association with fetal pulmonary hypoplasia. *Am J Obstet Gynecol* 1987; 157:764–769.
37. Bracero LA, Baxi LV, Rey HR, et al: Use of ultrasound in antenatal diagnosis of large-for-gestational age infants in diabetic gravid patients. *Am J Obstet Gynecol* 1985; 152:43–47.
38. Hadlock FP, Deter RL, Harrist RB, et al: A date-independent predictor of intrauterine growth retardation: Femur length/abdominal circumference ratio. *AJR* 1983; 141:979–984.

39. Ott WJ: Fetal femur length, neonatal crown-heel length, and screening for intrauterine growth retardation. *Obstet Gynecol* 1985; 65:460–464.

40. Vintzileos AM, Neckles S, Campbell WA, et al: Three fetal ponderal indexes in normal pregnancy. *Obstet Gynecol* 1985; 6:807–811.

41. Brown HL, Miller JM Jr, Gabert HA, et al: Ultrasonic recognition of the small-for-gestational-age fetus. *Obstet Gynecol* 1987; 69:631–635.

42. Benson CB, Doubilet PM, Saltzman DH, et al: FL/AC ratio: Poor predictor of intrauterine growth retardation. *Invest Radiol* 1985; 20:727–730.

43. Divon MY, Chamberlain PF, Sipos L, et al: Identification of the small for gestational age fetus with the use of gestational age-independent indices of fetal growth. *Am J Obstet Gynecol* 1986; 155:1197–2101.

44. Hays D, Patterson RM: A comparison of fetal biometric ratios to neonatal morphometrics. *J Ultrasound Med* 1987; 6:71–73.

45. Hadlock FP, Harrist RB, Fearneyhough TC, et al: Use of femur length/abdominal circumference ratio in detecting the macrosomic fetus. *Radiology* 1985; 154:503–505.

46. Benson CB, Doubilet PM, Saltzman DH, et al: Femur length/abdominal circumference ratio. Poor predictor of macrosomic fetuses in diabetic mothers. *J Ultrasound Med* 1986; 5:141–144.

47. Pap G, Szoke J, Pap L: Intrauterine growth retardation: ultrasonic diagnosis. *Acta Paediatr Hung* 1983; 24:7–15.

48. Vintzileos AM, Neckles S, Campbell WA, et al: Ultrasound fetal thigh-calf circumferences and gestational age—independent fetal ratios in normal pregnancy. *J Ultrasound Med* 1985; 4:287–292.

49. DeVore GR, Siassi B, Platt LD: The use of the abdominal circumference as a means of assessing M-mode ventricular dimensions during the second and third trimesters of pregnancy in the normal human fetus. *J Ultrasound Med* 1985; 4:175–182.

50. DeVore GR, Siassi B, Platt LD: Use of femur length as a means of assessing M-mode ventricular dimensions during second and third trimesters of pregnancy in normal fetus. *J Clin Ultrasound* 1985; 13:619–625.

51. Li DFH, Woo JSK: Fractional spine length: A new parameter for assessing fetal growth. *J Ultrasound Med* 1986; 5:379–383.

52. Vintzileos AM, Lodeiro JG, Feinstein SJ, et al: Value of fetal ponderal index in predicting growth retardation. *J Ultrasound Med* 1986; 5:379–383.

53. Jordaan HVF: Cardiac size during prenatal development. *Obstet Gynecol* 1987; 69:854–858.

54. Campbell J, Henderson A, Campbell S: The fetal femur/foot length ratio: A new parameter to assess dysplastic limb reduction. *Obstet Gynecol* 1988; 72:181–184.

55. Castillo RA, Devoe LD, Falls G, et al: Pleural effusions and pulmonary hypoplasia. *Am J Obstet Gynecol* 1987; 157:1252–1255.

56. Oman SD, Wax Y: Estimating fetal age by ultrasound measurements: an example of multivariate calibration. *Biometrics* 1984; 40:947–960.

57. Hadlock FP, Deter RL, Harrist RB, et al: Computer assisted analysis of fetal age in the third trimester using multiple fetal growth parameters. *J Clin Ultrasound* 1983; 11:313–316.

58. Hadlock FP, Deter RL, Harrist RB, et al: Estimating fetal age: computer-assisted analysis of multiple fetal growth parameters. *Radiology* 1984; 152:497–501.

59. Hadlock FP, Harrist RB, Shah YP, et al: Estimating fetal age using multiple parameters: A prospective evaluation in a racially mixed population. *Am J Obstet Gynecol* 1987; 156:955–957.

60. Ott WJ: Accurate gestational dating. *Obstet Gynecol* 1985; 66:311–315.

61. Smazal SF, Weisman LE, Hoppler KD, et al: Comparative analysis of ultrasonographic methods of gestational age assessment. *J Ultrasound Med* 1983; 2:147–150.

62. Weiner SN, Flynn MJ, Kennedy AW, et al: A composite curve of ultrasonic biparietal diameters for estimating gestational age. *Radiology,* 1977; 122:781–786.

63. Kurtz AB, Wapner RJ, Kurtz RJ, et al: Analysis of biparietal diameter as an accurate indicator of gestational age. *J Clin Ultrasound* 1980; 8:319–326.

64. Levi S, Erbsman F: Antenatal fetal growth from the nineteenth week: ultrasonic study of 12 head and chest dimensions. *Am J Obstet Gynecol* 1975; 121:262–268.

65. Weinraub Z, Schneider D, Langer R, et al: Ultrasonographic measurement of fetal growth parameters for estimation of gestational age and fetal weight. *Isr J Med Sc* 1979; 15:829–832.

66. Parker AJ, Davies P, Mayho AM, et al: The ultrasound estimation of sex-related variations of intrauterine growth. *Am J Obstet Gynecol* 1984; 149:665–669.

67. Wittman BK, Robinson HP, Aitchison T, et al: The value of diagnostic ultrasound as a screening test for intrauterine growth retardation: comparison of nine parameters. *Am J Obstet Gynecol* 1979; 134:30.

68. Neilson JP, Whitfield CR, Aitchison TC: Screening for the small-for-dates fetus: A two-stage ultrasonic examination schedule. *Br Med J* 1980; 280:1203–1206.

69. Neilson JP, Munjanja SP, Whitfield CR: Screening for small for dates fetuses: a controlled trial. *Br Med J* 1984; 289:1179–1182.

70. Neilson JP, Munjanja SP, Mooney R, et al: Product of fetal crown-rump length and trunk area: ultrasound measurement in high-risk pregnancies. *Br J Obstet Gynaecol* 1984; 91:756–761.

71. Sabbagha RE, Turner H, Rockett H, et al: Sonar BPD and fetal age: definition of the relationship. *Obstet Gynecol* 1974; 43:7–14.

72. Campbell S, Dewhurts CJ: Diagnosis of the small-for-dates fetus by serial ultrasonic cephalometry. *Lancet* 1971; 2:1002–1006.

73. Sabbagha RE, Barton BA, Barton FA, et al: Sonar biparietal diameter II. Predictive of the three fetal growth patterns leading to a closer assessment of gestational age and neonatal weight. *Am J Obstet Gynecol* 1976; 126:485–490.

74. Persson PH, Grennert L, Gennser G: Diagnosis of intrauterine growth retardation by serial ultrasonic cephalometry. *Acta Obstet Gynecol Scand [Suppl]* 1978; 78:40–48.

75. Sabbagha RE, Hughey M, Depp R: Growth adjusted sonographic age: a simplified method. *Obstet Gynecol* 1978; 51:383–386.

76. Sabbagha RE: Intrauterine growth retardation: antenatal diagnosis by ultrasound. *Obstet Gynecol* 1978; 52:252–256.

77. Kopta MM, Tomich PG, Crane JP: Ultrasonic methods of predicting the estimated date of confinement. *Obstet Gynecol* 1981; 57:657–660.

78. Dubowitz LMS, Goldberg C: Assessment of gestation by ultrasound in various stages of pregnancy in infants differing in size and ethnic origin. *Br J Obstet Gynaecol* 1981; 88:255–259.

79. Simon NV, Levisky JS, Siegle JC, et al: Evaluation of the dating of gestation via the growth adjusted sonographic age method. *J Clin Ultrasound* 1984; 12:195–199.

80. Arias F: The diagnosis and management of intrauterine growth retardation. *Obstet Gynecol* 1977; 49:293–298.

81. Crane JP, Kopta MM, Welt SI, et al: Abnormal fetal growth patterns. Ultrasonic diagnosis and management. *Obstet Gynecol* 1977; 50:205–211.

82. Persson PH, Grennert L, Gennser G, et al: Normal range curves for the intrauterine growth of the biparietal diameter. *Acta Obstet Gynecol Scand* 1978; 78:15–20.

83. Hohler CW, Inglis J, Collins H, et al: Ultrasound biparietal diameter defining relationships in normal pregnancy. *NY State J Med* 1976; 76:373–376.

84. Queenan JT, Kubarych SF, Cook LN, et al: Diagnostic ultrasound for detection of intrauterine growth retardation. *Am J Obstet Gynecol* 1976; 124:865–873.

85. Yiu-Chiu V, Chiu L: Ultrasonographic evaluation of normal fetal anatomy and congenital malformations. *CT* 1981; 5:367–381, 508–509.

86. Deter RL, Harrist RB, Hadlock FP, et al: Longitudinal studies of fetal growth with the use of dynamic image ultrasonography. *Am J Obstet Gynecol* 1982; 143:545.

87. Varma TR: Prediction of delivery date by ultrasound cephalometry. *J Obstet Gynaecol Br Commw* 1973; 80:316–319.

88. Osefo NJ, Chukudebelu WO: Sonar cephalometry and fetal age relationship in the Nigerian woman. *East Afr Med J* 1983; 98–102.

89. Sholl JS, Woo D, Rubin JM, et al: Intrauterine growth retardation risk detection for fetuses of unknown gestational age. *Am J Obstet Gynecol* 1982; 144:709–714.

90. Santos-Ramos R, Deunhoelter JH, Reisch JS, et al: Reliability of sonar fetal cephalometry in the estimation of gestational age and in the diagnosis of fetal growth retardation, in *Ultrasound in Medicine*, ed 4. New York, Plenum Press, 1977, pp 247–251.

91. Nyberg DA, Maek LA, Laing FC, et al: Distinguishing normal from abnormal gestational sac growth in early pregnancy. *J Ultrasound Med* 1987; 6:23–27.

92. Jeanty P, Cousaert E, deMaertelaer V, et al: Sonographic detection of smoking-related decreased fetal growth. *J Ultrasound Med* 1987; 6:13–18.

93. Martin RH, Higginbottom J: A clinical and radiological assessment of fetal age. *J Obstet Gynaecol Br Commw* 1971; 78:155–162.

94. O'Brien GD, Queenan JT: Growth of the ultrasound fetal femur length during normal pregnancy. Part I. *Am J Obstet Gynecol* 1981; 141:833–837.

95. Usher R, McLean F: Intrauterine growth of live-born Caucasian infants at sea level: standards obtained from measurements in 7 dimensions of infants born between 25 and 44 weeks of gestation. *Pediatrics* 1969; 74:901–910.

96. Babson SG, Benda GI: Growth graphs for the clinical assessment of infants of varying gestational age. *Pediatrics* 1976; 89:814–820.

97. Lubchenco LO, Hansman C, Dressler M, et al: Intrauterine growth as estimated from liveborn birth-weight data at 24 to 42 weeks of gestation. *Pediatrics* 1963; 32:793–800.

98. Gruenwald P: Growth of the human fetus, parts I & II. *Am J Obstet Gynecol* 1966; 94:1112–1132.

99. Thomson AM, Billewicz WZ, Hytten FE: The assessment of fetal growth. *J Obstet Gynaecol Br Commw* 1968; 75:903–916.

100. Brenner WE, Edelman D, Hendricks CH: A standard of fetal growth for the United States of America. *Am J Obstet Gynecol* 1976; 126:555–564.

101. Naeye RL, Dixon JB: Distortions in fetal growth standards. *Pediatr Res* 1978; 12:987–991.

102. Freeman MG, Graves WL, Thompson AB: Indigent Negro and Caucasian birth weight–gestational age tables. *Pediatrics* 1970; 46:9–15.

103. Williams RL, Creasy RK, Cunningham GC, et al: Fetal growth and perinatal viability in California. *Obstet Gynecol* 1982; 59:624–632.

104. Wong KS, Scott KE: Fetal growth at sea level. *Biol Neonate* 1972; 20:175–188.

105. Hern WA: Correlation of fetal age and measurements between 10 and 26 weeks of gestation. *Obstet Gynecol* 1984; 63:26–32.

106. Golbus MS, Berry LC Jr: Human fetal development between 90 and 170 days postmenses. *Teratology* 1976; 15:103–108.

107. Secher NJ, Hansen PK, Lenstrup C, et al: Birthweight-for-gestational age charts based on early ultrasound estimation of gestational age. *Br J Obstet Gynaecol* 1986; 93:128–134.

108. Patterson RM, Prihoda TJ, Gibbs CE, et al: Analysis of birth weight percentile as a predictor of perinatal outcome. *Obstet Gynecol* 1986; 68:459–463.

109. McMormick MC: The contribution of low birth weight to infant mortality and childhood morbidity. *N Engl J Med* 1985; 312:82–89.

110. Kitchen WH, Yu VYH, Orgill AA, et al: Collaborative study of very-low-birth-weight infants. *Am J Dis Child* 1983; 137:555–559.

111. Boyd ME, Usher RH, McLean FH: Fetal macrosomia: Prediction, risks, proposed management. *Obstet Gynecol* 1983; 61:715–722.

112. Acker DB, Sachs BP, Friedman EA: Risk factors for shoulder dystocia. *Obstet Gynecol* 1985; 66:762–768.

113. Deter RL, Hadlock FP: Use of ultrasound in the detection of macrosomia: A review. *J Clin Ultrasound* 1985; 13:519–524.

114. Donaldson SW, Cheney W: Prenatal estimation of birth weight by pelvicephalometry. *Radiology* 1948; 50:666–667.

115. Stockland L, Stanton AM: A new method of fetal weight determination. *Am J Roentgenol Radiat Ther Nucl Med* 1961; 86:425–431.

116. Kohorn EI: An evaluation of ultrasonic fetal cephalometry. *Am J Obstet Gynecol* 1967; 97:553–559.

117. Campbell S, Newman GB: Growth of the fetal biparietal diameter during normal pregnancy. *J Obstet Gynaecol Br Commw* 1971; 78:518–519.

118. Bartolucci L: Biparietal diameter of the skull and fetal weight in the second trimester: an allometric relationship. *Am J Obstet Gynecol* 1975; 122:439–445.

119. Ojala A, Ylostalo P, Jouppila P, et al: Fetal cephalometry by ultrasound in normal and complicated pregnancy. *Ann Chir Gynaecol Fenn* 1970; 59:71–75.

120. Pathak DR, Skipper BE, Munsick RA: Estimation of fetal or neonatal weight from the biparietal diameter. *J Reprod Med* 1977; 18:87–89.

121. Stocker J, Mawad R, Deleon A, et al: Ultrasonic cephalometry: Its use in estimating fetal weight. *Obstet Gynecol* 1975; 45:275–278.

122. Ianniruberto A, Gibbons JM: Predicting fetal weight by ultrasonic B-scan cephalometry: An improved technic with disappointing results. *Obstet Gynecol* 1971; 37:689–694.

123. Jordaan HVF: Fetal biparietal diameter and birth weight: An interpopulation comparison. *S Afr Med J* 1976; 50:1166–1170.

124. Sabbagha RE, Turner JH: Methodology of B-scan sonar cephalometry with electronic calipers and correlation with fetal birth weight. *Obstet Gynecol* 1972; 40:74–81.

125. Gonzales AC, Dale E, Byers RH, et al: Limitations in predictions of gestational age and birth weight by ultrasonographic methods. *J Clin Ultrasound* 1978; 6:233–238.

126. Jordaan HVF: Biological variation in the biparietal diameter and its bearing on clinical ultrasonography. *Am J Obstet Gynecol* 1978; 131:53–59.

127. Divon MY, Chamberlain MC, Sipos L, et al: Underestimation of fetal weight in premature rupture of membranes. *J Ultrasound Med* 1984; 3:529–531.

128. Kosar WP, Steer CM: The relation of body weight to the biparietal diameter in the newborn. *Am J Obstet Gynecol* 1956; 71:1232–1234.

129. Weinraub Z, Schneider D, Langer R, et al: Ultrasonographic measurement of fetal growth parameters for estimation of gestational age and fetal weight. *Isr J Med Sc* 1979; 15:829–832.

130. Campbell S, Wilkin D: Ultrasonic measurement of fetal abdomen circumference in the estimation of fetal weight. *Br J Obstet Gynaecol* 1975; 82:689–697.

131. Kurjak A, Breyer B: Estimation of fetal weight by ultrasonic abdominometry. *Am J Obstet Gynecol* 1976; 125:962–965.

132. Poll V, Kasby CB: An improved method of fetal weight estimation using ultrasound measurements of fetal abdominal circumference. *Br J Obstet Gynaecol* 1979; 86:922–928.

133. Higginbottom J, Slater J, Porter G, et al: Estimation of fetal weight from ultrasonic measurement of trunk circumference. *Br J Obstet Gynaecol* 1975; 82:698–701.

134. McCallum WD, Brinkley JF: Estimation of fetal weight ultrasonic measurements. *Am J Obstet Gynecol* 1979; 133:195–200.

135. Rossavik IK, Deter RL: The effect of abdominal profile shape changes on the estimation of fetal weight. *J Clin Ultrasound* 1984; 12:57–59.

136. Finikiotis F, MacLennan AH, Verco PW, et al: An evaluation of two methods of antenatal ultrasonic fetal weight estimation. *Aust NZ J Obstet Gynaecol* 1980; 20:135–138.

137. Thompson HE, Holmes JH, Gottesfeld KR, et al: Fetal development as determined by ultrasonic pulse echo techniques. *Am J Obstet Gynecol* 1965; 92:44–52.

138. Pap G, Pap L: Ultrasonic estimation of gestational age and fetal weight. *Paediatr Acad Sci Hung* 1979; 20:119–135.

139. Hansmann M: A critical evaluation of the performance of ultrasonic diagnosis in present-day obstetrics. *Gynakologe* 1974; 7:26–35.

140. Shepard MJ, Richard VA, Berkowitz RL, et al: An evaluation of two equations for predicting fetal weight by ultrasound. *Am J Obstet Gynecol* 1982; 142:47–54.

141. Warsof SL, Gohari P, Berkowitz RL, et al: The estimation of fetal weight by computer-assisted analysis. *Am J Obstet Gynecol* 1977; 128:881–892.

142. Jeanty P, Cantraine F, Romero R, et al: A longitudinal study of fetal weight growth. *J Ultrasound Med* 1984; 3:321–328.

143. Thompson HE, Makowski EL: Estimation of birth weight and gestational age. *Obstet Gynecol* 1971; 37:44–47.

144. Timor-Tritsch IE, Itskovitz J, Brandes JM: Estimation of fetal weight by real-time sonography. *Obstet Gynecol* 1981; 57:653–656.

145. Ott WH, Doyle S: Ultrasonic diagnosis of altered fetal growth by use of a normal ultrasonic fetal weight curve. *Obstet Gynecol* 1984; 63:201–204.

146. Ott WJ: Clinical application of fetal weight determination by real-time measurements. *Obstet Gynecol* 1981; 57:758–762.

147. Weinberger E, Cyr DR, Jirsch JH, et al: Estimating fetal weights less than 2000 g: An accurate and simple method. *AJR* 1984; 141:937–977.

148. Tamura RK, Sabbagha RE, Dooley SL, et al: Real-time ultrasound estimations of weight in fetuses of diabetic gravid women. *Am J Obstet Gynecol* 1985; 153:57–60.

149. Eik-Nes SH, Grottum P, Andersson NJ: Clinical evaluation of two formulas for estimation of fetal weight. *Acta Obstet Gynecol Scand* 1981; 60:567–573.

150. Eik-Nes SH, Grottum P: Estimation of fetal weight by ultrasound measurement: Development of a new formula. *Acta Obstet Gynecol Scand* 1982; 61:299–305.

151. Eik-Nes SH, Grottum P, Andersson NJ: Estimation of fetal weight by ultrasound measurement: Clinical application of a new formula. *Acta Obstet Gynecol Scand* 1982; 61:307–312.

152. Eik-Nes SH, Persson PH, Grottum P, et al: Prediction of fetal growth deviation by ultrasonic biometry: Clinical application. *Acta Obstet Gynecol Scand* 1983; 62:117–123.

153. Lunt R, Chard T: A new method for estimation of fetal weight in late pregnancy by ultrasonic scanning. *Br J Obstet Gynaecol* 1976; 83:1–5.

154. Rossavik IK, Bjoro K: The prenatal determination of fetal weight by dynamic scanning. *Early Hum Dev* 1981; 5:133–138.

155. Thurnau GR, Tamura RK, Sabbagha R, et al: A simple estimated fetal weight equation based on real-time ultrasound measurements of fetuses less than thirty-four weeks' gestation. *Am J Obstet Gynecol* 1983; 145:557–561.

156. Campogrande M, Todros T, Brizzolara M: Prediction of birth weight by ultrasound measurements of the fetus. *Br J Obstet Gynaecol* 1977; 84:175–178.

157. Jordaan HVF, Clark WB: Prenatal determination of fetal brain and somatic weight by ultrasound. *Am J Obstet Gynecol* 1980; 138:54–59.

158. Jordaan HVF: Estimation of fetal weight by ultrasound. *J Clin Ultrasound* 1983; 11:59–66.

159. Birnholz JC: Ultrasound characterization of fetal growth. *Ultrasonic Imaging* 1980; 2:135–149.

160. Sampson MB, Thomason JL, Kelly SL, et al: Prediction of intrauterine fetal weight using real-time ultrasound. *Am J Obstet Gynecol* 1982; 142:554–556.

161. Dornan KJ, Hansmann M, Redord DHA, et al: Fetal weight estimation by real-time ultrasound measurement of biparietal and transverse diameter. *Am J Obstet Gynecol* 1982; 142:652–657.

162. Secher NJ, Djursing H, Hansen PK, et al: Estimation of fetal weight in the third trimester by ultrasound. *Eur J Obstet Gynecol Reprod Biol* 1987; 24:1–11.

163. Weiner CP, Sabbagha RE, Vaisrub N, et al: Ultrasonic fetal weight prediction: Role of head circumference and femur length. *Obstet Gynecol* 1985; 65:812–816.

164. Hadlock FP, Deter RL, Roecker E, et al: Relation of fetal femur length to neonatal crown-heel length. *J Ultrasound Med* 1984; 3:1–3.

165. Roberts AV, Lee AJ, James AG: Ultrasonic estimation of fetal weight: A new predictive model incorporating femur length for the low-birth-weight fetus. *J Clin Ultrasound* 1985; 13:555–559.

166. Hadlock FP, Harrist RB, Carpenter RJ, et al: Sonographic estimation of fetal weight. The value of femur length in addition to head and abdomen measurements. *Radiology* 1984; 150:535–540.

167. Campbell WA, Vintzileos AM, Neckkles S, et al: Use of the femur length to estimate weight in premature infants: Preliminary results. *J Ultrasound Med* 1985; 4:583–590.

168. Hadlock FP, Harrist RB, Sharman RS, et al: Estimation of fetal weight with the use of head, body, and femur measurements—A prospective study. *Am J Obstet Gynecol* 1985; 151:333–337.

169. Hill LM, Breckle R, Gehrking WC, et al: Use of femur length in estimation of fetal weight. *Am J Obstet Gynecol* 1985; 152:847–852.

170. Woo JSK, Wan CW, Cho KM: Computer-assisted evaluation of ultrasonic fetal weight prediction using multiple regression equations with and without the fetal femur length. *J Ultrasound Med* 1985; 4:65–67.

171. Woo JSK, Wan MCW: An evaluation of fetal weight prediction using a simple equation containing the fetal femur length. *J Ultrasound Med* 1986; 5:453–457.

172. Warsof SL, Wolf P, Coulehan J, et al: Comparison of fetal weight estimation formulas with and without head measurements. *Obstet Gynecol* 1986; 67:569–573.

173. Benson CB, Doubilet PM, Saltzman DH: Sonographic determination of fetal weights in diabetic pregnancies. *Am J Obstet Gynecol* 1987; 156:441–444.

174. Yarkoni S, Reece A, Wan M, et al: Intrapartum fetal weight estimation: A comparison of three formulae. *J Ultrasound Med* 1986; 5:707–710.

175. Picker RH, Saunders DM: A simple geometric method for determining fetal weight in utero with the compound gray scale ultrasonic scan. *Am J Obstet Gynecol* 1976; 124:493–494.

176. Morrison J, McLennan MJ: The theory, feasibility and accuracy of an ultrasonic method of estimating fetal weight. *Br J Obstet Gynaecol* 1976; 83:833–837.

177. Thompson TR, Manning FA: Estimation of volume and weight of the perinate: Relationship to morphometric measurement by ultrasonography. *J Ultrasound Med* 1983; 2:113–116.

178. Brinkley JF, McCallum WD, Muramatsu SK, et al: Fetal weight estimation from lengths and volumes found by three-dimensional ultrasonic measurements. *J Ultrasound Med* 1984; 3:163–168.

179. Rossavik IK, Torjusen GO, Deter RL, et al: Efficacy of mathematical methods for ultrasound examinations in diabetic pregnancies. *Am J Obstet Gynecol* 1986; 155:638–644.

180. Eden RD, Frederick RJ, Kodack LD, et al: Accuracy of ultrasonic fetal weight prediction in pre-term infants. *Am J Obstet Gynecol* 1983; 147:43–48.

181. Deter RL, Hadlock FP, Harrist RB, et al: Evaluation of three methods for obtaining fetal weight estimates using dynamic image ultrasound. *J Clin Ultrasound* 1981; 9:421–425.

182. Chervenak FA, Romero R, Berkowitz RL, et al: Use of sonographic estimated fetal weight in the prediction of intrauterine growth retardation. *Am J Perinatol* 1984; 1:298–301.

183. Ott WJ, Doyle S: Ultrasonic diagnosis of altered fetal growth by use of a normal ultrasonic fetal weight curve. 1984; 63:201–204.

184. Key RC, Dattel BJ, Resnik R: The ultrasonographic estimation of fetal weight in the very-low-birth-weight infant. *Am J Obstet Gynecol* 1983; 145:574–578.
185. Sampson MB, Beckmann CRB, Thomason JL, et al: Single ultrasonic estimation of fetal weight in utero compared with birth weight. *J Reprod Med* 1985; 30:28–29.
186. Patterson RM: Estimation of fetal weight during labor. *Obstet Gynecol* 1985; 65:330–332.
187. Miller JM Jr, Korndorffer FA III, Gabert HA: Fetal weight estimates in late pregnancy with emphasis on macrosomia. *J Clin Ultrasound* 1986; 14:437–442.
188. Hill LM, Breckle R, Wolfgram KR, et al: Evaluation of three methods for estimating fetal weight. *J Clin Ultrasound* 1986; 14:171–178.
189. Wong F, Rogers M, Chang A: An evaluation of three ultrasound equations for fetal weight prediction. *Aust NZ J Obstet Gynaecol* 1985; 25:271.
190. Miller JM, Kissling GE, Korndoffer FA III, et al: A cross-sectional study of in utero growth of the above average sized fetus. *Am J Obstet Gynecol* 1986; 155:1052–1055.

Chapter 27 _____

Uterine Measurements
Alfred B. Kurtz, M.D.
Barry B. Goldberg, M.D.

UTERINE VOLUME

The volume of the pregnant uterus, initially termed the *total intrauterine volume*, or TIUV, was first calculated in the late 1970s.[1–3] All three articles computed the volume using a prolate ellipse formula (TIUV = 0.523 × the maximum uterine length × width × height), all giving their data in graph form with a standard deviation range. Gohari et al.[1] presented their data from +1 to −2 SD. Phillips et al.[2] gave a 1-SD range and showed the difference between singleton, twin, and triplet gestations, and Levine et al.[3] gave a range from the upper to the lower 2.5th percentile. All three articles showed a linear relationship with the TIUV increasing as both the weeks of gestation and biparietal diameter increased to term. The articles, however, differed markedly in their values. At 24 weeks, with a biparietal diameter of 61 mm, the TIUV ranged from 1,400 to 3,800 cc. By 40 weeks, with a biparietal diameter of 95 mm, variation was even larger, 4,200 to 7,800 cc. Despite these discrepancies, the initial success in the detection of growth retardation was found to be good, with Gohari et al.[1] reporting a sensitivity of 75%, a specificity of 100%, and a predictive accuracy of 100% when a threshold of 1.5 SD below the mean was used. This accuracy, however, could not be reproduced.[4] In a group of 252 patients, using a threshold of abnormality at the lower 10% tolerance limit, growth retardation was only detected with a predictive accuracy of 41%!

Conceptually, the idea of the total uterine volume is sound. It should be a good indicator of not only the size of the pregnant uterus but also of its three main components—the fetus, the amniotic fluid, and the placenta. The reasons for the marked discrepancies between studies and the poor predictive accuracy in the detection of growth retardation are therefore puzzling. Three studies[5–7] found that the major source of error was not in the concept of uterine volume but rather in the use of the prolate ellipse formula for its calculation. When the uterine volume was calculated instead from a stepped area-to-volume technique with comparison to known volumes, the stepped area method was accurate to within 5% of the true volume while the prolate ellipse method was inaccurate by as much as 55%. As a result, it was recommended that the stepped area-to-volume method be used to calculate the uterine volume[6, 7] and that the name be changed from TIUV to *total uterine volume,* or TUV, since the measurement encompassed not just the intra-uterine contents but also the myometrium.[7]

One additional article suggested an entirely different method of measuring the uterus.[8] It stated that the addition of the maximum longitudinal and transverse uterine areas (LTUA) gave less of an error than the multiplication of the three linear measurements used in the prolate ellipse formula. While this may be true, and while greater reproducibility in measurements might be obtained, the two areas do not relate to uterine volumes except in very specific and unusual situations.[7] For this reason, the LTUA technique is not of clinical value.

Two different groups evaluated the stepped area-to-volume TUV technique.[9, 10] Both used similar technique with a static scanner. Transverse scans were obtained at specific intervals from the bottom to the top of the uterus. The area of each transverse image was computed from an equation for an ellipse ($\pi\, d_1/2 \times d_2/2$) and all the areas added together to obtain the TUV. Geirsson et al.[10] presumably scanned at 1 to 2 cm intervals, as proposed in their previous article.[6] Kurtz et al.[9] found that obtaining scans at 3-cm intervals closely approximated the volumes obtained at 1-cm intervals with an average error of only 3.5%.[7] Both articles[9, 10] stated their results in graph and numeric form. Kurtz et al.[9] presented a range of values at 200-cc increments from mean gestational ages of 15.4 to 38.7 weeks and from mean biparietal diameters of 35.3 to 91.1 mm, while Geirsson et al.[10] gave their results from 20 to 40 weeks in 5-week increments. Both had standard deviation ranges, Kurtz et al.[9] from the upper and lower first, fifth, and tenth percentile, and Geirsson et al.[10] from the upper and lower third percentile. Both had reasonably sized series, Kurtz et al.[9] evaluating 260 normal pregnancies cross-sectionally, almost all patients scanned only once, while Geirsson et al.[10] examined 147 women longitudinally on four separate occasions. Geirsson et al.,[10] eliminated 32 patients (over 21% of their cases) for clinical reasons.

Kurtz et al.[9] also examined 26 abnormal cases, 14 large uteri and 12 small uteri. All the large and 10 of the 12 small uteri fell outside the upper or lower 90% confidence limit. Because of the apparent clinical usefulness of their data, the two tables of TUV versus both biparietal diameter and gestational age by Kurtz et al.[9] are recommended (Fig 27–1, Tables 27–1 and 27–2). More work is necessary for further evaluation of this technique, since only a small number of abnormal patients had been studied. For the appropriate measurements to be taken, static images are necessary. Since more and more emphasis is being placed on real-time examinations, and less on static scanning, it is not certain whether this technique, although presumably valuable, will ever by fully evaluated.

PLACENTA

Placental weight and thickness have been analyzed pathologically. In two series on delivered placentas,[11, 12] the weight was measured in one series from 23 to 43 weeks[11] and in the other at term.[12] The results at term matched closely, both articles finding a placental weight of approximately 420 g. In addition, one of the articles measured the thickness of the placenta at term and found it to be 1.64 ±0.5 cm.[12] The exact place for measuring placental thickness, however, was never indicated.

Ultrasound evaluated the placental thickness and volume. Two articles[13, 14] measured placental thickness at various stages of gestation. Grannum et al.,[13] without

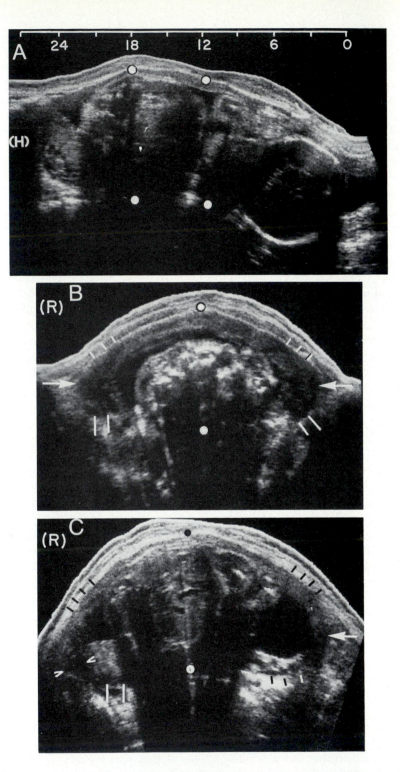

FIG 27-1.
Calculation of total uterine volume. **A,** long-axis midline static scan of the pregnant uterus. The *centimeter scale* at the top demonstrates the uterus divided into 3-cm intervals. *Dots* represent the anterior and posterior uterine margins of scans at 12 and 18 cm above the maternal bladder. **B** and **C,** transverse static scans at **(B)** 12 cm and **(C)** 18 cm above the maternal bladder. The outer uterine walls are denoted by *dots* anteriorly and posteriorly, by *dashes* anterolaterally and posterolaterally, and by *arrows* laterally. *(H)* = toward patient's head; *(R)* = toward patient's right. (From Kurtz AB, Kurtz RJ, Rifkin MD, et al: *J Ultrasound Med* 1984; 3:229–308. Used by permission.)

TABLE 27–1.
Comparison of Total Uterine Volume (TUV) to Biparietal Diameter*

	Biparietal Diameter (mm)						
	Lower Percentile Limits of Normal				Upper Percentile Limits of Normal		
TUV (cc)	99th	95th	90th	Mean	90th	95th	99th
600	18.9	22.8	24.8	35.3	45.7	47.8	51.7
800	23.4	27.3	29.3	39.7	50.2	52.2	56.1
1,000	27.6	31.5	33.6	44.0	54.4	56.5	60.4
1,200	31.7	35.6	37.6	48.1	58.5	60.6	64.4
1,400	35.6	39.5	41.5	52.0	62.4	64.5	68.3
1,600	39.3	43.2	45.3	55.7	66.1	68.2	72.1
1,800	42.9	46.7	48.8	59.2	69.7	71.7	75.6
2,000	46.2	50.1	52.1	62.6	73.0	75.1	79.0
2,200	49.4	53.3	55.3	65.7	76.2	78.2	82.1
2,400	52.4	56.2	58.3	68.7	79.2	81.2	85.1
2,600	55.2	59.0	61.1	71.5	82.0	84.0	87.9
2,800	57.8	61.7	63.7	74.1	84.6	86.6	90.5
3,000	60.2	64.1	66.1	76.6	87.0	89.1	93.0
3,200	62.5	66.3	68.4	78.8	89.3	91.3	95.3
3,400	64.5	68.4	70.5	80.9	91.3	93.4	97.3
3,600	66.4	70.3	72.3	82.8	93.2	95.3	99.1
3,800	68.1	72.0	74.0	84.5	95.0	97.0	100.8
4,000	69.6	73.5	75.6	86.0	96.4	98.5	102.4
4,200	71.0	74.9	76.9	87.3	97.8	99.8	103.7
4,400	72.1	76.0	78.0	88.5	98.9	101.0	104.9
4,600	73.1	77.0	79.0	89.5	99.9	101.9	105.8
4,800	73.9	77.8	80.0	90.2	100.7	102.7	106.6
5,000	74.5	78.4	80.4	90.8	101.3	103.3	107.2
5,200	74.9	78.8	80.8	91.3	101.7	103.7	107.6
5,400	75.1	79.0	81.1	91.5	101.9	104.0	107.9
5,600	75.2	79.1	81.1	91.6	102.0	104.0	107.9
5,800	75.1	78.9	81.0	91.4	101.9	103.9	107.8
6,000	74.7	78.6	80.7	91.1	101.6	103.6	107.5

*From Kurtz AB, Kurtz RJ, Rifkin MD, et al: *J Ultrasound Med* 1984; 3:299–308. Used by permission.

stating where the measurement was taken, found placental thickness to decrease gradually in the mid- to late third trimester. At 30 to 32 weeks, 32 to 34 weeks, and 34 to 36 weeks, the placental thickness averaged 38 mm, 36.6 mm, and 34.8 mm, respectively. Hoddick et al.[14] measured the midportion of the placenta with static scans from 10 weeks until term, excluding the myometrium and subplacental veins. Without using the umbilical cord insertion or any other anatomic landmark, they found the placenta to increase in thickness with advancing menstrual age, never exceeding 40 mm. Presenting their numbers in graph form, they found the placenta to have a mean value of 10 ±5 mm at 10 weeks, increasing to 20 ±10 mm at 20 weeks. At 30 and 40 weeks, respectively, the placenta measured 28 ±6 mm and 33 ±7 mm. These upper and lower limits could be of value in the future in evaluating small and large placentas if a landmark can be established to make the measurements reproducible. It is recommended that the umbilical cord insertion be used as the anatomic landmark, measurements taken perpendicularly from the chorionic plate to the decidua basalis (the edge of the myometrium). While it may be difficult to identify the myometrium, neither the myometrium nor the retroplacental zone should be included in the measurement (Fig 27–2).

TABLE 27–2.
Comparison of Total Uterine Volume (TUV) to Average Gestational Age*

| | Average Gestational Age (wk) | | | | | | |
| | Lower Percentile Limits of Normal | | | | Upper Percentile Limits of Normal | | |
TUV (cc)	99th	95th	90th	Mean	90th	95th	99th
600	8.7	10.3	11.1	15.4	19.7	20.5	22.1
800	10.5	12.1	12.9	17.2	21.5	22.3	23.9
1,000	11.9	13.5	14.3	18.6	22.9	23.7	25.3
1,200	13.3	14.9	15.7	20.0	24.3	25.1	26.7
1,400	14.6	16.2	17.0	21.3	25.6	26.5	28.0
1,600	15.9	17.5	18.3	22.6	26.9	27.7	29.3
1,800	17.1	18.7	19.6	23.9	28.1	29.0	30.6
2,000	18.3	19.9	20.8	25.1	29.3	30.2	31.8
2,200	19.5	21.1	21.9	26.2	30.5	31.3	32.9
2,400	20.6	22.2	23.0	27.3	31.6	32.4	34.0
2,600	21.6	23.2	24.0	28.3	32.6	33.5	35.1
2,800	22.6	24.2	25.0	29.3	33.6	34.5	36.0
3,000	23.6	25.2	26.0	30.3	34.6	35.4	37.0
3,200	24.5	26.1	26.9	31.2	35.5	36.3	37.9
3,400	25.3	26.9	27.8	32.0	36.3	37.2	38.8
3,600	26.1	27.7	28.6	32.8	37.1	38.0	39.6
3,800	26.9	28.5	29.3	33.6	37.9	38.7	40.3
4,000	27.6	29.1	30.0	34.3	38.6	39.4	41.0
4,200	28.3	29.8	30.7	35.0	39.3	40.1	41.7
4,400	28.9	30.5	31.3	35.6	39.9	40.7	42.3
4,600	29.4	31.0	31.9	36.1	40.4	41.3	42.9
4,800	29.9	31.5	32.4	36.7	40.9	41.8	43.4
5,000	30.4	32.0	32.8	37.1	41.4	42.2	43.8
5,200	30.8	32.4	33.3	37.5	41.8	42.7	44.3
5,400	31.2	32.8	33.6	37.9	42.2	43.0	44.6
5,600	31.5	33.1	34.0	38.2	42.5	43.4	45.0
5,800	31.8	33.4	34.2	38.5	42.8	43.6	45.2
6,000	32.0	33.6	34.5	38.7	43.0	43.9	45.5

*From Kurtz AB, Kurtz RJ, Rifkin MD, et al: *J Ultrasound Med* 1984; 3:299–308. Used by permission.

Three additional ultrasound articles evaluated with static scans the volumetric growth of the human placenta,[10, 15] two giving their results in numeric and graph form[10, 16] and the other in graph form only.[15] Different techniques were used. Geirsson et al.,[10] scanning at 1- to 2-cm intervals, calculated the placental volume in 115 pregnant women as the difference between the total uterine volume and the intraamniotic volume. Bleker et al.[16] obtained one long-axis and then three transverse scans of the placenta, approximating the area between slices and comparing it to 10 delivered placentas. While close correlation was detected, placental volume was found to decrease after birth due to the loss of the fetal blood to the neonate. Wolf et al.[15] produced transverse images at 1- to 2-cm intervals, tracing the placental outline with a digitizer to calculate an area for each slice. The volume was estimated by a modified rectangular formula. Close correlation was obtained with six placentas measured shortly after birth. While all three articles showed an initial increase in placental volume early in the pregnancy, Bleker et al.[16] stated that in 10 of 12 patients the placental volume reached its maximum by approximately 32 gestational weeks and thereafter either leveled off or decreased. Geirsson et al.[10] and Wolf et al.[15] showed an increasing placental volume throughout pregnancy, with the incremental growth either greatest prior to 35 weeks with very little additional growth thereafter[10] or increasing steadily to term.[15] Geirrson et al.[10] gave a standard deviation, while the other two did not.

The numbers between studies varied considerably. Geirsson et al.[10] showed a steady increase in placental volumes from 259 to 800 cc from 20 weeks to term while Wolf et al.[15] revealed a steady increase from 200 to greater than 1,000 cc over the same period of time. Bleker et al.[16] revealed variable numbers throughout gestation

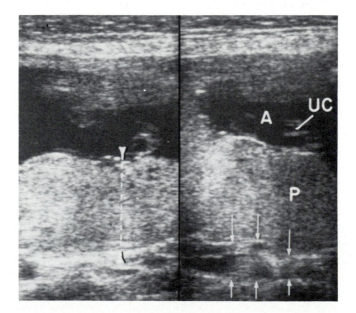

FIG 27–2.
Dual image scan of an early third trimester uterus. **Right image,** scan of the placenta *(P)* at the point of umbilical cord *(UC)* insertion. *A* = amniotic fluid; *arrows* denote hypoechoic retroplacental zone. **Left image,** measurement of the placenta obtained perpendicularly at the origin of the umbilical cord, denoted by *arrowheads* and *dashed line.* Note that the measurement is taken from the thin hyperechoic chorionic plate (at the cord insertion) through the placenta, not including the retroplacental area.

with some of their cases changing by only 100 cc between 20 and 40 weeks. While the technique by Wolf et al.[15] would seem to be the more accurate in measuring placental volumes, more work on a much larger group of patients is necessary to establish its validity and clinical usefulness.

AMNIOTIC FLUID

The amount of amniotic fluid surrounding the fetus is important during fetal development and affects perinatal outcome.[17] Oligohydramnios (decreased amniotic fluid) has been associated with fetal dysmaturity syndromes, fetal congenital anomalies, particularly renal abnormalities, and, if prolonged, with hypoplasia of the fetal lungs. Polyhydramnios or hydramnios (increased amniotic fluid) has been associated with maternal factors (such as diabetes mellitus, Rh isoimmunization) and fetal anomalies (mostly upper gastrointestinal or neurologic).

Amniotic fluid can be evaluated either qualitatively (subjectively) or quantitatively (objectively with measurements). Whether analyzed subjectively or objectively, the determination of both normal and decreased amniotic fluid was found to be accurate with little intra- or interobserver variation and regardless of the experience of the observer.[18] Crowley[19] further used the subjective criteria that amniotic fluid could be considered normal if it could be demonstrated between fetal limbs and the uterine wall anteriorly or between fetal limbs and the fetal trunk posteriorly (Fig 27–3). When determined to be normal, she found the incidence of meconium staining, fetal acidosis, fetal distress, and the Apgar scores was significantly reduced or nonexistent. Hashimoto et al.[20] and Goldstein and Filly[21] also found that the subjective diagnosis of decreased amniotic fluid was accurate.

Six groups in seven studies[20, 22–27] attempted to quantitate amniotic fluid by measuring its largest pocket and setting a lower limit for normal (see Fig 27–3). Manning et al.[22] decided that the amniotic fluid could be considered normal if one pocket measured 10 mm or greater in its broadest diameter. Mercer et al.[23] defined amniotic fluid as normal if the largest pocket were greater than 10 mm in size, moderately decreased if the pocket were 5 to 10 mm in size, and markedly decreased if less than 5 mm. Chamberlain et al.[24, 25] used scans perpendicular to the maternal abdomen and measured both transverse and vertical pockets of fluid. They defined the amniotic fluid as decreased if the largest pocket were less than 10 mm in both vertical and transverse dimensions and marginal if between 10 and 20 mm in vertical and 10 mm in transverse dimensions. Patterson et al.[26] took an average of the vertical and the two horizontal diameters of the largest pocket of fluid and determined this measurement to be more reproducible than that of a single vertical measurement. They felt that a number of 30 mm was probably the best screening threshold below which decreased fluid and growth retardation could be detected. Hashimoto et al.[20] measured the length, width, and depth of the largest pocket of fluid and multiplied the three numbers together. An arbitrary number of 60 was found to be the dividing line between a normal amount of amniotic fluid above and oligohydramnios below. Phelan and co-workers[27] divided the uterus into four quadrants, measuring the vertical diameter of the largest pocket in each quadrant and adding them together. A number of 12.9 ±4.9 cm separated normal from decreased amniotic fluid.

Manning et al.[22] found that by using his 10-mm definition, later termed the 1-cm rule, a diagnosis of normal amniotic fluid could accurately predict a normal fetus in

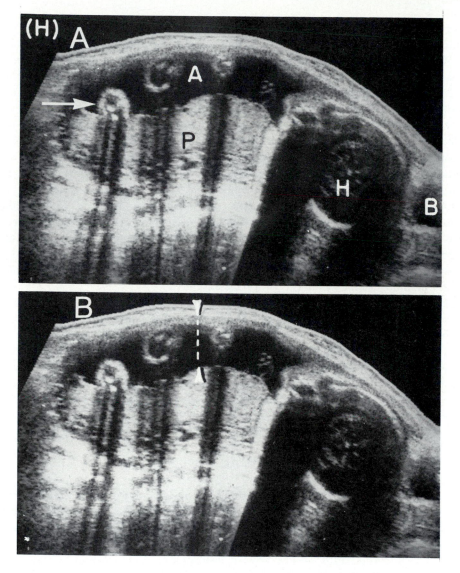

FIG 27–3.
Long-axis midline scan of a 28-week pregnancy. The amount of amniotic fluid *(A)* is normal by both objective and subjective criteria. **A,** the fetus is in vertex presentation with its head *(H)* immediately superior to the maternal bladder *(B)*. *Arrow* denotes fetal limb; *P* = placenta. **B,** same image as **A** measuring an AP pocket of fluid greater than 3 cm in size, denoted by *arrowheads* and *dashed line*. *(H)* = toward patient's head.

93.4% of cases while a diagnosis of decreased amniotic fluid meant growth retardation in 89.9% of cases with a significant tenfold increase in perinatal morbidity. Mercer et al.,[23] using his own 5-mm rule, found that when cases of ruptured membranes were discarded, 7% of neonates with less than a 5-mm pocket of amniotic fluid had congenital malformations, lower Apgar scores at 1 and 5 minutes, increased fetal distress and meconium, and if detected prior to 27 weeks, had significantly poorer neonatal outcome. Chamberlain et al.[24, 25] also found the same significant relationship between decreased amniotic fluid volume and the incidence of both major congenital anomalies (9.37%) and growth retardation (38.6%). Patterson et al.[26] and Rutherford and co-workers[28] similarly found that amniotic fluid measurements below their lower limits were associated with decreased fluid and adverse perinatal outcome.

A reevaluation of the 1-cm rule was performed in two studies.[29, 30] When this rule was used as the sole criterion for the diagnosis of growth retardation,[29] only five of 125 small-for-date fetuses were detected and it was concluded that the 1-cm rule was not of significant value in the prediction of growth retardation.[29] In addition, in three of six small-for-date fetuses, the correct diagnosis of oligohydramnios was made subjectively although the largest pocket of fluid was greater than 1 cm[30] (Fig 27–4). Therefore, while it is important that decreased amniotic fluid be detected, it is not important whether this diagnosis is made qualitatively or quantitatively. Furthermore, an observer who subjectively thinks that there is decreased amniotic fluid should not be dissuaded from making that diagnosis on the basis of the quantitative measurement of a fluid pocket. It has now also been shown that the same subjective decision can be used to differentiate most cases of polyhydramnios (increased amniotic fluid) from normal[21] (Fig 27–5). An actual number, regardless of the method employed, would seem to be of value only if follow-up examinations to evaluate changes in the amount of amniotic fluid were contemplated.

An attempt at determining intraamniotic fluid volumes has also been performed. Geirsson[10, 31] measured intraamniotic fluid volume by use of the stepped area-to-volume method. The intraamniotic number encompasses both the fluid and the fetus. In the second and early third trimester, there is more fluid than fetus, with the reverse present near term. While specific numbers were given and there was correlation with dye dilution techniques performed on the amniotic fluid, this method does not seem to offer any more information than the amniotic fluid analyses described above.

UMBILICAL CORD AND UMBILICAL VEIN

Studies have been performed on newborn infants, born prematurely from as early as 20 weeks until term, to evaluate the length and width of the umbilical cord.[12, 32–35] The normal umbilical cord was found to increase in length from the early gestational age to term, a mean and 1 SD of 32 ± 8 mm at 20 weeks to 60 ± 13 mm at 40 weeks.[12] The width has also been measured and at term found to have a mean number of 14 mm in preterm and 16 mm in term gestations.[12] While it has been determined that a short umbilical cord is associated with psychomotor abnormalities from either early intrauterine constraint or fetal limb dysfunction,[32, 33] there is a low predictive value in determining fetal abnormality because the normal cord length has such a wide range of normal values.

The number and size of the blood vessels within the umbilical cord has also been studied in newborn infants.[36, 37] While there is usually one vein and two arteries, occasionally only one vein and one artery is detected. This finding of a single umbilical artery has been reviewed extensively in an autopsy series.[37] In singleton gestations, a single artery has been found in 20% of cases and when detected coexists with a higher incidence of fetal malformations (approximately 20%, many major and multiple), stillbirths, spontaneous abortions, and increased perinatal mortality. It should be remembered, however, that while abnormalities are high, 80% of fetuses with a single umbilical artery are still normal. Of interest is the additional finding that a single umbilical artery occurs much more commonly in twin gestations and that in

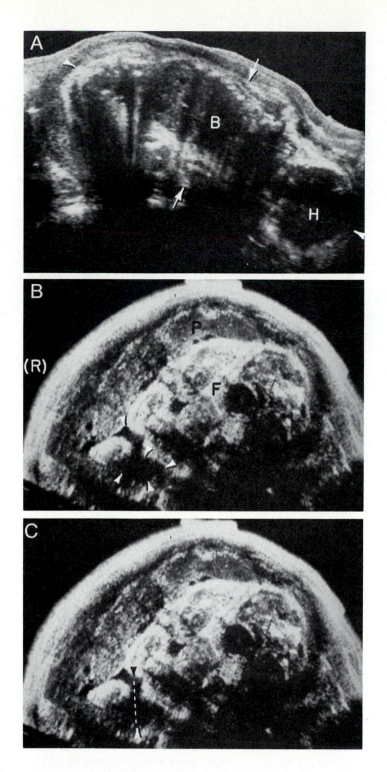

FIG 27–4.
Static scans of a 34-week fetus with subjectively marked decrease in amniotic fluid. Objectively, and incorrectly, the fluid measured within the normal range. **A,** long-axis midline scan showing the uterus (outlined by *arrows* and *arrowheads*) without any demonstrable fluid surrounding the fetus. *H* = fetal head; *B* = fetal body. **B,** transaxial scan at upper portion of uterus, showing the only demonstrable pocket of amniotic fluid *(arrowheads)*, adjacent to the fetal body *(F)*. *P* = placenta with grade II changes. **C,** same image as **B**. The pocket of amniotic fluid, measured in its broadest dimension, is over 1 cm in size, denoted by *arrowheads* and *dashed line*. Although objectively the fluid measures normal in amount, severe oligohydramnios is present. *(R)* = toward patient's right.

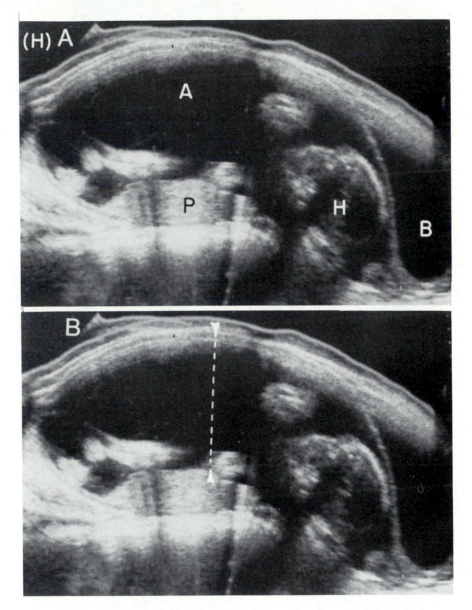

FIG 27–5.
Static scans of a 30-week pregnancy with subjectively increased amniotic fluid (polyhydramnios). No objective measurements are available at present. **A,** long-axis midline scan showing increased amniotic fluid *(A). H* = fetal head; *P* = placenta; *B* = maternal bladder; *(H)* = toward patient's head. **B,** same image as **A** showing AP measurement, denoted by *arrowheads* and *dashed line.*

this setting does not have any increased incidence of malformations or mortality. To detect a single umbilical artery, multiple places along the cord should be evaluated.[37] Particularly at the distal end where the cord inserts into the placenta, two umbilical arteries may normally fuse into a single trunk. In another article,[36] the mean and minimum diameters of the umbilical artery and veins were evaluated at time of delivery. Within 5 seconds after delivery, the mean and minimum diameter measurements of the vein were 6.6 and 2.4 mm, and of the artery 5.4 and 1.1 mm.

To date there have been no ultrasound studies of the umbilical cord. It would be difficult to evaluate the length of the umbilical cord because of the cord's variable placement and coiled configuration within the amniotic fluid (Fig 27–6). Nevertheless, an umbilical cord of less than 30 mm would be strongly suggestive of abnormal shortening. In addition, it would not be easy to image multiple places along the cord to evaluate for the number of umbilical arteries (Fig 27–7). Even if a single artery were diagnosed, however, the finding would have limited value since the fetus would most likely still be normal.

It has been suggested in two articles from the same institution[38, 39] that the size of the umbilical vein may be of value in the detection of Rh isoimmunization. These articles found that the umbilical vein diameters were normally slightly different in the amniotic fluid and within the liver, and at different times in gestational life. From 18 to 37 weeks, the diameters were shown to increase slightly in the amniotic fluid from 7 to 11.6 mm and within the liver from 6.6 to 10 mm. When larger diameters were detected, the authors of both articles felt that this was strongly suggestive of Rh sensitization. While they felt that the umbilical vein within the cord had more of a tendency to dilate than that within the liver, both were found to be increased in a small but significant number of Rh-isoimmunized fetuses. In fact, they stated that this dilatation sometimes preceded the optical density changes of the amniotic fluid. However, in two more recent articles,[40, 41] the umbilical vein diameter was found to be relatively insensitive. Vintzileos et al.[40] detected an increase in the vein diameter in only one of 16 cases (eight of which were severe) of isoimmunized fetuses. Witter and Graham[41] evaluated 24 fetuses with Rh isoimmunization and found all cases to overlap the normal range. Therefore, while the umbilical vein

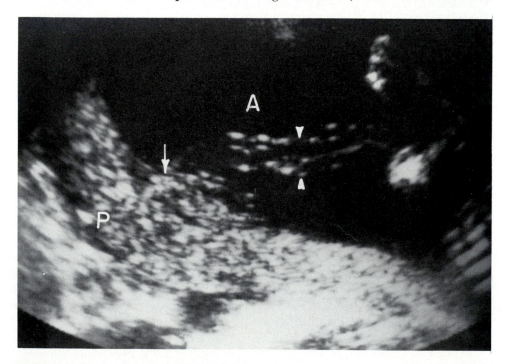

FIG 27–6.
Ultrasound scan of a 36-week pregnancy showing an 8-cm portion of the umbilical cord (denoted by *arrowheads*) from its insertion *(arrow)* into the placenta *(P)*. Due to the coiled configuration of the cord within the amniotic fluid *(A)*, it would be very difficult to measure its full length.

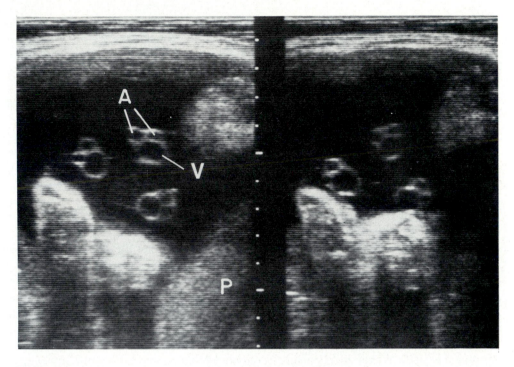

FIG 27–7.
Ultrasound dual image of a 30-week pregnancy showing multiple cross sections of the umbilical cord. The labeled scan on the left shows the normal two arteries *(A)* and one vein *(V)* of each segment. Note that the vein is slightly larger than the arteries. *P* = placenta.

diameter is an interesting measurement, it does not appear to be as promising as originally proposed for the detection of affected Rh-isoimmunized fetuses, even when severe. At present, the measurement is therefore not recommended.

CERVIX

In the pregnant uterus, the exact location of the cervix, and in particular the internal cervical os, is important. When a low-lying placenta is detected, it allows for a determination of whether the placenta covers the internal cervical os, termed a *placenta previa*. The overall length and width of the cervical canal would also be helpful in diagnosing effacement due to either an incompetent cervix or premature onset of labor.

There have been nine ultrasound articles that have evaluated the cervical dimensions,[42–50] two of these by the same group of authors.[43, 44] Four studies[42–44, 47] were performed using static scanners. In eight,[42–49] the authors relied on a markedly distended bladder to evaluate the cervix. The ninth study[50] employed real-time ultrasound with the maternal bladder at first completely or partially filled, and then completely emptied.

In the four studies performed with static scans[42–44, 47] and one using real-time,[45] the exact anatomy of the cervix was not well defined. The area of the external cervical os was identified; the endocervical canal was not clearly imaged. It was claimed in three of the articles[42–44] that the region of the internal cervical os could be identified by an "isthmus," a point of narrowing at the upper part of the cervix. This particular landmark might be correct but is questionable because of the distortion of the cervix by its compression between the distended bladder and the sacrum. As proof that this narrowing is not a consistent finding, images with the bladder partially empty did not show the isthmus. The other study, using a static scanner,[47] failed to show the exact places to measure, citing previous work presented at the 1978 Nordic Congress of Obstetrics and Gynecology. These data were never published in a peer-reviewed journal. One of the real-time articles[45] also failed to show the precise places to measure. These authors also cited previous work but failed to reference the prior study. As a result, these three studies[43–45, 47] will not be considered further.

The remaining three studies using a full urinary bladder technique[46, 48, 49] showed the exact landmarks measured. The cervical length from the external to internal os was measured in two,[46, 48] the width of the cervical (endocervical) canal in one,[46] and the thickness of the anterior wall of the lower uterine segment in one[46] (Fig 27–8). The width of the cervix at the internal cervical os, while a potentially important measurement, was only evaluated by the three studies cited in the previous paragraph[43–45, 47] and will not be discussed further.

The cervical length (see Fig 27–8) was found by two observers to be always normal if greater than 40 mm in length. Podobnik and co-workers[46] divided their examinations into 4-week increments from 10 to 36 weeks. In the 10- to 14-week block, the cervical length was 49.7 ±3.1 mm (1 SD), decreasing gradually by 33 to 36 weeks to 44.2 ±4.1 mm (1 SD). There were only slight statistical differences between the increments, none at greater than $P<.05$. Their cases of incompetent cervix[46] were significantly below these normal lengths, all less than 40 mm from 10 to 28 weeks. Ayers et al.[48] evaluated the cervical length from 8 to 34 weeks and found a normal length of 52 ±12 mm (2 SD). Measurements were not taken after 34 weeks because of potentially normal cervical effacement. While there appears to be some errors in the article, that is, the abstract stated that "only 60% of women with a normal uterine cavity showed cervical lengths of *less than* 40 mm" (a statement not borne out by the remainder of the article) and their figure 1B showed an abnormal cervical length but measured at incorrect landmarks, the remainder of the article appears to be correct. They found no differences between the primigravida and multigravida cervix. In 88 abnormal cases, 70 patients had cervical lengths below 40 mm.

The width of the cervical (endocervical) canal and the thickness of the anterior wall of the lower uterine segment were evaluated in one article[46] (Figs 27–8 and 27–9). Using the same increments from 10 to 36 weeks, the normal endocervical canal was never dilated above 6.3 mm, with a maximum width at 25 to 28 weeks of 5.2 ±1.1 mm (1 SD). The remainder of the incremental widths were below 6.0 mm. The thickness of the anterior wall of the lower uterine segment also remained relatively constant throughout the same 10- to 36-week range, 18.8 ±0.2 mm (1 SD) at 10 to 14 weeks to 17.6 ±2.3 mm (1 SD) at 33 to 36 weeks. Using the lowest limit from the 29- to 32-week range of 14.5 mm, it was found that all abnormal cases of cervical incompetence were well below this number.

From their study, Podobnik and co-workers[46] found that 36 of 80 patients (45%) with cervical incompetence exhibited ultrasound findings *before* developing clinical signs. Furthermore, these authors stated that in many cases of an incompetent cervix, the cervical length and thickness of the anterior wall of the lower uterine segment became abnormal before obvious widening of the cervical canal took place. These findings are potentially important. By the time cervical canal widening is present,

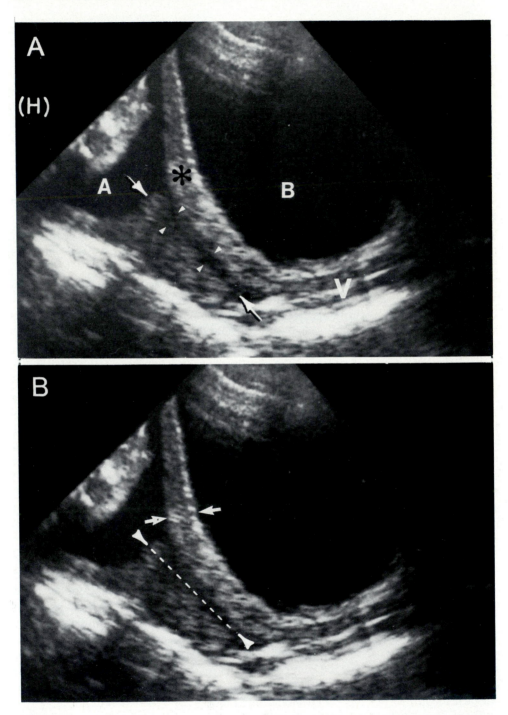

FIG 27–8.
Real-time long-axis midline scan of the normal lower uterine segment performed through a partially distended maternal urinary bladder *(B)*. **A,** the cervix is defined in length *(arrows)* from the external cervical os to the flattened internal cervical os, the latter toward the patient's head *(H)*. Note the hypoechoic endocervical canal between the two arrows. The endocervical width is denoted by *arrowheads*. Asterisk shows the anterior wall of the lower uterine segment. *V* = vagina; *A* = amniotic fluid. **B,** same image as **A** showing the length measurement of the cervix and its endocervical canal, denoted by *arrowheads* and *dashed line. Arrows* show the place to measure the width of the anterior wall lower uterine segment.

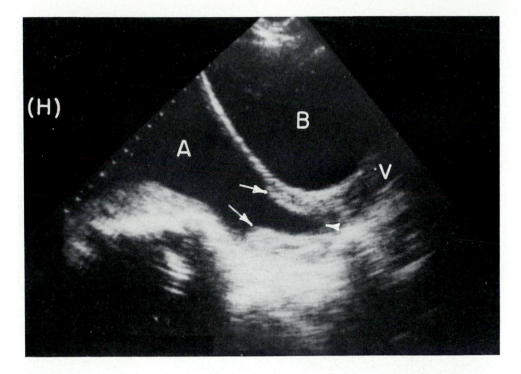

FIG 27–9.
Incompetent cervix. Real-time long-axis midline scan of the lower uterine segment performed through a distended maternal urinary bladder *(B)* showing an open endocervical canal from the internal cervical os *(arrows)* to the external cervical os *(arrowhead)*. The overall width of the cervix, especially at the level of the internal os, is markedly enlarged. *A* = amniotic fluid; *V* = vagina; *(H)* = toward patient's head.

there is frequently prolapse of fetal parts and the umbilical cord. Detection prior to the stage of incompetence is therefore of clinical importance. While the cervical length has been corroborated by Ayers et al.,[48] the other two measurements have not. Nevertheless, all three measurements—the cervical length, endocervical canal width, and anterior lower uterine segment wall thickness—are recommended[46] (Table 27–3).

Michaels and co-workers[49] showed the importance of imaging and measuring the cervical length and endocervical dilatation in patients with cervical incompetence who are then treated by cerclage. As expected, with treatment the cervical length

TABLE 27–3.
Cervix Measurements

Maternal Bladder	Cervical Length (mm) Mean	Cervical Length (mm) Lower Limits of Normal	Anterior Wall Width of Lower Uterine Segment (mm) Mean	Anterior Wall Width of Lower Uterine Segment (mm) Lower Limits of Normal	Endocervical Canal Width (mm) Upper Limits of Normal
Distended (10–36 wk)*	47	40	18	14.5	6.3
Empty (8–40 wk)†	32.5	23	—	—	—

*Data from Podobnik M, Bulic M, Smiljanic N, et al: *J Clin Ultrasound* 1988; 13:383–391.
†Data from Bowie JD, Andreotti RF, Rosenberg ER: *AJR* 1983; 140:737–740.

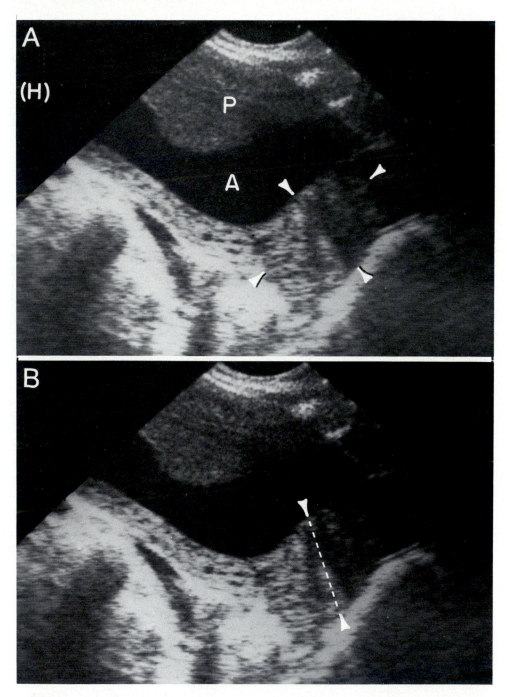

FIG 27–10.
Real-time long-axis midline scan of the lower uterine segment. **A,** the maternal urinary bladder is completely empty so that the image is obtained by scanning through the amniotic fluid *(A). Arrowheads* outline the cervix which is much more squared-off than when distorted by a distended bladder. P = placenta; *(H)* = toward patient's head. **B,** same image as **A.** The hyperechoic endocervical canal is positioned more anteroposteriorly when the bladder is empty. Both the endocervical and cervical measurements are denoted by *arrowheads* and *dashed line.*

increased and the endocervical canal decreased toward their normal limits. These data also showed the importance of determining these measurements after treatment.

The major problem with all of these studies is the use of a distended maternal urinary bladder which can narrow and distort both the cervix and lower uterine segment. Bowie et al.,[50] using a real-time scanner and different degrees of maternal bladder distention, were able to detect the endocervical canal as either a hyper- or hypoechoic band within the cervix and define the internal cervical os as either flat or very slightly funnel-shaped (without an "isthmus") from 8 to 40 weeks (Fig 27–8,A). In a group of 50 pregnant patients, 30 (60%) could be visualized. This visualization varied with the stage of gestation, caused by differences in the size and position of the fetus relative to the cervix. Prior to 20 weeks, the cervix could be clearly imaged in 100% of patients, decreasing to 68% between 20 to 30 weeks, and to 18% between 30 weeks and term. When the urinary bladder was partially distended, the mean cervix and its endocervical canal measured 46 mm with a range of 34 to 61 mm (Fig 27–10). The mean number corresponds to the work by Podobnik et al.[46] and Ayers et al.,[48] but the range appears to be large. When the urinary bladder was emptied, however, the mean length of the cervix was significantly decreased to 32.5 mm with a range of 23 to 45 mm (Fig 27–10). These measurements support the finding that a distended urinary bladder distorts the cervix. As with Ayers et al.,[48] Bowie et al.[50] also found that the number of previous pregnancies did not cause a difference in the cervical length. Width measurements were not taken. Measurements of cervical length when the urinary bladder is empty is also recommended (see Table 27–3).

REFERENCES

1. Gohari P, Berkowitz RL, Hobbins JC: Prediction of intrauterine growth retardation by determination of total intrauterine volume. *Am J Obstet Gynecol* 1977; 127:255–260.
2. Phillips JF, Goodwin DW, Thomason SB, et al: The volume of the uterus in normal and abnormal pregnancy. *J Clin Ultrasound* 1976; 5:107–110.
3. Levine SC, Filly RA, Creasy RK: Identification of fetal growth retardation by ultrasonographic estimation of total intrauterine volume. *J Clin Ultrasound* 1979; 7:21–26.
4. Chinn DH, Filly RA, Callen PW: Prediction of intrauterine growth retardation by sonographic estimation of total intrauterine volume. *J Clin Ultrasound* 1981; 9:175–179.
5. Grossman M, Flynn JJ, Aufrichtig D, et al: Pitfalls in ultrasonic determination of total intrauterine volume. *J Clin Ultrasound* 1982; 10:17–20.
6. Geirsson RT, Christie AD, Patel N: Ultrasound volume measurements comparing a prolate ellipsoid method with a parallel planimetric area method against a known volume. *J Clin Ultrasound* 1982; 10:329–332.
7. Kurtz AB, Shaw WM, Kurtz RJ, et al: The inaccuracy of total uterine volume measurements: Sources of error and a proposed solution. *J Ultrasound Med* 1984; 3:289–297.
8. Middleton WD, Bowie JD, Welt SI: LTUA—A new and more reproducible method of estimating intrauterine size. *J Ultrasound Med* 1982; 1:123–127.
9. Kurtz AB, Kurtz RJ, Rifkin MD, et al: Total uterine volume: A new graph and its clinical applications. *J Ultrasound Med* 1984; 3:299–308.
10. Geirsson RT, Ogston SA, Patel NB, et al: Growth of total intrauterine, intra-amniotic and placental volume in normal singleton pregnancy measured by ultrasound. *Br J Obstet Gynaecol* 1985; 92:46–53.
11. Molteni RA, Stys SJ, Battaglia FC: Relationships of fetal and placental weight in human beings: Fetal/placental weight ratio at various gestational ages and birth weight distributions. *J Reprod Med* 1978; 21:327–334.
12. Younoszai MK, Haworth JC: Placental dimensions and relations in preterm, term, and growth-retarded infants. *Am J Obstet Gynecol* 1969; 103:265–271.

13. Grannum PAT, Berkowitz RL, Hobbins JC: The ultrasonic changes in the maturing placenta and their relation to fetal pulmonic maturity. *Am J Obstet Gynecol* 1979; 133:915–922.
14. Hoddick WK, Mahony BS, Callen PW, et al: Placental thickness. *J Ultrasound Med* 1985; 4:479–482.
15. Wolf H, Oosting H, Treffers PE: Placental volume measurement by ultrasonography: Evaluation of the method. *Am J Obstet Gynecol* 1987; 156:1191–1194.
16. Bleker OP, Kloosterman GJ, Breur W, et al: The volumetric growth of the human placenta: A longitudinal ultrasonic study. *Am J Obstet Gynecol* 1977; 127:657–661.
17. Chamberlain P: Amniotic fluid volume: Ultrasound assessment and clinical significance. *Semin Perinatol* 1985; 9:163–167.
18. Halperin ME, Fong KW, Zalev AH, et al: Reliability of amniotic fluid volume estimation from ultrasonograms: intraobserver and interobserver variation before and after the establishment of criteria. *Am J Obstet Gynecol* 1985; 153:264–267.
19. Crowley P: Non-quantitative estimation of amniotic fluid volume in suspected prolonged pregnancy. *J Perinat Med* 1980; 8:249–251.
20. Hashimoto B, Filly RA, Belden C, et al: Objective method of diagnosing oligohydramnios in postterm pregnancies. *J Ultrasound Med* 1987; 6:81–84.
21. Goldstein RB, Filly RA: Sonographic estimation of amniotic fluid volume. Subjective assessment versus pocket measurements. *J Ultrasound Med* 1988; 7:363–369.
22. Manning FA, Hill LM, Platt LD: Qualitative amniotic fluid volume determination by ultrasound: Antepartum detection of intrauterine growth retardation. *Am J Obstet Gynecol* 1981; 139:254–258.
23. Mercer LJ, Brown LG, Petres RE, et al: A survey of pregnancies complicated by decreased amniotic fluid. *Am J Obstet Gynecol* 1984; 149:355–361.
24. Chamberlain PF, Manning FA, Morrison I, et al: Ultrasound evaluation of amniotic fluid volume. I. The significance of marginal and decreased amniotic fluid volumes to perinatal outcome. *Am J Obstet Gynecol* 1984; 150:245–249.
25. Chamberlain PF, Manning FA, Morrison R, et al: Ultrasound evaluation of amniotic fluid volume. II. The significance of increased amniotic fluid volume to perinatal outcome. *Am J Obstet Gynecol* 1984; 150:250–254.
26. Patterson RM, Prihoda TJ, Pouliot MR: Sonographic amniotic fluid measurement and fetal growth retardation: A reappraisal. *Am J Obstet Gynecol* 1987; 157:1406–1410.
27. Phelan JP, Smith CV, Broussard P, et al: Amniotic fluid volume assessment with the four-quadrant technique at 36–42 weeks' gestation. *J Reprod Med* 1987; 32:540–542.
28. Rutherford SE, Phelan JP, Smith CV, et al: The four-quadrant assessment of amniotic fluid volume: An adjunct to antepartum fetal heart rate testing. *Obstet Gynecol* 1987; 70:353–356.
29. Hoddick WK, Callen PW, Filly RA, et al: Ultrasonographic determination of qualitative amniotic fluid volume in intrauterine growth retardation: Reassessment of the 1 cm rule. *Am J Obstet Gynecol* 1984; 149:758–762.
30. Hill LM, Breckle R, Wolfgram KR, et al: Oligohydramnios: Ultrasonically detected incidence and subsequent fetal outcome. *Am J Obstet Gynecol* 1983; 147:407–410.
31. Geirsson RT, Patel NB, Christie AD: In-vivo accuracy of ultrasound measurements of intrauterine volume in pregnancy. *Br J Obstet Gynaecol* 1984; 91:37–40.
32. Naeye RL: Umbilical cord length: Clinical significance. *J Pediatr* 1985; 107:278–281.
33. Miller ME, Higginbottom M, Smith DW: Short umbilical cord: Its origin and relevance. *Pediatrics* 1981; 67:618–621.
34. Malpas P: Length of the human umbilical cord at term. *Br Med J* 1964; 1:673–674.
35. Walker CW, Pye BG: The length of the human umbilical cord: A statistical report. *Br Med J* 1960; 1:546–548.
36. Moinian M, Meyer WW, Lind J: Diameters of umbilical cord vessels and the weight of the cord in relation to clamping time. *Am J Obstet Gynecol* 1969; 105:604–611.
37. Heifetz SA: Single umbilical artery: A statistical analysis of 237 autopsy cases and review of the literature. *Perspect Pediatr Pathol* 1984; 8:345–378.
38. Mayden KL: The umbilical vein diameter in Rh isoimmunization. *Med Ultrasound* 1980; 4:119–125.
39. DeVore GR, Mayden K, Tortora M, et al: Dilation of the fetal umbilical vein in rhesus hemolytic anemia: A predictor of severe disease. *Am J Obstet Gynecol* 1981; 141:464–466.
40. Vintzileos AM, Campbell WA, Storlazzi E, et al: Fetal liver ultrasound measurements in isoimmunized pregnancies. *Obstet Gynecol* 1986; 68:162–167.
41. Witter FR, Graham D: The utility of ultrasonically measured umbilical vein diameters in isoimmunized pregnancies. *Am J Obstet Gynecol* 1983; 146:225–226.

42. Zemlyn S: The length of the uterine cervix and its significance. *J Clin Ultrasound* 1981; 9:267–269.
43. Brook I, Feingold M, Schwartz A, et al: Ultrasonography in the diagnosis of cervical incompetence in pregnancy—A new diagnostic approach. *Br J Obstet Gynaecol* 1981; 88:640–643.
44. Feingold M, Brook I, Zakut H: Detection of cervical incompetence by ultrasound. *Acta Obstet Gynecol Scand* 1984; 63:407–410.
45. Varma TR, Patel RH, Pillai U: Ultrasonic assessment of cervix in "at risk" patients. *Acta Obstet Gynecol Scand* 1986; 65:147–152.
46. Podobnik M, Bulic M, Smiljanic N, et al: Ultrasonography in the detection of cervical incompetency. *J Clin Ultrasound* 1988; 13:383–391.
47. Vaalamo P, Kivikoski A: The incompetent cervix during pregnancy diagnosed by ultrasound. *Acta Obstet Gynecol Scand* 1983; 62:19–21.
48. Ayers JWT, DeGrood RM, Compton AA, et al: Sonographic evaluation of cervical length in pregnancy: Diagnosis and management of preterm cervical effacement in patients at risk for premature delivery. *Obstet Gynecol* 1988; 71:939–944.
49. Michaels WH, Montgomery C, Karo J, et al: Ultrasound differentiation of the competent from the incompetent cervix: prevention of preterm delivery. *Am J Obstet Gynecol* 1986; 154:537–546.
50. Bowie JD, Andreotti RF, Rosenberg ER: Sonographic appearance of the uterine cervix in pregnancy: The vertical cervix. *AJR* 1983; 140:737–740.

Chapter 28

Mathematical Growth Models

Alfred B. Kurtz, M.D.
Barry B. Goldberg, M.D.

Recently, a number of authors have analyzed fetal growth mathematically. By the use of equations that were linear, quadratic, cubic, or even more complicated, fetal parameters have been studied in small populations of fetuses. While some of the theoretical approaches are novel, none appear to offer practical advantages over existing tables. Nevertheless, the fetal parameters that have been evaluated and the articles that have studied them are listed in Table 28–1.

TABLE 28–1.
Mathematical Growth Models

Parameter	No. of Articles	(Reference)
Biparietal diameter	5	(1–5)
Head circumference	4	(1,2,4,5)
Head area	2	(5,6)
Head volume	3	(5,7,8)
Abdominal circumference	4	(1,2,4,5)
Abdominal area	2	(5,9)
Abdominal volume	3	(5,7,8)
Femur length	1	(10)
Head to abdominal volume ratio	1	(8)
Total fetal volume	1	(11)
Fetal weight	2	(2,12)

REFERENCES

1. Adam AH, Robinson HP, Dunlop C: A comparison of crown-rump length measurements using a real-time scanner in an antenatal clinic and a conventional B-scanner. *Br J Obstet Gynaecol* 1979; 86:521–524.
2. Deter RL, Harrist RB, Hadlock FP, et al: Longitudinal studies of fetal growth with the use of dynamic image ultrasonography. *Am J Obstet Gynecol* 1982; 143:545.
3. Wexler S, Fuchs C, Golan A, et al: Tolerance intervals for standards in ultrasound measurements: Determination of BPD standards. *J Clin Ultrasound* 1986; 14:243–250.
4. Todros T, Ferrazzi E, Groli C, et al: Fitting growth curves to head and abdomen measurements of the fetus: A multicentric study. *J Clin Ultrasound* 1987; 15:95–105.

5. Deter RL, Rossavik IK, Harrist RB, et al: Mathematic modeling of fetal growth: Development of individual growth curve standards. *Obstet Gynecol* 1986; 68:156–161.
6. Rossavik IK, Deter RL, Hadlock FP: Mathematical modeling of fetal growth. III. Evaluation of head growth using the head profile area. *J Clin Ultrasound* 1987; 15:23–30.
7. Rossavik IK, Deter RL: Mathematical modeling of fetal growth. I. Basic principles. *J Clin Ultrasound* 1984; 12:529–533.
8. Rossavik IK, Deter RL: Mathematical modeling of fetal growth. II. Head cube (A), abdominal cube (B) and their ratio (A/B). *J Clin Ultrasound* 1984; 12:535–545.
9. Rossavik IK, Deter RL, Hadlock FP: Mathematical modeling of fetal growth. IV. Evaluation of trunk growth using the abdominal profile area. *J Clin Ultrasound* 1987; 15:31–35.
10. Deter RL, Rossavik IK, Hill RM, et al: Longitudinal studies of femur growth in normal fetuses. *J Clin Ultrasound* 1987; 15:299–305.
11. Deter RL, Harrist RB, Hadlock FP, et al: Longitudinal studies of fetal growth using volume parameters determined with ultrasound. *J Clin Ultrasound* 1984; 12:313–324.
12. Rossavik IK, Torjusen GO, Deter RL, et al: Efficacy of mathematical methods for ultrasound examinations in diabetic pregnancies. *Am J Obstet Gynecol* 1986; 155:638–644.

PART VIII

Multiple Gestations

Chapter 29

Twins

Alfred B. Kurtz, M.D.

Barry B. Goldberg, M.D.

Many articles have been published evaluating twin gestations. At birth, the mean weight and duration of the gestations are less for twin than for singleton pregnancies,[1,2] with birth weights and pregnancy durations even shorter for triplet and quadruplet pregnancies. Twins occur approximately 1 in every 85 births, varying in incidence in different racial groups and in different nations. The incidence of triplet and quadruplet pregnancies is much more uncommon, 1 in 7,600 and 1 in 670,000, respectively. The remainder of this chapter is therefore confined to the analysis of twin gestations since adequate series have not been compiled on larger-sized multiple pregnancies.

There are two types of twinning: dizygotic and monozygotic. Dizygotic twins occur in about 80% of cases and are caused by the production of two ova and their subsequent fertilization. Monozygotic twins arise from the division of one ovum after fertilization. This occurs in the remaining 20% of cases. Twinning can be evaluated in another way, that is, by the types of membranes separating the twins. In dizygotic twins, each fetus is in a totally separate sac surrounded by its own chorion and amnion, and is therefore termed dichorionic-diamniotic. In a certain percentage of monozygotic twins, approximately 20% to 30%, the ovum divides within the first day after fertilization. This division is early enough that these twins too are in their own separate sacs and are also dichorionic-diamniotic. Most monozygotic twins, however, are not. In about 70% to 75% of cases, the ovum divides between the first and seventh days and, while the twins are in their own amniotic sac, they share a common chorionic sac and are called monochorionic-diamniotic twins. A smaller percentage, approximately 3%, divide even later, 7 to 13 days after fertilization, so that the twins are within the same sac, share the same amnion and chorion, and are termed monochorionic-monoamniotic. Rarely, if the division is after the 13th day, the twins only partially separate, a situation leading to conjoined or Siamese twinning.

The type of twinning is important. All twins have the same increased complication rate of prematurity and smallness in size, and all have the same problems at birth with the second-born twin having increased perinatal mortality, usually from anoxia and prolapsed cord.[3] In addition, monochorionic twins, whether in one or two amniotic sacs, have further potential complications.[4] They may have a twin-twin transfusion caused by placental vascular shunting which can lead to one small growth-retarded and one plethoric hydropic fetus. In addition, monochorionic-monoamniotic twins may be further complicated by umbilical cord entanglement.

It is the purpose of the ultrasound evaluation of twin gestations to establish if there are multiple gestations, to analyze the gestational age of the twins, and to determine if physical and growth abnormalities exist. While physical abnormalities are the same as those in singleton gestations and will not be discussed further, the in utero growth of twin gestations is unique.

In addition to the number of pregnancies, the determination of dichorionicity and monochorionicity is of predictive value in the assessment of the potential risk factors described above. Two recent articles[5, 6] have stated that separate placentas and different fetal genders assures dichorionicity. In addition, a thick separation membrane comprised of two layers of chorion and two layers of amnion would favor the same diagnosis, while a thin membrane of two layers of amnion would favor the diagnosis of monochorionic-diamniotic twinning[6–8] (Fig 29–1). This membrane and its thickness is more definitively defined in the first trimester. By the third trimester, the membrane is more difficult to image and technical factors can influence thickness.[8] If a membrane cannot be identified, even when good technique has been used, monochorionic-monoamniotic twinning is probable.

The most common measurement for twin gestations, as with singleton gestations, has been the biparietal diameter which has been evaluated in 13 articles.[9–21] Nine presented numeric data,[9–15, 20, 21] all except one[14] giving a standard deviation and all except another[9] also showing their results in graph form. Two articles[16, 17] presented their results only in graph form, one giving a standard deviation.[17] The last two articles[18, 19] stated their results only in their conclusions without giving any numbers or graphs. These latter two articles will therefore not be considered further in the analysis of the biparietal diameters.

Of the remaining 11,[9–17, 20, 21] nine also evaluated the biparietal diameter growth of the twin gestations in comparison to similar growth for singleton gestations.[9–12, 14–16, 19, 21] In addition, four of the articles evaluated the biparietal diameter growth of one twin against the other.[9, 14–16] From a composite of all these articles, it can be stated that the growth of the biparietal diameter of both twins closely parallels the biparietal diameter growth of singleton gestations until at least 28 to 30 weeks. After that time, the predominant opinion is that there is some decrease in the growth of the biparietal diameters with most articles still showing an overlap with singleton gestations at 2 SD even as late as 38 weeks. As a result, the biparietal diameter measurement tables of singleton gestations can be used for twin gestations until at least the mid–third trimester. Nevertheless, a table of biparietal diameter measurements in twin gestations is presented[20] (Fig 29–2) (Table 29–1). While it is based on much smaller numbers and therefore has a large standard deviation, its mean values are accurate. This table serves as a reminder of the slowing in biparietal diameter growth after 30 weeks.

The growth of the biparietal diameter of each twin closely paralleled the other. Approximately 1 to 3 mm may normally separate the two biparietal diameters throughout gestation,[9, 10, 14, 15, 17, 22, 23] with two of these articles considering the twins normal even when the biparietal diameters showed a difference of 5 mm or more.[14, 17] There were, however, discrepancies between studies. Authors disagreed on whether the biparietal diameter growth is similar for both dichorionic and monochorionic twins. Two articles found dichorionic twins to be larger[16, 18] with one study finding them equal in size.[11] It is possible that the discrepancies in head size may be related

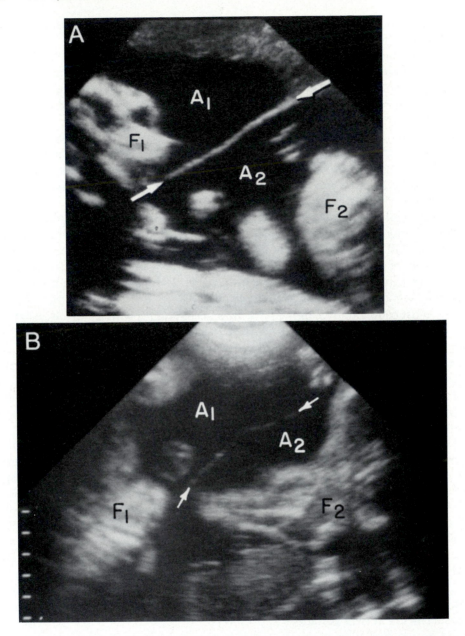

FIG 29–1.
Membrane characteristics separating twin gestations. **A,** the dichorionic-diamniotic membrane *(arrows)* is thick and well defined. One fetus (F_1) and its amniotic fluid (A_1) is separated from the other fetus (F_2) and its amniotic fluid (A_2). **B,** the monochorionic-diamniotic membrane *(arrows)* is much thinner and "wispy" in appearance. The fetuses $(F_1$ and $F_1)$ and their amniotic fluid $(A_1$ and $A_2)$ are separate.

to unusually shaped heads caused by the crowding of the twins against each other rather than true differences in growth. Although this cannot be proved since no articles measured the fronto-occipital diameter, cephalic index, or calculated a head circumference, it can be suggested from the following two observations. Socol et al.[13] stated that although there was slowing of twin biparietal diameter growth, the

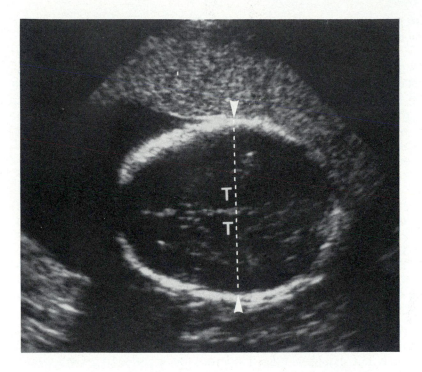

FIG 29–2.
The biparietal diameter measurement is taken in transaxial view with the thalamus *(T)* or midbrain in the midline. The measurement, denoted by *arrowheads* and *dotted line,* is taken from leading edge (outer margin) to leading edge (inner margin).

newborn twin head circumferences were comparable to singleton gestations. Persson and Grennert[16] found in 80% of cases that the twin in vertex presentation (with the head in the pelvis) had a consistently larger biparietal diameter measurement. Since the larger fetus should be randomly placed in either the lower or upper part of the uterus, the detection of most of the "larger" heads in the lower uterine segment implies that different head shapes rather than true differences in head size are responsible for the discrepancies in the biparietal diameter.

When discrepancies do exist, however, there is also disagreement about the value of divergent biparietal diameters in establishing the diagnosis of growth retardation. Four authors[14, 17, 22, 23] felt that if a discrepancy between the two biparietal diameters was either more than 5 mm or 5%[17] or increased 3 mm or more over at least a 2-week period, growth retardation should be suggested. Using these criteria, two series[14, 22] detected 53% and 77% of growth-retarded fetuses, respectively. Three other articles, however, felt that the biparietal diameter difference alone was not enough to permit the detection of growth retardation in twins since on occasion both fetuses could be growth-retarded, thus invalidating the differences in the biparietal diameters.[9, 18, 19] One of the articles[9] found that even when a difference of 5 mm or more existed between the biparietal diameters, the weight difference of the infants at birth was only infrequently 25% or greater. The other two,[18, 19] without showing tables or graphs, concluded that the biparietal diameter growth was not adequate for detection of growth retardation. Nevertheless, although perhaps not accurate in all cases, twin gestations do share the same environment. A discrepancy of greater

TABLE 29–1.
Fetal Measurements in Twin Gestations*†

Gestational Age (wk)	Biparietal Diameter (mm)		Abdominal Circumference (mm)	
	Predicted Mean	Range From 5th to 95th Percentile	Predicted Mean	Range From 5th to 95th Percentile
27	69	61–78	236	202–273
28	74	66–82	239	185–293
29	74	66–82	249	199–299
30	74	64–84	253	215–291
31	78	68–88	269	231–307
32	79	71–87	272	236–308
33	81	73–89	271	229–313
34	82	76–88	289	251–327
35	84	76–92	296	262–330
36	85	79–91	298	266–330
37	85	79–91	292	240–344

*From Grumbach K, Coleman BG, Arger PH, et al: *Radiology* 1986; 158:237–241. Used by permission.
†Data obtained on 103 twin parts.

than 5 mm or an increasing discrepancy between the biparietal diameters cannot be taken casually but should be judged as a warning of potential growth retardation in the smaller twins or for a twin-twin transfusion syndrome in both.

Evaluation of the fetal body in twin gestations has been performed in four articles.[13, 19, 20, 24] Secher et al.[24] measured the twin abdominal diameters and found them to grow normally throughout gestation. Socol et al.[13] and Grumbach et al.,[20] however, found the abdominal circumference to decrease slightly in the later part of the third trimester. Nevertheless, the curves for normal singleton and twin gestations overlapped at 2 SD, even at term. Neilson[19] determined the product of the crown-rump length and the trunk area of twins at 34 to 36 weeks. Using static scans, the long axis of the fetus was measured from the top of the head to the bottom of the urinary bladder and the abdominal area measurement was taken at the level of the liver. In a prospective study, this product detected all 15 of 21 twin pairs that were small-for-dates with a 22% false-positive rate. A follow-up study by Neilson[25] similarly detected all 19 small-for-date twin fetuses of the 62 studied. Of the additional 43 babies that were normal at birth, there were 11 falsely predicted to be small-for-gestational-age. While this work has a high degree of accuracy, it is oversensitive and further work will be necessary prior to its routine use. A table of abdominal circumference is included as a reminder of the slightly different growth of twins[20] (Fig 29–3) (see Table 29–1). The mean numbers, when compared to the abdominal circumferences of singleton gestations, shows a decrease in abdominal growth after 32 weeks, somewhat similar but less in degree than the decrease that occurs in the biparietal diameter. The standard deviation is relatively large because of the small number of cases in the series.

It would therefore seem that all twin parameters should decrease after the mid–third trimester. If so, this would be consistent with the newborn findings that twin gestations are smaller than singleton gestations. Surprisingly, Grumbach et al.[20] found that the femur length remained normal, equal to that of singleton gestational measurements, until the end of their study at 37 weeks (Fig 29–4). While this work

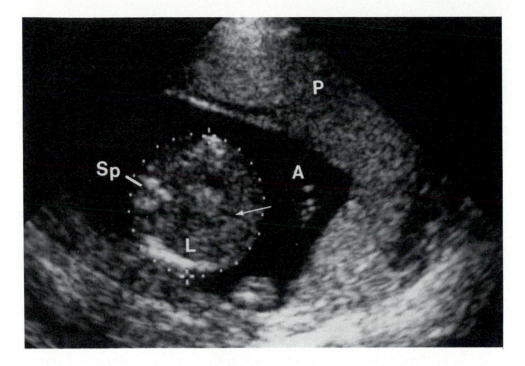

FIG 29–3.
Abdominal circumference. Transaxial image of the upper abdomen at the region of the liver *(L)*. The umbilical portion of the left portal vein *(arrow)* is situated within the liver in the midline. The circumference is traced with a digitizer or map reader *(dotted line)* or can be calculated from an equation. *P* = placenta; *Sp* = spine; *A* = amniotic fluid.

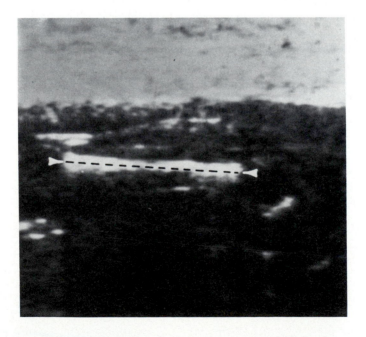

FIG 29–4.
Femur length measurement. The long axis of the hyperechoic femoral shaft is measured, denoted by *arrowheads* and *dashed line,* disregarding the hypoechoic nonossified epiphyseal cartilages.

needs further corroboration, it implies that the twin fetal parameters may not be smaller in the late third trimester. Instead, the femur may be normal because it is the only major parameter which is not distorted by the crowding of the enlarging twins. It is therefore recommended, based on this work,[20] that when there are discrepancies in the head and body measurements of either twin, the femur length be used to date the pregnancy and evaluate appropriate growth.

Articles on aborted fetuses[26] and on live newborn infants[2, 3, 27] have shown that in the first and second trimester the fetal weights of twins closely approximate those of singleton gestations (similar to the biparietal diameter findings). After approximately 27 weeks, the weights of twin gestations decreased in relation to singleton twin gestations, an effect which was more pronounced in monochorionic than in dichorionic twins. Asymmetric growth retardation usually occurs after 34 weeks. A discrepancy of at least 15%, and more likely 25%, in body weight between the two fetuses strongly suggests that the smaller of the two is growth-retarded.[23, 28]

Three articles have evaluated fetal weight in twin gestations.[29–31] These series consisted of 35,[29] 43,[30] and 116[31] twin pairs. Two articles[29, 31] used a weight chart based on biparietal and abdominal circumference. In one,[29] curvilinear growth was detected and the values were presented in number and graph form with a 2 SD range. In the third trimester there was a slowing in fetal weight caused by slowing in the biparietal diameter growth. The abdominal circumference growth remained constant and the weights of the twins remained close. The other[31] found that the abdominal circumference was more sensitive than the biparietal diameter at detecting dissimilar weight. The last article[30] evaluated twin fetal weights using the biparietal diameter, abdominal circumference, and femur length. While no numbers were given, the authors found that fetal weight was the most sensitive predictor of discordant fetal growth and also found that this was caused by an abdominal circumference difference of 20 mm or more.

The weights of twin gestations were not significantly different at 2 SD from singleton gestations, although the mean numbers are less than for singleton gestations.[29] While it is important that this work be substantiated, Table 29–2 will give the reader an understanding of expected fetal weight in twins.[29] The weight is calculated using the biparietal diameter (see Fig 29–2) and abdominal circumference (see Fig 29–3) from the weight table[32] discussed in the fetal weight chapter.

TABLE 29–2.

Estimated Fetal Weight in Twin Pregnancies*†

Gestational Age (wk)	Weight (g)				
	Percentile				
	5th	25th	50th	75th	95th
16	132	141	154	189	207
17	173	194	215	239	249
18	214	248	276	289	291
19	223	253	300	333	412
20	232	259	324	378	534
21	275	355	432	482	705
22	319	452	540	586	876
23	347	497	598	684	880
24	376	543	656	783	885
25	549	677	793	916	1,118
26	722	812	931	1,049	1,352
27	755	978	1,087	1,193	1,563
28	789	1,145	1,244	1,337	1,774
29	900	1,266	1,395	1,509	1,883
30	1,011	1,387	1,546	1,682	1,992
31	1,198	1,532	1,693	1,875	2,392
32	1,385	1,677	1,840	2,068	2,793
33	1,491	1,771	2,032	2,334	3,000
34	1,597	1,866	2,224	2,601	3,208
35	1,703	2,093	2,427	2,716	3,336
36	1,809	2,321	2,631	2,832	3,465
37	2,239	2,540	2,824	3,035	3,679
38	2,669	2,760	3,017	3,239	3,894

*From Yarkoni S, Reece EA, Holford T, et al: *Obstet Gynecol* 1987; 69:636–639. Used by permission.

†Weight calculated from formula by Shepard MJ, Richards VA, Berkowitz RL, et al: *Am J Obstet Gynecol* 1982; 142:42–54.

REFERENCES

1. Guttmacher AF, Kohl SG: The fetus of multiple gestations. *Obstet Gynecol* 1985; 12:528–541.
2. Gruenwald R: Growth of the human fetus. II. Abnormal growth in twins and infants of mothers with diabetes, hypertension, or isoimmunization. *Am J Obstet Gynecol* 1966; 94:1120–1132.
3. Tamura RK, Sabbagha RE, Pan WH, et al: Ultrasonic fetal abdominal circumference: Comparison of direct versus calculated measurement. *Obstet Gynecol* 1986; 67:833–835.
4. Naeye RL, Tafari N, Judge D, et al: Twins: Causes of perinatal death in 12 United States cities and one African city. *Am J Obstet Gynecol* 1978; 131:267–272.
5. Mahony BS, Filly RA, Callen PW: Amnionicity and chorionicity in twin pregnancies: Prediction using ultrasound. *Radiology* 1985; 155:205–209.
6. Barss VA, Benacerraf BR, Frigoletto FD Jr: Ultrasonographic determination of chorion type in twin gestation. *Obstet Gynecol* 1985; 66:779–783.
7. Hertzberg BS, Kurtz AB, Choi HY, et al: Significance of membrane thickness in the sonographic evaluation of twin gestations. *AJR* 1987; 148:151–153.

8. Townsend RR, Simpson GF, Filly RA: Membrane thickness in ultrasound prediction of chorionicity of twin gestations. *J Ultrasound Med* 1988; 7:326–332.

9. Erkkola R, Ala-Mello S, Piiroinen O, et al: Growth discordancy in twin pregnancies: A risk factor not detected by measurements of biparietal diameter. *Obstet Gynecol* 1985; 66:203–206.

10. Leveno KJ, Santos-Ramos R, Duenhoelter JH, et al: Sonar cephalometry in twins: A table of biparietal diameters for normal twin fetuses and a comparison with singletons. *Am J Obstet Gynecol* 1979; 135:727–730.

11. Divers WA, Hemsell DL: The use of ultrasound in multiple gestations. *Obstet Gynecol* 1979; 53:500–504.

12. Gottlicher S, Madjaric J, Krone HA: Der biparietale Durchmesser des fetalen Kopfes bei Zwillingen und Einlingen im Verlauf der Schwangerschaft. Eine vergleichende Studie. *Geburtshilfe Frauenheilkd* 1977; 37:762–767.

13. Socol ML, Tamura RK, Sabbagha RE, et al: Diminished biparietal diameter and abdominal circumference growth in twins. *Obstet Gynecol* 1984; 64:235–238.

14. Houlton MCC: Divergent biparietal diameter growth rates in twin pregnancies. *Obstet Gynecol* 1977; 49:542–545.

15. Grennert L, Persson PH, Genser F: Intrauterine growth of twins judged by BPD measurements. *Acta Obstet Gynecol Scand [Suppl]* 1978; 78:28–32.

16. Persson PH, Grennert L: The intrauterine growth of the biparietal diameter of twins. *Acta Genet Med Gemellol (Roma)* 1979; 28:273–277.

17. Crane JF, Tomich PG, Kopta M: Ultrasonic growth patterns in normal and discordant twins. *Obstet Gynecol* 1980; 55:678–683.

18. Schneider L, Bessis R, Tabaste JL, et al: Foetal twin biometry. *Acta Genet Med Gemellol (Roma)* 1979; 28:299–301.

19. Neilson JP: Detection of the small-for-dates twin fetus by ultrasound. *Br J Obstet Gynaecol* 1981; 88:27–32.

20. Grumbach K, Coleman BG, Arger PH, et al: Twin and singleton growth patterns compared using US. *Radiology* 1986; 158:237–241.

21. Shah YG, Graham D, Stinson SK, et al: Biparietal diameter growth in uncomplicated twin gestation. *Am J Perinatol* 1987; 4:229–232.

22. Houlton MCC, Marivate M, Philpott RH: The prediction of fetal growth retardation in twin pregnancy. *Br J Obstet Gynaecol* 1981; 88:264–273.

23. Haney AF, Crenshaw MC, Dempsey PJ: Significance of biparietal diameter differences between twins. *Obstet Gynecol* 1978; 51:609–613.

24. Secher NF, Kaern J, Hansen PK: Intrauterine growth in twin pregnancies: Prediction of fetal growth retardation. *Obstet Gynecol* 1985; 66:63–67.

25. Neilson JP: Detection of the small-for-gestational age twin fetus by a two stage ultrasound examination schedule. *Acta Genet Med Gemellol (Roma)* 1982; 31:235–240.

26. Iffy L, Lavenhar MA, Jakobovits A, et al: The rate of early intrauterine growth in twin gestation. *Am J Obstet Gynecol* 1983; 146:970–972.

27. Naeye RL, Benirschke K, Hagstrom JWC, et al: Intrauterine growth of twins as estimated from liveborn birth-weight data. *Pediatrics* 1966; 37:409–416.

28. O'Brien WF, Knuppel RA, Scerbo JC, et al: Birth weight in twins: An analysis of discordancy and growth retardation. *Obstet Gynecol* 1986; 67:483–486.

29. Yarkoni S, Reece EA, Holford T, et al: Estimated fetal weight in the evaluation of growth in twin gestations: A prospective longitudinal study. *Obstet Gynecol* 1987; 69:636–639.

30. Storlazzi E, Vintzileos AM, Campbell WA, et al: Ultrasonic diagnosis of discordant fetal growth in twin gestations. *Obstet Gynecol* 1987; 69:363–367.

31. Brown CEL, Guzick DS, Leveno KJ, et al: Prediction of discordant twins using ultrasound measurement of biparietal diameter and abdominal perimeter. *Obstet Gynecol* 1987; 70:677–681.

32. Shepard MJ, Richards VA, Berkowitz RL, et al: An evaluation of two equations for predicting fetal weight by ultrasound. *Am J Obstet Gynecol* 1982; 142:47–54.

Index